Stress, Shock, and Adaptation in the Twentieth Century

Rochester Studies in Medical History

ISSN 1526-2715

Additional Titles of Interest

The Origins of Organ Transplantation: Surgery and Laboratory Science, 1880–1930
Thomas Schlich

Communities and Health Care: The Rochester, New York, Experiment
Sarah F. Liebschutz

The Neurological Patient in History
Edited by L. Stephen Jacyna and Stephen T. Casper

The Birth Control Clinic in a Marketplace World
Rose Holz

Bacteriology in British India: Laboratory Medicine and the Tropics
Pratik Chakrabarti

Barefoot Doctors and Western Medicine in China
Xiaoping Fang

Beriberi in Modern Japan: The Making of a National Disease
Alexander R. Bay

The Lobotomy Letters
Mical Raz

Plague and Public Health in Early Modern Seville
Kristy Wilson Bowers

Medicine and the Workhouse
Edited by Jonathan Reinarz and Leonard Schwarz

A complete list of titles in the Rochester Studies in Medical History series may be found on our website, www.urpress.com.

Stress, Shock, and Adaptation in the Twentieth Century

Edited by David Cantor
and Edmund Ramsden

University of Rochester Press

First published 2014

University of Rochester Press
668 Mt. Hope Avenue, Rochester, NY 14620, USA
www.urpress.com
and Boydell & Brewer Limited
PO Box 9, Woodbridge, Suffolk IP12 3DF, UK
www.boydellandbrewer.com

ISBN-13: 978-1-58046-476-5
ISSN: 1526-2715

Library of Congress Cataloging-in-Publication Data

Stress, shock, and adaptation in the twentieth century / edited by David Cantor and Edmund Ramsden.
p. ; cm. — (Rochester studies in medical history, ISSN 1526-2715)
Includes bibliographical references and index.
ISBN 978-1-58046-476-5 (hardcover : alk. paper)
I. Cantor, David, 1957– editor of compilation. II. Ramsden, Edmund, editor of compilation. III. Series: Rochester studies in medical history. 1526-2715
[DNLM: 1. Stress, Psychological—history—Great Britain. 2. Stress, Psychological—history—United States. 3. Adaptation, Psychological—Great Britain. 4. Adaptation, Psychological—United States. 5. History, 20th Century—Great Britain. 6. History, 20th Century—United States. 7. Life Style—history—Great Britain. 8. Life Style—history—United States. WM 11 AA1]
RC49
616.08—dc23

2013043804

A catalogue record for this title is available from the British Library.

This publication is printed on acid-free paper.
Printed in the United States of America.

Contents

Part Four: Work

Part Five: Managing Stress

Part Six: Surveilling Stress

Acknowledgments

The embryo of this book was a workshop—"Stress, Trauma, and Adaptation in the Twentieth Century"—held at the National Institutes of Health (NIH) on November 9–10, 2010, the offspring of three sponsors: the Office of History at the NIH, the History of Medicine Division of the National Library of Medicine (NLM), and the Centre for Medical History at Exeter University. The conception of the workshop and this book could not have happened without the help of many people at these parent organizations: Mark Jackson, Joseph Melling, and Claire Keyte at Exeter; Robert Martensen and Sharon Mathis in the Office of History; and Donald Lindberg, Elizabeth Fee, Paul Theerman, Jeffrey Reznick, Mike Sappol, and Ba Ba Chang at the NLM. Exeter's paternity was assisted by a Wellcome Trust–funded project on the history of stress directed by Mark and Jo and by a further Wellcome Trust conference grant. Ted Brown, Suzanne Guiod, and Julia Cook at the University of Rochester Press were admirable midwives to the book, and two anonymous referees donated seminal and germinal advice. The exhausted but happy editors would like to thank all of them for their help.

Introduction

DAVID CANTOR AND EDMUND RAMSDEN

Forty years ago American sociologist Alvin Toffler predicted that the rate of change in modern civilization would accelerate to such a degree that it would be impossible for individuals to adapt. Toffler would famously call this anxiety "Future Shock": shattering stress and disorientation leading to social, psychological, even physiological breakdown.[1] He had based his predictions on scientific studies, most notably the work of the physiologist Hans Selye. An architect of the modern concept of "stress," Selye argued that adaptations such as corticosteroids could be maladaptive when the body was under constant distress. He described a "general adaptation syndrome" comprising three stages: an initial alarm or shock phase; a stage of adaptation in which physiological resistance allowed normal function; and a final stage of exhaustion, collapse, even death, when adaptive mechanisms failed.[2] While Selye focused on nonspecific physiological responses to harmful agents, others widened this perspective, looking at the relationship between a huge variety of environmental stressors and a range of chronic diseases—hypertension, gastric ulcers, arthritis, allergies, cancer, and a variety of mental illnesses.

In many ways, Toffler and Selye were giving a coherent social and physiological basis to something that had long seemed intuitive: that the health of an individual and society required a degree of order, balance, and equilibrium. Modernity and its concomitant (and unnatural) processes of rapid population growth, industrialization, urbanization, and technological complexity threatened these requirements. In 1881 the American neurologist George M. Beard (1839–83) argued that many Americans were suffering from nervous exhaustion or neurasthenia, the consequence of rapid social and technological transformations.[3] In Britain the medical officer John Hawkes was similarly concerned that the advancing speed of social and intellectual pursuits in the nineteenth century led to increased "pressure" on the mind.[4] By the early twentieth century, with increasing levels of fatigue and traumatic neurosis among industrial workers and shell shock among soldiers, it seemed that people were ill-prepared for the strains of advanced civilization.

This volume explores what happens when stress enters the discourse around modernity. While there have long been associations made between modern life and mental and physiological illness, the concept of stress has intensified and refocused such debates. It has contributed to a gradual displacement of nervous explanations and to the emergence of hormonal and biochemical accounts of mental illness that not only involve psychological disorder but physical and biological disease. While stress carries on much of the cultural work of neurasthenia and fatigue, it has also proven critical to the refinement and expansion of notions of psychopathology in the postwar era. As stress is shared by all, there has, one could argue, taken place a further democratization of mental-health problems. All individuals, irrespective of gender, race, or class, suffer in some way from the various trials and tribulations of modern life.[5]

The problem of stress is perhaps becoming *the* most widely utilized medical concept in contemporary constructions and expressions of personal identity, the built environment, and the complexities of the competitive capitalist economy. Even at the level of Selye's clinical physiology lies the fundamental paradox of modernity—that the very efficiency and rationality of the body as machine or system, giving us strength, power, and the ability to respond to shock and disease, can also destroy the individual. The concept of stress therefore unites major themes in the historical study of modernity—the problems of individuality; the group and mass; social disorder and conformity; the effects of the urban environment on behavior and well-being; industrial methods of work, leisure, and recreation; the complexities and dangers of technological systems; the breakdown of traditional cultural institutions; and the emergence of increasingly fractured social roles. Some have even perceived stress to be the essence of a postmodern existence in which social stability and coherence, order, and meaning have been undermined and overwhelmed. Postmodern culture, it has been argued, is inherently traumatic.[6]

Stress also unites scientific disciplines and traverses boundaries between laboratory and field and between individual, society, and population. It therefore serves as a vehicle for uniting themes within the history of science. The rapid spread of the concept throughout the social, biological, medical, even natural sciences is reflective of its ability to inspire research, often of a holistic and interdisciplinary nature. Some scientific communities are, perhaps, more predisposed to the concept, attracted to ideas of equilibrium or feedback, and concerned with pressures on social, psychological, and ecological systems.[7] Others have struggled with the concept, often seeking to redefine it in their own terms.[8] Stress has been subject to intense debate over its precise meaning and its significance to the individual and society.

Exploring such controversies—over, for example, stress as a physiological object to be studied in the laboratory or a psychological process demanding the skills of the social scientist—allows us to explore interests at stake as stress comes into the mix.

The subject of stress also shows how the history of science can inform historical scholarship concerned with health, work, the city, public policy, class, race, gender, and social, economic, and political change. Indeed, public and medical concern with stress has only intensified, evident in the burgeoning stress "industry" that seeks to provide us with the tools to adapt to a rapidly changing world. In the United States alone, the cost of stress to the economy has been estimated to be $300 billion annually.[9] The worldwide prevalence and socioeconomic impact of stress have led to suggestions that stress now constitutes a global epidemic, and claims that we are now living in an age of stress have become a common cliché across the media. The promised future of recumbent ease offered by the networked age of the Global Village is seen to have instead been attended by increased anxiety, mental illness, and stress. Across the media spectrum, self-help jostles with confessional autobiography. When faith in the "talking cure" wanes, remedial action falls under the ambit of the clinical sciences. DuPont's "better living through chemistry" has been achieved through the development of "mood drugs"—pharmacological cures promising the abolition of mental anguish and feeding aspirations for becoming what Peter D. Kramer has called "better than well."[10] So pervasive is the discourse of stress that it is even used to explain ailments and interventions that are often incompatible. For some, smoking and alcohol consumption are the pathological consequences of stress; for others (Selye included) they are necessary and useful therapeutic agents.

This volume is the first major collection of historical studies on stress and its place in modernity. While there is a vast historical literature on neurasthenia in the nineteenth century, shell shock during World War I, and a growing body of academic literature focused on post-traumatic stress disorder following World War II, there are surprisingly few studies of the history of stress in modern societies, in spite of its impact as a concept on science and medicine.[11] Cary L. Cooper and Philip J. Dewe's *Stress: A Brief History* provides an overview of conceptual developments, particularly in the psychology of stress, but does not explore debates about the biology and pathology of stress in any depth or analyze the sociocultural contexts that shaped stress discourse. Robert Kugelmann adopts the idea of an age of stress but provides a largely internalist account, aiming, like Cooper and Dewe, to promote stress as a subject of popular and medical concern. There is also some historical discussion in the more polemical works by Angela Patmore, Serge Doublet, and Dana Becker.[12] A much-awaited historical treatment of stress has recently been published by Mark Jackson, a contributor to this volume. Focusing considerable attention on the critical role of Hans Selye in the development and promotion of the stress concept, Jackson argues that it is necessary to understand how it was that stress emerged as such a key indicator of psychosocial well-being; how it served as such an effective conceptual framework for understanding and managing social, political, and environmental systems and personal experiences; and how in turn its influence helped generate a range of methods for relaxation and happiness. Jackson argues that stress is a manifestation of the quest for stability, balance, and meaning in a secular world, and for this reason, "stress is no myth as some scholars have suggested."[13]

This book provides a close contextual reading of the proliferation of stress as an explanation for the problems of the modern world from a number of different historical perspectives.[14] It seeks to shift attention from stress as a biological and psychological entity and toward its historical construction as a discourse, a family of related concepts, and social and scientific practices. Such an approach is sorely needed. In much of the historical literature, stress is treated as a given, something that exists unproblematically in the outside world.[15] This book will historicize it as an explanation for many of the perceived problems of modernity, to explain how it has proliferated so widely since World War II and how it has forged connections between different areas of science and life.

The Proliferation of Stress

Stress was not the first signifier of a troubled modernity. In different ways neurasthenia, depression, hysteria, melancholia, anxiety, and suicide have provided ways of talking about modern problems, as have physical conditions such as cancer, heart disease, ulcers, consumption, and constipation. Stress has joined the pantheon of diseases of modernity and has displaced some such as neurasthenia from the 1940s, although this process of displacement was neither immediate nor uniform across different nations.[16] Whereas those who suffered from neurasthenia were chronically exhausted and depleted of nerve force, those who suffered from the later condition of stress were chronically overwrought, pushed beyond their ability to cope with modern life.[17]

This is not to say that neurological explanations were ever entirely abandoned. On the contrary, they became incorporated into new ways of seeing the correlation of the bodily organs and were embodied in new specialties, such as neuroendocrinology. From such a perspective, psychological and neurological mediators were followed by a cascade of neurohormonal events. Nerves thus continued to play a part in scientific formulations of the pathophysiological processes involved, and they also remained important in popular accounts of stress. The term "displacement" should, therefore, not be confused with "replacement." Stress displaced neurasthenia in two senses of the term: first, the discourse of stress tended to be used more commonly than nerves or neurasthenia in both popular and scientific literature, and, second, the persistence of nervous explanations was often subordinated to new ways of thinking about stress, incorporated into a broader discourse about stress. Thus, not only has stress displaced neurasthenia in complex and unpredictable ways, it has also linked this and other diseases of civilization together, as cause or consequence.[18] Crucially, stress has provided a common discourse about modern life. Although it has a multitude of meanings, its very diversity and flexibility help explain why it has become so prevalent.

The antecedents of stress are not only in the science and practice of psychiatry, physiology, and the social and biological sciences more generally but also in older forms of knowledge about the self and the relationship between mind and body. As Anne Harrington argues, the perceived importance of a healthy mind for a healthy body has long been with us, yet its various formulations in terms of hypnotic suggestion, confessional ritual, psychoanalysis, placebo effects, and self-help movements have been continually debunked and reinvented. The concept of stress was able to reformulate older ideas in a way that secured them in the rigorous sciences of the laboratory and tied them to influential theories of evolutionary adaptation. Older concepts and ideas were redefined not only by innovative laboratory studies of physiological stability or homoeostasis but by wider social, cultural, and intellectual currents: Walter B. Cannon saw his concept of homeostasis as offering solutions to the problems of the economic depression, for example, while commitments to social reform and the protection of the environment focused attention on the dangers of stress to social and ecological systems.[19] Concerns about the consequences of military conflict, anxieties about political instability, urban unrest, the threat of terrorism, and the dangers of the lifestyles driven by modern consumer capitalism have all helped focus attention on the problem of stress in various ways, particularly when allied to popular theories of cybernetics, sociobiology, and holistic medicine. The science of stress that emerged was driven and shaped by, and served to structure and direct, the search for individual and collective stability in a seemingly volatile and unbalanced world.

World War II plays a particularly important part in this story. As Theodore M. Brown and Tulley Long show in this volume it was during the war that psychologists first began to explore how the abnormal conditions of war affected normal people. Whereas at the beginning of the war, attention had focused on people with pathological predispositions to mental illness, by its end there was a new interest in how ordinary people, not obviously predisposed to neuroses, were affected. Unlike studies of earlier notions of neurasthenia and shell shock, where the focus was on the depletion of a limited nerve force that differed among individuals, stress research came to focus attention on how the body's adaptation to wartime conditions was itself destructive. The effects of various environmental conditions and the factors that tipped normal bodily reactions into pathological processes were now subject to study.

After the war this new interest in the role of stress in the normal population was extended to a variety of other psychological and behavioral conditions. In the first place stress seems to have been associated with psychological responses to extreme conditions such as grief, loss, or the discovery of deadly illnesses such as cancer. Caregivers found, for example, that conditions of extreme stress could provide a cathartic moment, which allowed otherwise reticent people to talk about life events and so begin a process of coming to terms with them.[20] In the second place, and building on earlier insights from psychosomatic medicine, it also came to be perceived as both the cause of a wide range of less traumatic, yet chronic, physiological and behavioral conditions and as a means of managing and coping with them.

Stress was taken up by a growing number of disciplines and professions, including social and industrial psychology, ecology, sociology, social work, nursing, and urban planning. An ever-increasing number of life situations came to be explained through the lens of stress: housing, work, unemployment, migration, racial and gender discrimination, and life in the total institution. Critical analyses of such practices were intimately bound up with the emergent social and political upheavals of the 1960s. The proliferation of stress was thus aided by an increased concern with social and economic disadvantage and with the perceived isolation and alienation of certain populations in modern urban environments, such as women in suburbia, the worker in the regimented factory or partitioned office, or children and the elderly in high-rise apartment buildings.[21] Yet it should not be supposed that stress was entirely the property of the Left. In the 1950s, for example, the Johns Hopkins psychobiologist Curt Richter attacked the welfare state on the grounds that it made people unable to cope with even the most trivial of life stresses.[22] Others would argue that stress was the inevitable and necessary consequence of a competitive industrial economy—that it functioned to limit the numbers of those at the bottom of the social hierarchy or that it was most common among the most successful, thus serving to remove the stigma of mental illness by associating it with the high-achieving, competitive, and masculine type A personality.[23]

Stress was also taken up by others to account for personal experiences and problems. The psychological gaze was extended into everyday life, while at the same time the public was increasingly pushed to psychologize and individualize its gaze. For example, Thomas Holmes and Richard Rahe and

Barbara and Bruce Dohrenwend encouraged people to measure their own responses to life events.[24] Thus, while experts were increasingly expanding the range of events that stress could usefully explain, the public was also encouraged to take up the language of stress to describe events that they perceived as meaningful. With such a proliferation in the usage of the concept of stress, many scientists and practitioners were concerned that stress may have lost its meaning as a diagnostic category. Stress, it is commonly noted, seems to involve anything and everything.

Stress also came to be seen as both the cause and the consequence of a wide range of *physical* ills. Stress—be it physiological or psychological—was implicated as a cause of cancer, heart disease, panic disorder, ulcers, hypertension, angina, migraines, colitis, constipation, diarrhea, diabetes, allergy, backaches, headaches, arthritis, busman's bowel, and many other physical ailments.[25] The new interest in stress was linked to the growing postwar concern about chronic and degenerative conditions. Selye himself highlighted the ways in which constant attacks on the body—stressors, as he came to call them in 1950—prompted its adaptive response to become maladaptive. Diseases such as arthritis were sometimes explained in terms of long-term chronic irritation, and the new wonder drug of cortisone, used to treat rheumatoid arthritis, gave added impetus to a linkage between stress and chronic and degenerative conditions.[26] Stress helped to blur the distinction between physical and psychological illness. Old ideas about the how people responded to serious illnesses were recast in the language of stress, as were concerns about how people responded to medical and surgical interventions against these conditions.

Critical to the success of stress was the way that it lent itself to physical measurement. It was first grounded in efforts to link behavior and psychology to biophysiology and thus had clearly identifiable effects on the physical body. In the animal laboratory this was easily measured through adrenal hypertrophy, atrophy of the lymphatic structures, and the ulceration of stomach and duodenum. In humans its measurement was more complicated, but, nevertheless, through the physical measures of cortisol levels, catecholamines, and even palmar sweating, it was considerably easier than other mental processes and disorders. It was also particularly amenable to survey techniques, respondents responding to a straightforward series of questions involving stressful life events, which could then be calibrated. While, indeed, questions emerged regarding the degree to which stress functioned as a symptom or a cause, particularly when measures such as blood pressure were used as markers, once again, it was the ability of stress to tie such a range of illnesses and symptoms together within a coherent whole that made it such a useful concept. As such, stress can be seen to have provided a wide variety of tools for intervening in the material world.[27]

Connectivity

Stress, we have argued, has developed a multiplicity of meanings, sometimes conflicting, sometimes blurring, into those of other diseases of civilization. This diversity and flexibility helps to explain why its use has proliferated since World War II. We would argue, however, that its success as a concept is also due to its ability to connect different domains. Stress links the body to the population, laboratory to field, physiology to behavior, animal to human. Stress has become a conceptual space in which the study of clinical medicine, biology, physiology, endocrinology, neurology, biochemistry, psychology, psychiatry, behavior, and ethics can enter into dialogue. In a sense it is a boundary object, to the degree that these different domains do not necessarily share a common meaning of stress, but that it provides an opportunity for the exchange of ideas and practices, for the development of new scientific networks and subdisciplines, and for public and disciplinary engagement and disagreement.

This book is organized around a series of connections. It does not claim to be comprehensive but instead builds on a growing body of scholarship that has begun to open up possibilities for further research. Let's take, for example, the discipline of ecology. As Gregg Mitman, Sharon Kingsland, and Robert Kohler have all shown, ecology was steeped in organismic analogy and metaphors of balance and, we would argue, was primed to engage with ideas of stress when they emerged in the 1940s and 1950s.[28] It is in 1950, the same year that Selye redefined the term "stress" and began to aggressively promote it as a state or condition, that the first paper in ecology was published that uses stress as a mechanism that regulates animal populations.[29] Building on the organismic analogy, stress provided ecologists with a way of uniting the skills of the theoretician and field scientist with those of the endocrinologist, showing how behavior is determined by, and determining of, physiological systems. Emphasizing the shared evolutionary history of human and nonhuman animals, stress was also a means for ecologists to comment on the problems facing human society.

Another area is the growing influence of systems theory and cybernetics, which deserves far more attention than we can give it here. We need to understand the degree to which the language of systems helped to prepare for the reception of the concept of stress or, alternatively, how ideas of physiological dynamics and equilibrium aided the development of systems theory. What is certain is that their histories are closely intertwined. The concept of stress allowed for physiological, behavioral, populational, and ecological systems to be connected into a functional, self-regulating whole. For example, Roy Grinker argued in 1956 for the existence of five systems—enzymatic, organ, nervous, psychological, and sociocultural—all interdependent, linked through circular processes of transaction.[30] Stress in one system may have effects on another or be compensated for by adjustments in others. The integration within each system and the defenses against disintegration constitute the forces that tend to maintain a steady state. For Grinker, an understanding of the system allows for intervention. Stress functioned, therefore, as a mechanism that connects these systems, allowing for the possibility of a unified theory of human (and presumably animal) behavior.

Finally, while we pay particular attention to particular groups within society, we are less specific about stress in relation to gender and race.[31] There is, of course, a very significant racial dimension to debates and policies in urban planning, in which stress plays an important role. For example, the anthropologist Edward Hall's influential studies of urban life promoted the idea that different races and cultural groups were more susceptible to different types of stresses. Hall's work can be usefully compared to Gerald Grob's nineteenth-century studies of the mental illness in African American populations. Where Grob's account identifies how the perceived inability of the African American to cope with life in the competitive industrial economy was used to condone slavery, Hall's account of the resilience of urban minority populations to crowding stress could be used to condone high-density public housing. With regard to gender, Ali Haggett's book on British homemakers explores the role of stress in the postwar domestic environment, while Elianne Riska's work has focused on the ideals of masculinity contained in the definition of the type A personality.[32] The history of stress can thus contribute not only to our understanding of the ways in which mental and psychosomatic illnesses are often regarded as more prevalent among certain populations but also to how these perceptions of populations were structured by broader anxieties about race, gender, and class. The problem of stress became central to debates regarding differences and similarities between groups and proved particularly useful in justifying a range of planning and policy decisions. Stress, therefore, not only connects medical and scientific theories, concepts, disciplines, and professions but is also critical to making connections between the social, behavioral, and biomedical sciences and the public domain.

Rationale of Organization

This book is divided into six sections that explore how stress proliferated and the different connections it facilitated.

Part One: Packaging Stress

The book begins with two chapters that explore how stress was packaged in different ways that allowed it to proliferate. Mark Jackson explores how the important figure of Selye constructed the notion of stress, picking up ideas and practices from other scientists and molding stress into a bodily condition or state. While (as we shall see in this book) scholars have complicated Selye's place within the history of stress, Jackson argues that Selye retains a significant role. He suggests that Selye's notion of stress can be seen as what he calls a "conceptual matrix" for communication across disciplines and communities, both within science and without. In Jackson's formulation Selye was an industry unto himself, publishing numerous articles and books and giving interviews to media. He was also someone who was able to take very complex ideas and make them accessible to a broader audience. Selye's formulation of the stress concept raised as many questions as answers. Nevertheless, even among those who disagreed with his conceptualization of stress, it served to stimulate both discussion and scientific work. Selye might have packaged stress in particular ways, but this did not mean that others always accepted his interpretation.[33]

In Elizabeth Siegel Watkins's account, stress not only is packaged but serves as a metaphorical packaging for the sale of a variety of products, from antidepressants to life-management courses. In her chapter Watkins shows that stress has a multiplicity of different meanings and uses, which helps to explain its proliferation in late twentieth-century America. In particular she shows how porous the boundary was between popular and scientific conceptions of stress. Popular conceptions of stress shaped scientific work and ideas as much as scientific conceptions of stress shaped popular discourse. Thus, this is not a story about how stress moves unidirectionally from the scientific domain to the popular; the movement was two-way. Furthermore, Watkins argues that stress gave a physical, biochemical basis to a variety of illness (such as anxiety and depression) that previously lacked such a basis, which was important to the sale of a variety of products to combat these conditions. Stress thus came to be part of the marketing of mental-health products: packaging in the sense that it presented these products to potential customers in ways designed to encourage them to purchase or demand them.

Part Two: Trauma and Acute Stress

The following two chapters take one of Watkins's points further, critically analyzing the series of movements by which shock, fear, and trauma were give a crucial neurophysiological foundation. In Allan Young's account of post-traumatic stress disorder (PTSD), he shows how the concept of stress worked to bring together Sigmund Freud's ideas of traumatic neurosis with Hughlings Jackson's model of the brain into a coherent and persuasive whole. Stress allowed for the identification of the cause, consequence, and the treatment of PTSD, which in turn became a universal phenomenon, because a hugely heterogeneous collection of symptoms were given homogeneity and coherence. Young's account thus highlights one of the more general points of this book about the complex ways in which stress comes to displace older concepts, incorporating aspects of older ideas and at times subordinating them to a broader discourse about PTSD.

Otniel E. Dror's chapter adds to this complex story of displacement and incorporation, showing how stress reformulated older ideas of Freud's and Walter Cannon's regarding balance and homeostasis.[34] Again identifying its power to encapsulate a broad range of ills, Dror shows how stress focused not only on chronic conditions but also on acute episodes that lead to illness and death. The post–World War II modeling of states of *acute* stress (sudden unexpected death) drew on and internalized interwar models of "voodoo death." This process entailed the reframing of what had been conceived and construed as a "primitive" and extreme form of *fear*, which was confined to "primitive" people, into the everyday and pervasive *stress* experience of "civilized" peoples in modern Western societies. Both Young's and Dror's analyses highlight the role of stress as a signifier of the problems of modernity and civilization; but while Young shows how stress allowed for PTSD to become a common consequence of the trials and tribulations of everyday life, Dror argues that modern problems have not merely become chronic, progressive, debilitating, and degenerative but remain sudden, acute, intensive, and unexpected.

Part Three: War

The third section highlights the important role of war and the state in facilitating stress research. Theodore M. Brown's account of stress in World War II examines major transformations in the ways in which psychiatrists employed by the US military approached the problem of war-related stress. Although they began by seeking to screen out those predisposed to neuroses, they increasingly shifted attention to focus on how normal populations responded to the abnormal conditions of war. Brown argues that psychiatrists came to emphasize stress as an external condition acting on the body, something that was able to explain the increasing number of psychiatric disorders they detected, while simultaneously expanding the role of psychiatry as a discipline with explanatory power. Stress thus had value as an explanatory tool, a means of professional advancement, and a service to the wartime state, something deployed to improve military efficiency. Brown goes on to argue that psychiatrists' insights into stress in wartime were later transferred to civilian populations. The war provided them with an opportunity, a laboratory in which to refine tools that could be used to explore the psychological and behavioral problems of civilians.

Tulley Long extends this account into the early Cold War. Specifically, she examines three episodes that highlight how, in the context of the Korean War and its aftermath, psychiatrists and physiologists sought to manage the psychiatric problems faced by servicemen, to maintain and improve military efficiency. Long highlights how the military facilitated interdisciplinary research between physiologists, endocrinologists, psychologists, and others, and, indeed, how stress research in the 1950s demanded interdisciplinarity. At the same time she highlights the difficulties of relying on physiological measurements of stress because of the difficulty of surveying populations and collecting samples under "stressful" wartime conditions. Long's account thus highlights not only the ways in which the American military shaped the organization of stress research in the 1950s but how the conditions of war shaped the practice of stress research.

Part Four: Work

The extension of the concept of stress into the study and management of civilian populations was by no means straightforward. The workplace is generally considered to have been the most conducive to the study of the relationship between the environment and mental and physical health. However, as Joseph Melling shows, stress coexisted with a variety of other terms such as strain, anxiety, distress, nerves, and fatigue, gradually emerging as the dominant concept as the result of workers' diminished tolerance of working practices, trade union agitation, and the falling away of alternative concepts. He argues that the concern with stress in the workplace has been a recent historical development in both Britain and the United States—the consequence of social and institutional needs more than scientific developments. While Melling's study is focused on Britain, it suggests that further comparative research that carefully identifies when and why stress enters into the discourse of occupational health in different nations would be of great value. Just as in the military, stress helped focus attention on the role of intolerable conditions in shaping the responses of normal people to industrial environments more than ideas of nerves and fatigue, which focus on individual failings and weaknesses.

This idea of a shift from individual variation to the stress-inducing workplace is further explored in Junko Kitanaka's study of Japan from the 1990s to the present day.[35] Kitanaka argues that depression has recently emerged as a much-politicized biomedical category used by workers for claiming sick leave and economic compensation. Japanese psychiatrists, she claims, have played a pivotal role in creating this new form of biosociality by providing powerful testimonies for depressed workers, showing how depression is rooted in workplace conditions and consequently elevating depression to a symbol of collective distress faced by many Japanese in times of economic uncertainty. But psychiatrists also occupy a problematic place between workers, government, and industry. If, in Kitanaka's account, psychiatrists have provided opportunities for workers to portray depression and a symbol of collective distress, they have also been called on by the government and industry to cultivate a system of psychiatric surveillance and a new science of measuring work stress and to scrutinize the psychopathology of workers. Her chapter therefore provides us with a much-needed understanding of the ways in which workplace stress is manipulated in different ways by psychiatry in the service of the state, the employer, and the individual worker.

Part Five: Managing Stress

War and work were not the only environments in which stress came to be monitored and managed. The following two chapters explore the management of stress in two quite different institutional environments. Robert G. W. Kirk's chapter examines how the language of stress operated within developing discourses of animal welfare in Britain. In the three decades following the close of World War II, "animal welfare" emerged as a powerful discourse that, alongside the new behavioral science of ethology, worked to broaden the perceived properties of animals, opening up new territories of intervention. Animal experiences of suffering, once confined to physiological pain, now came to include mental suffering, encompassing states of discomfort, distress, fear, frustration, and boredom. The conceptual landscape of stress made these factors, together with other pathologies detrimental to welfare, explicable through the animals' inability to cope within their environment. Welfare, thereby, became a matter of management. Kirk pays particular attention to the laboratory and the farm as two sites where animal welfare discourse was prominent in determining new managerial approaches to relating with animals. In both cases the development of animal welfare discourse worked to bring into being a distinct, materialized approach to welfare in which the concept of stress operated to construe suffering as animals failing to manage their relationship to the environment in which they lived. Within this logic the promotion of animal productivity became, in practice, indistinguishable from the promotion of animal welfare.

David Cantor's chapter explores how psychiatrists in the 1950s sought to manage patients' reactions to cancer and its treatments. Focusing on the physician Arthur M. Sutherland and his work at Memorial Hospital, Cantor shows how stress was deployed as an explanatory tool in understanding why potential patients delayed seeking help, how they responded to treatment, and how recovery progressed or did not. Cantor situates this interest in the response of patients to therapy within the broader context of long-standing concerns that patients delayed too long in seeking appropriate help for what might be cancer, a new post–World War II interest in the process of postoperative recovery, the growth of radical surgery at Memorial, and emergent critiques by patients of postoperative care. As in Kirk's chapter, psychological well-being was deemed critical to physical health. However, Cantor also argues that Sutherland's work served to defend radical surgery at a time when patients were increasingly dissatisfied with postoperative care. More broadly, and in common with Melling's chapter, he highlights the limitations of the appeal of stress in the 1950s. While Sutherland's research on the psychology of cancer was widely adopted, his use of stress was only patchily taken up by others seeking to manage patients with cancer, despite its centrality to his own understanding of patient psychology.

Part Six: Surveilling Stress

The final two chapters are about stress research in the field—the use of stress as a concept and measurement in examining the effects of the urban environment on populations and groups. Edmund Ramsden focuses on a network of psychologists, sociologists, architects, and city planners who, from the late 1950s, turned their attention to the role of the *physical* environment in determining behavior, health, and well-being. Disillusioned with the methods and theories of their parent disciplines, they were also united by concerns that urban environments were damaging to individuals and society. Interdisciplinary collaborations were founded on the basis of the language of stress, and solutions to urban problems identified through the understanding and control of various environmental stressors. Stress came to be operationalized both as a tool of urban renewal and as its critique.

The last chapter in this volume, Rhodri Hayward's, focuses more specifically on methods and in particular on the use of questionnaires and rating scales for measuring psychopathology, personal distress, and life events. Hayward explores the problems of participants being active in the reconstruction of narratives, in which stress becomes privileged as an aspect of everyday life and personal identity. What Hayward's study does—complementing that of Tulley Long's—is to highlight the problems of undertaking stress research in populations from the 1950s. But where Long focuses on the problems of doing physiological research under conditions of war, Hayward's focus is on the use of questionnaires and rating scales for populations in suburban Camberwell. In concluding with this article, we can see how far stress, as a theory, concept, and measure, has traveled from the physiological laboratory. It has been adapted to sites as diverse as the battlefield, factory, office, animal laboratory, suburban neighborhood, slum, and apartment building. While the contributions of this volume have emphasized its flexibility, adaptability, and connectivity as a concept, its success, as Hayward's chapter makes clear, also lies in its ability to connect with, translate, and give voice to so many of our experiences and concerns with modern living.

Notes

1. Alvin Toffler, *Future Shock* (New York: Bantam Books, 1970).

2. Hans Selye, "A Syndrome Produced by Diverse Nocuous Agents," *Nature* 138 (July 4, 1936): 32.

3. George M. Beard, *American Nervousness: Its Causes and Consequences* (New York: Putnam's Sons, 1881); Charles E. Rosenberg, "The Place of George M. Beard in Nineteenth-Century Psychiatry," *Bulletin of the History of Medicine* 36 (1962): 245–59; Barbara Sicherman, "The Uses of a Diagnosis: Doctors, Patients, and Neurasthenia," *Journal of the History of Medicine and Allied Sciences* 32 (January 1977): 33–54.

4. Hawkes, 1857, quoted in George Rosen, "Social Stress and Mental Disease from the Eighteenth Century to the Present: Some Origins of Social Psychiatry," Milbank Memorial Fund Quarterly 37 (1959): 21.

5. For earlier efforts to democratize mental illness, see Arthur Brock, who saw neurasthenia as the normal condition of the pre–World War I mind. *Health and Conduct* (London: Williams and Norgate, 1923), xv. For more on Brock, see David Cantor, "Between Galen, Geddes and the Gael: Arthur Brock, Modernity and Medical Humanism in Early-Twentieth-Century Scotland," *Journal of the History of Medicine and Allied Sciences* 60 (2005): 1–41.

6. Patrick J. Bracken, "Post-modernity and Post-traumatic Stress Disorder," *Social Science and Medicine* 53 (2001): 733–43.

7. In sociology and social psychology, ideas of "cultural lag" and "stimulus overload" have long been popular; see William F. Ogburn, *On Culture and Social Change* (Chicago: University of Chicago Press, 1964); and Georg Simmel, "The Metropolis and Mental Life," in *The Sociology of Georg Simmel*, trans. Kurt Wolff (1903; repr., New York: Free Press, 1950). For studies of stress in ecological and natural systems, see John J. Christian, "The Adreno-Pituitary System and Population Cycles in Mammals," *Journal of Mammalogy* 31 (1950): 247–59; and Charles C. Adams, "The Relation of General Ecology to Human Ecology," *Ecology* 16 (1935): 316–35; in cybernetics, see Peter Galison, "The Ontology of the Enemy: Norbert Wiener and the Cybernetic Vision," *Critical Inquiry* 21 (1994): 228–66; in genetics, see Julian Huxley, Ernst Mayr, and Humphry Osmond, "Schizophrenia as a Genetic Morphism," *Nature* 204 (1964): 220–21.

8. See Russell Viner, "Putting Stress in Life: Hans Selye and the Making of Stress Theory," *Social Studies of Science* 29, no. 3 (1999): 391–410.

9. Paul J. Rosch, "The Quandary of Job Stress Compensation," *Health and Stress* 3 (2001): 1–4.

10. Peter D. Kramer, *Listening to Prozac* (New York. Viking, 1993).

11. For a selection of the literature, see Ben Shephard, *A War of Nerves: Soldiers and Psychiatrists, 1914–1994* (London: Cape, 2000); Peter Leese, *Shell Shock:*

Traumatic Neurosis and the British Soldiers of the First World War (Basingstoke: Palgrave, 2002); Allan Young, *The Harmony of Illusions: Inventing Post-traumatic Stress Disorder* (Princeton, NJ: Princeton University Press, 1995); Edgar Jones and Simon Wessely, *Shell Shock to PTSD: Military Psychiatry from 1900 to the Gulf War* (New York: Psychology Press, 2005); Janet Oppenheim, *"Shattered Nerves": Doctors, Patients, and Depression in Victorian England* (New York: Oxford University Press, 1991); Marijke Gijswijt-Hofstra and Roy Porter, *Cultures of Neurasthenia: From Beard to the First World War* (Amsterdam: Rodopi, 2001); Francis G. Gosling, *Before Freud: Neurasthenia and the American Medical Community, 1870–1910* (Urbana: University of Illinois Press, 1987); David G. Schuster, *Neurasthenic Nation: America's Search for Health, Happiness, and Comfort, 1869–1920* (New Brunswick, NJ: Rutgers University Press, 2011); Ruth Leys, *Trauma: A Genealogy* (Chicago: University of Chicago Press, 2000); Michael J. Cowan, *Cult of the Will: Nervousness and German Modernity* (University Park: Pennsylvania State University Press, 2007); and Joanna Bourke, *Fear: A Cultural History* (London: Virago, 2005).

12. Cary L. Cooper and Philip J. Dewe, *Stress: A Brief History* (Malden, MA: Blackwell, 2004); Robert Kugelmann, *Stress: The Nature and History of Engineered Grief* (Westport, CT: Praeger, 1992); Angela Patmore, *The Truth about Stress* (London: Atlantic Books, 2006); Serge Doublet, *The Stress Myth* (Chesterfield, MO: Science and Humanities Press, 2000); and Dana Becker, *One Nation under Stress: The Trouble with Stress as an Idea* (New York: Oxford University Press, 2013). See in particular Becker's sociologically informed study that while questioning the formulation of stress as a disease, interprets it as a powerful metaphor for contemporary social ills.

13. Mark Jackson, *The Age of Stress: Science and the Search for Stability* (Oxford: Oxford University Press, 2013), 268.

14. For an indication of the possibilities of such a history, see Anne Harrington's valuable chapter on stress in *The Cure Within: A History of Mind-Body Medicine* (New York: Norton, 2008).

15. For an example of how stress is treated as a real entity, see Gregg Mitman, *The State of Nature: Ecology, Community, and American Social Thought, 1900–1950* (Chicago: University of Chicago Press, 1992), 7.

16. In eastern Europe, the Soviet Union, and China, neurasthenia persisted much longer than in the West; see Vladan Starcevic, "Neurasthenia in European Psychiatric Literature," *Transcultural Psychiatry* 31 (1994): 125–36. Moreover, as Kuriyama has shown, when stress entered the discourse of Japanese medicine, it took on some of the aspects of neurasthenia; see "Sutoresu no kokogaku [The archaeology of stress]," in *Karada no dento to kindai* [Tradition and modernity in the body], ed. Kitazawa Kazutoshi and Kuriyama Shigehisa (Tokyo: Seikyusha, 2004), 390–420.

17. Harrington, *Cure Within*, 142. On neurasthenia and exhaustion, see Anson Rabinbach, *The Human Motor: Energy, Fatigue, and the Origins of Modernity* (New York: Basic Books, 1990).

18. While stress may not have displaced cancer or heart disease as a way of talking about modernity, it has been viewed as the cause or consequence of both and thus helped to shape how these physical diseases have been imagined as diseases of modernity.

19. Harrington, *Cure Within*. See also Edward Shorter, *From the Mind into the Body: The Cultural Origins of Psychosomatic Symptoms* (New York: Free Press, 1994);

on Cannon, see Stephen J. Cross and William R. Albury, "Walter B. Cannon, L. J. Henderson, and the Organic Analogy," *Osiris* 3 (1987): 165–92.

20. See, for example, Virginia Dericks, "Periods of Stress," teaching notes, [1960s?], folder 14, Virginia Dericks Papers, Center for Nursing Historical Inquiry, Health Care Product Evaluation Center, University of Virginia School of Nursing, Charlottesville, Virginia.

21. Gary W. Evans, ed., *Environmental Stress* (Cambridge: Cambridge University Press, 1982).

22. Curt P. Richter, "Rats, Man, and the Welfare State," *American Psychologist* 14 (1959): 18–28.

23. Denis Stott, "Abnormal Mothering as a Cause of Mental Subnormality: II. Case Study and Conclusions," *Journal of Child Psychology* 3 (1962): 133–48; Elianne Riska, "From Type A Man to the Hardy Man: Masculinity and Health," *Sociology of Health and Illness* 24 (2002): 347–58.

24. Thomas H. Holmes and Richard H. Rahe, "The Social Readjustment Rating Scale," *Journal of Psychosomatic Research* 11 (1967): 213–18; Barbara Snell Dohrenwend and Bruce Philip Dohrenwend, eds., *Stressful Life Events: Their Nature and Effects* (New York: Wiley, 1973). For an analysis of the influence of life events in the popular realm, see Steve D. Brown, "The Worst Things in the World: Life Events Checklists in Popular Stress Management Texts," in *Ordinary Lifestyles: Popular Media, Consumption and Taste*, ed. David Bell and Joanne Hollows (Buckingham: Open University Press, 2005), 231–42.

25. See Carsten Timmermann, "Appropriating Risk Factors: The Reception of an American Approach to Chronic Disease in the Two German States, c. 1950–1990," *Social History of Medicine* 24 (2011): 157–74; Rhodri Hayward, *Psychiatry in Modern Britain* (forthcoming); Mark Jackson, *Allergy: The History of a Modern Malady* (London: Reaktion Books, 2006); Robert A. Aronowitz, *Making Sense of Illness: Science, Society and Disease* (Cambridge: Cambridge University Press, 1998); James C. Whorton, *Inner Hygiene: Constipation and the Pursuit of Health in Modern Society* (New York: Oxford University Press, 2000); Jackie Orr, *Panic Diaries: A Genealogy of Panic Disorder* (Durham, NC: Duke University Press, 2006).

26. On cortisone, see Harry M. Marks, "Cortisone, 1949: A Year in the Political Life of a Drug," *Bulletin of the History of Medicine* 66 (1992): 419–39; David Cantor, "Cortisone and the Politics of Drama, 1949–55," in *Medical Innovations in Historical Perspective*, ed. John V. Pickstone (Basingstoke: Macmillan, 1992), 165–84; Cantor, "Cortisone and the Politics of Empire: Imperialism and British Medicine, 1918–1955," *Bulletin of the History of Medicine* 67 (1993): 463–93; Lea Haller, "Stress, Cortison und Homöostase: Künstliche Nebennierenrindenhormone und physiologisches Gleichgewicht, 1936–1960," *NTM Zeitschrift für Geschichte der Wissenschaften, Technik und Medizin* 18 (2010): 169–95.

27. Nancy Cartwright, Towfic Shomar, and Mauricio Suarez, "The Tool Box of Science: Tools for the Building of Models with a Superconductivity Example," *Poznan Studies in the Philosophy of the Sciences and the Humanities* 44 (1995): 137–49.

28. Mitman, *State of Nature*; Sharon E. Kingsland, *The Evolution of American Ecology, 1890–2000* (Baltimore: Johns Hopkins University Press, 2005); Robert E. Kohler, *Landscapes and Labscapes: Exploring the Lab-Field Border in Biology* (Chicago: University of Chicago Press, 2002).

29. Christian, "Adreno-Pituitary System."

30. Roy R. Grinker, "The Intrapersonal Organization: A Model for Relationships among Systems," in *Toward a Unified Theory of Human Behavior: An Introduction to General Systems Theory*, ed. Roy R. Grinker and Helen MacGill Hughes (New York: Basic Books, 1956), 11.

31. Nevertheless, in this volume Elizabeth Siegel Watkins highlights the role of stress in relation to white-collar illnesses, while Edmund Ramsden also discusses the role stress has played in the relations between class and urban planning.

32. Edward T. Hall, *The Hidden Dimension* (Garden City, NY: Doubleday, 1966); Gerald N. Grob, "Class, Ethnicity, and Race in American Mental Hospitals, 1830–75," *Journal of the History of Medicine and Allied Sciences*, 28 (1973): 207–29; Ali Haggett, *Desperate Housewives: Neuroses and the Domestic Environment, 1945–1970* (London: Pickering and Chatto, 2012); Elianne Riska, "The Rise and Fall of the Type A Man," *Social Science and Medicine* 51 (2000): 1665–74.

33. Jackson discusses this topic further in *The Age of Stress.*

34. On Freud and homeostasis, see Nigel Walker, "Freud and Homeostasis," *British Journal for the Philosophy of Science* 7 (1956): 61–72; Daniel Pick, "Freud's Group Psychology and the History of the Crowd," *History Workshop Journal* 40 (1995): 39–62; David Bakan, *Disease, Pain, and Sacrifice: Toward a Psychology of Suffering* (Chicago: University of Chicago Press, 1968).

35. She expands on these points in Junko Kitanaka, *Depression in Japan: Psychiatric Cures for a Society in Distress* (Princeton, NJ: Princeton University Press, 2012).

Part One

Packaging Stress

Chapter One

Evaluating the Role of Hans Selye in the Modern History of Stress

Mark Jackson

> This is the philosophical point of view which alters our concept of disease. . . . Medical men who recognize the revolutionary and shattering nature of these developments realize that a great adjustment in our thinking has to be made. Here is the pool of Bethesda.
>
> J. S. L. Browne, "New Pool of Bethesda"

> Some years ago, Hans Selye postulated a general adaptation syndrome due to stress, but this concept has been of doubtful value in advancing the understanding of maladies.
>
> John W. Todd, "Plain Words in Medicine"

According to many stress researchers, as well as historians, modern biological formulations of stress can be traced back to a brief and rather speculative article written by the Austrian-born Hungarian scientist Hans Selye (1907–82) in 1936. The article set out what appeared to be a characteristic triphasic pattern of nonspecific physiological responses to injury: the "general adaptation syndrome" comprised an initial alarm phase that was followed by a stage of resistance or adaptation, leading eventually to a stage of exhaustion and death.[1] Within traditional narratives of stress history, which have often been written by researchers themselves and which portray the origins and development of scientific understandings of stress as relatively unproblematic and progressive, it was the general adaptation syndrome, or what Selye sometimes referred to rather ostentatiously as "Selye's syndrome," that provided a conceptual framework for Selye and his colleagues to develop a complex neurohormonal model of stress that implicated pituitary and adrenal function in the etiology of many chronic diseases, such as hypertension, peptic ulceration, renal disease, arthritis, asthma, and cancer.[2]

In later reflections on the intellectual origins of the general adaptation syndrome, Selye claimed that his insights into biological stress were not only the serendipitous product of a series of laboratory experiments performed on rats in the Department of Biochemistry at McGill University in Montreal, during which he had been attempting to isolate a new ovarian hormone. They were also the result of his clinical experiences as a medical student in Prague during the 1920s, when he had been struck by the similar sickly appearance of patients suffering from diverse chronic conditions such as tuberculosis, cancer, and burns: "All five patients, whatever their disease . . . had something in common," he wrote in his autobiography many years later. "*They all looked and felt sick.*"[3] It was primarily these personal encounters with patients in the clinic and observations in the laboratory, Selye insisted, that had led him to suggest that many clinical features of disease were the result of a failure in the nonspecific adaptive mechanisms of the body.

Selye's emphasis on his own pioneering contributions to the field has been reiterated in other historical accounts, which have juxtaposed analysis of his scientific status with more controversial anecdotal evidence of his commitment and character to highlight his role in shaping and popularizing modern formulations of stress. In 1975 John W. Mason, a neuroendocrinologist at the Walter Reed Army Institute of Research in Washington, suggested that the importance of Selye's work had led many researchers to assume (wrongly, according to Mason) that "usage of the term 'stress,' in a biological sense, begins historically with Selye's publications."[4] Although Mason pointed to earlier usage of the term and parallel formulations of the links between emotional stress and disease, he nevertheless acknowledged that Selye's 1936 paper on adaptation and disease had become part of the canon of stress literature, constituting a primary point of reference for scholars throughout the world regardless of their disciplinary orientation or focus. Historians have often perpetuated the conviction that Selye's article constituted a turning point in the history of stress and have occasionally acclaimed Selye as the creator, or father, of stress.[5]

These assessments of Selye's impact on the development of stress research are not entirely misplaced. During the 1930s, 1940s, and 1950s, Selye and his colleagues authored an expansive number of articles and monographs that clearly shaped and energized biological, and indeed psychological, studies of stress. Not only did Selye's reputation attract scholars from around the world to his research institutes, but Selye himself also became a much sought-after speaker on stress and health in many countries. In recognition of his contributions to stress research, Selye was nominated for the Nobel Prize in Physiology or Medicine seventeen times between 1949 and 1953, particularly for his "work on endocrinology and the adaptation syndrome," for his contributions to the "isolation of steroid hormones," and for his formulation of "stress reactions."[6] Although influential, Selye's theories of adaptation and stress were not unequivocally accepted by his contemporaries or indeed by his students: on the contrary, his experimental methods, his conceptual framework, and his entrepreneurial style were all strongly challenged, and many of his findings were eventually discarded. Nevertheless, as many of the chapters in this book indicate, during the middle decades of the twentieth century, Selye's notion of biological stress and its impact on health was adopted and adapted by researchers in a variety of adjacent fields, including military medicine, veterinary medicine, clinical allergy, sociobiology, population studies, cybernetics, and psychiatry.[7]

In spite of Selye's apparent prominence in the history of stress research, there have been few critical evaluations of the intellectual and cultural determinants of Selye's theories, few challenges to Selye's self-composed narrative of creation and progress, and few attempts to explore the heterogeneity of scientific responses to his ideas. Biographical accounts of his life and historical overviews of his contributions to modern understandings of stress have been based predominantly on his popular, often superficial and self-promoting, publications rather than on his more detailed scientific endeavors or archival sources.[8] Previous studies have tended toward polarized interpretations: at one extreme, many of those who worked closely with him in Montreal have regarded Selye, rather uncritically, as the preeminent figure in the field, responsible almost single-handedly for constructing and promoting a link between adaptation, stress, and organic disease; at the other extreme, historians and social scientists, wary perhaps of the hagiographic tendencies of scientific biography, have been more openly skeptical, pointing to Selye's capacity for entrepreneurship and media manipulation and playing down his scientific credibility. Closer inspection of his extensive output on the physiology and biochemistry of stress and analysis of contemporary reactions to his ideas suggest a more complex, and more intriguing, story. By focusing in turn on his theories of adaptation, his studies of steroid hormones, and his growing preoccupations with the language and mastery of stress, this chapter argues that, although his work was rigorously contested, Selye provided an important methodological platform for scientists and clinicians interested in understanding the relationship between stressful modern lives and disease.

The General Adaptation Syndrome

Born in Austria in 1907, Hans Selye was brought up in Komárom, on the border between Czechoslovakia and Hungary. After completing his medical degree and a doctorate in organic chemistry at the German University of Prague, he received a Rockefeller Foundation fellowship to study at Johns Hopkins in Baltimore before he moved to the Department of Biochemistry

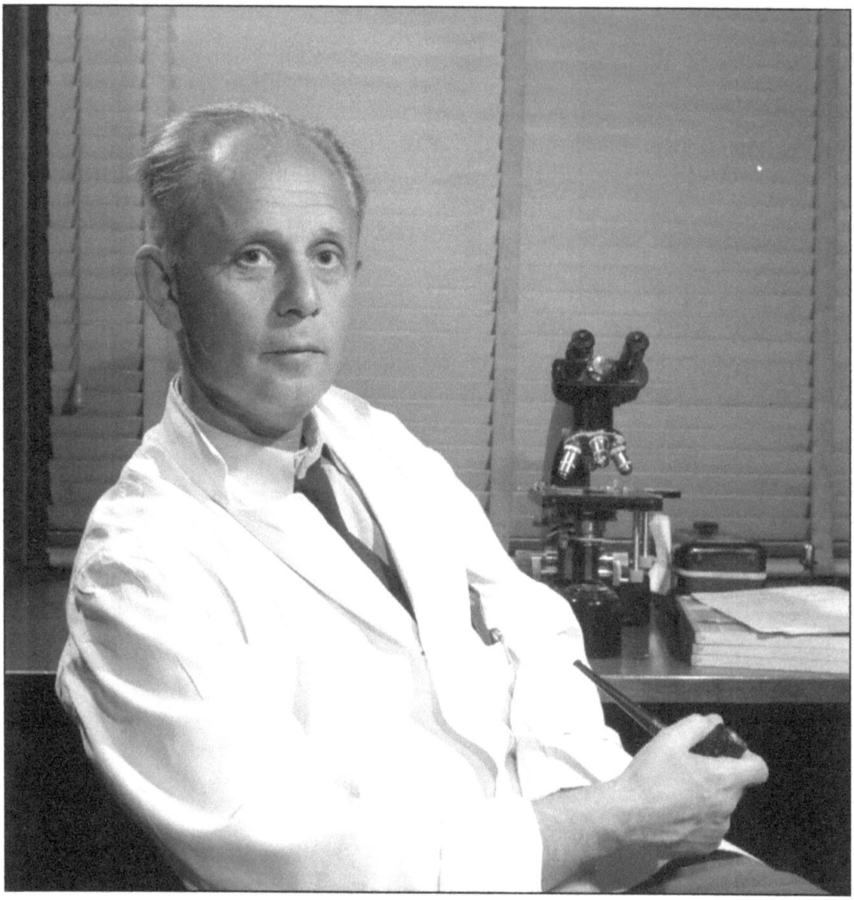

Figure 1.1. Hans Selye, 1956. Photograph by Chris Lund. National Film Board of Canada, Library and Archives Canada (PA-116671).

at McGill University in Montreal, under the sponsorship of James Bertram Collip (1892–1965), a biochemist who had discovered the parathyroid hormone and had been a member of the team responsible for isolating insulin in the 1920s. Selye's early work at McGill focused on the identification of ovarian hormones. It was in one of the papers emanating from this research in 1935, coauthored with Thomas McKeown (1912–88), who had been in Montreal between 1932 and 1934 as a National Research Council–funded doctoral student, that Selye first used the word "stress" to describe the adverse circumstances to which laboratory animals were subjected during experiments.[9] However, it was a brief article in *Nature* the following year that established a rudimentary framework for Selye's subsequent formulation of biological stress.

According to Selye, experiments on rats indicated that biological responses to "nocuous agents," such as cold, surgical injury, excessive exercise, or sublethal doses of drugs, demonstrated a stereotypical triphasic pattern irrespective of the nature of the injury: an initial alarm phase was followed by a stage of resistance that would lead eventually to exhaustion if exposure to the damaging agent persisted. Regarded by Selye as a form of defense similar to immunity, the general adaptation syndrome represented "a generalised effort of the organism to adapt itself to new conditions."[10] During the late 1930s and 1940s Selye explored the physiological stages of the general adaptation syndrome in more detail and clarified the central role of the adrenal glands in adaptive reactions.[11] In particular, he introduced the notion of "adaptation energy" to explain not only reduced tolerance to other forms of injury during the stage of resistance but also the eventual exhaustion and death suffered by laboratory animals after repeated exposure to environmental pressures. Using the weight of the thymus as an index of damage, Selye suggested that animals possessed only a finite capacity to adapt to injury: the cost of adaptation was the loss of "adaptation energy," a form of energy or resistance that was unrelated to calorific intake.[12] In subsequent formulations Selye referred to the loss of energy in terms of the "wear and tear" of life and drew a direct parallel between the stage of exhaustion on the one hand and processes of aging and dying on the other.[13]

Selye's most explicit exposition of his theory of adaptation and disease, at least prior to his wholesale adoption of the concept and language of stress, was an extended article published in 1946. More than one hundred pages long and containing nearly seven hundred references, this much-cited article established a model for Selye's regular overviews of the stress literature, which were published annually from 1950.[14] Selye situated his work primarily within studies of traumatic shock and toxicology, citing, for example, the work of the Harvard physiologist Walter Cannon (1871–1945), to whom the article was dedicated, and the American surgeon George W. Crile (1864–1943) on the physiological impact of surgical shock and the role of the nervous system in determining symptoms. Defining the general adaptation syndrome as "the sum of all non-specific, systemic reactions of the body which ensue upon long continued exposure to stress," Selye reviewed the biochemistry and pathological anatomy of adaptive responses, factors affecting the course of the general adaptation syndrome, and theoretical interpretations of the syndrome, including the pivotal role of hormones. He also set out the clinical implications of the general adaptation syndrome: "many of the most common maladies of man," he claimed, "are 'diseases of adaptation,' that is to say, the by-products of abnormal adaptive reactions to stress."[15]

Although Selye subsequently explained the genesis and parameters of the general adaptation syndrome primarily in terms of his personal endeavors, often relying largely on his own experimental results to substantiate his arguments and claiming a relatively smooth process of translation from laboratory findings to clinical implications, his scientific publications and archival records suggest a more complex heritage. In particular, his work echoed, and sometimes directly drew on, preceding and adjacent studies of physiological adaptation, contemporary accounts of fatigue and anxiety among modern populations, and psychosomatic understandings of disease. In the first place the overarching framework of Selye's syndrome resonated with wider contemporary interest in adaptation. During the 1920s and 1930s it was not unusual for clinicians to regard an apparent increase in chronic diseases in Western societies in terms of faulty adaptation or adjustment to the environment. In 1923, for example, the British physician Francis G. Crookshank (1873–1933) highlighted the pivotal role of adaptation to external circumstances in shaping health and disease: while health comprised successful adaptation to the environment, disease constituted "a dissociation of functional unity, or, maladjustment due to failure or incompleteness of adaptive response."[16]

For Crookshank and others, the need for effective adaptation was particularly prominent among modern populations: "The fact is that, at the present time, social change—industrial, economic, and the like—is everywhere modifying the conditions of life more rapidly than we care to admit;—far more rapidly for the exercise of the *natural* powers of adaptation of the human race."[17] Clinical preoccupations with the impact on health of adapting to physical and mental trauma were evident elsewhere during the late nineteenth and early twentieth centuries: in accounts of railway spine; in George Beard's explanation for the increased prevalence of nervous disorders, such as neurasthenia, among modern, sensitive American populations; and in Adolf Meyer's (1866–1950) psychobiology, according to which abnormal behavior was understood in terms of a failure of adaptive responses. As Rhodri Hayward has argued, in a world threatened by social, political, and economic instability, the notion of adaptation became increasingly central to Anglo-American psychiatric, psychological, and neurological theory and practice during this period.[18]

Concerns about the impact of social and technological change on human health and on the limits of adaptability were clearly shaped not only by developments in physiology, which allowed scientists to measure more directly the impact of everyday life on the function of cells and bodies, but also by fears about increasing levels of mental stress, fatigue, and traumatic neurosis among industrial workers and soldiers.[19] Preoccupations with nervous energy, stress, and fatigue and attempts to address them were expressed in a variety of locations. In the late nineteenth century, for example, both mesmerism and yoga were advocated on the basis that they could restore or more effectively channel depleted energy.[20] The sale and consumption of nerve tonics, such as Phosferine, Phyllosan, and Sanatogen, rested on claims that such proprietary preparations would help to combat what appeared to be an epidemic of anxiety, fatigue, nervous stress, and strain induced by the "modern conditions of high-pressure living." In a similar fashion, more orthodox physiological studies of shock, exhaustion, and the origins and nature of the emotions by George W. Crile, whose work was well known to Selye, highlighted the manner in which "noci-influences" operated to cause disease through the discharge of nervous energy.[21]

Similarities between Selye's and Crile's accounts of adaptation and disease are striking. At a general level Crile claimed that physiological systems were being driven at "an overwhelming rate of speed" by the "stress of our present-day life." Both acute and prolonged overstimulation by physical or emotional trauma placed the body "under stress," leading to the release of adrenaline and disturbing the previously "evenly balanced work" of the organs, especially those responsible for bearing "the stress of life," namely the brain, adrenal glands, and liver. Echoing previous discussions of neurasthenia and insanity, Crile implicated a variety of stresses in the etiology of chronic disease, including emotional strain, infection, physical labor, pregnancy, and "the stress of business or professional life." Cases of diabetes, like neurasthenia, were supposedly more prevalent among Jews, who were regarded as "especially emotional in character," and among businessmen concerned about the price of stocks. Although Crile acknowledged that adaptability, or the precise levels of "adaptive energy," varied between individuals (as well as between species) and although he accepted that different organs sometimes failed under stress, giving rise to different clinical manifestations, he emphasized what became a key feature of Selye's subsequent approach to stress and disease, namely the nonspecific nature of the pathological manifestations of responses to shock and trauma: "The essential pathology of shock," Crile insisted, "is identical whatever the cause."[22]

Energy, fatigue, and stress were also familiar motifs in accounts of the impact of work and war on the health and efficiency of what Anson Rabinbach has referred to as the "human motor." In his presidential address to the American Philosophical Society in 1906, the Harvard psychologist William James (1842–1910) encouraged colleagues to explore "the amount of energy" required and available for mental and moral activities and praised the ability of yoga to stabilize the nervous system and restore or unleash "unused reservoirs of power." Shortly after World War I, many of the witnesses to the British War Office inquiry into shell shock attributed the condition to prolonged and severe mental stress and fatigue: according to W. H. R. Rivers (1864–1922), for example, shell shock was largely the product of "stress, using stress as a wide term, including sleeplessness, anxiety, fatigue, responsibility."[23] Mental and physical disturbances associated with warfare in the air were similarly explained in terms of the strain, fatigue, and anxiety generated by prolonged flying and the conscious suppression of fear.[24] During the 1930s and 1940s much of the work at the Harvard Fatigue Laboratory, established in 1927 under the directorship of Lawrence J. Henderson (1878–1942), also concentrated on studying adaptive responses to physical stress and fatigue.[25]

It is not clear whether Selye was influenced directly by these studies of the fatigue and stress caused by modern life. In his discussions of adaptation energy and exhaustion he tended to cite the result of his own experiments rather than refer to any broader literature to support his arguments. It is clear, however, that Selye's formulation of the general adaptation syndrome did draw heavily on closely related interwar studies of physiological stability and self-regulation, on which scientific and clinical discussions of fatigue were partly based. Although stability constituted a crucial concept in contemporary debates about psychological health, scientific and medical interest in adaptive stability was most evident in the laboratory investigations of Walter Cannon.[26] During the 1920s Cannon published a number of key papers on the regulatory mechanisms by which organisms controlled a variety of internal conditions, such as blood glucose and salt concentrations, temperature, and acid-base balance. Cannon emphasized the manner in which these physiological processes were regulated by carefully coordinated cooperation between the autonomic nervous system and the endocrine glands, introducing the term "homeostasis" to describe the adaptive mechanisms that preserved functional stability in the face of environmental change.[27] In addition, he highlighted the clinical significance of these findings: deficient or uncontrolled hormonal secretion, particularly from the pituitary, thyroid, and adrenal glands, stimulated by "great emotional stress," he argued, could "play havoc with our internal adjustments" and generate disease.[28]

Cannon's account of self-regulatory adaptive processes clearly provided an important context for Selye's formulation of the general adaptation syndrome: Selye's 1946 article was dedicated to Cannon; Selye discussed Cannon's physiology at length in most of his books on adaptation and stress; and many of Cannon's publications appeared in Selye's extensive bibliographies. In 1975 Selye also contributed two chapters to a posthumous Festschrift for Cannon, in which he referred to Cannon as "one of the greatest physiologists not only of this century, but of all time" and suggested that, along with Claude Bernard, Cannon had exerted the greatest influence on his formulation of the general adaptation syndrome.[29] It may well be that Selye's subsequent adoption of the term "stress" also owes much to the work of Cannon, who had incorporated notions of stress in his accounts of homeostasis and emphasized the role of emotions in precipitating stresses and strains on the nervous system.[30] In addition, Cannon's elaboration of what he termed "social homeostasis" provided the blueprint for Selye's subsequent construction of a "natural philosophy of life," designed to maintain or restore individual happiness and social stability.[31]

Adjacent developments in clinical medicine may also have shaped Selye's preoccupation with adaptation and disease. Proponents of psychosomatic medicine, such as Franz Alexander (1891–1964) and Helen Flanders Dunbar (1902–59), for example, were not only exploring the impact of emotions and personality on mental and physical health during this period but also, like Selye, regularly describing health and disease in terms of energy, stability, homeostasis, the balance of the nervous and endocrine systems, and adjustment to shock.[32] There were also close similarities between the temporality of Dunbar's "delayed-action mines of childhood," in which an initial shock or persistent conflict eventually caused psychological or physical collapse, and the pattern of Selye's general adaptation syndrome.[33] Interactions between Selye's studies and those of Dunbar, Alexander, and others may have been direct. There is certainly some evidence for an exchange of concepts and approaches between Selye and proponents of psychosomatic medicine: not only did Selye publish his reflections on psychosomatic processes in *Psychosomatic Medicine,* a journal founded and initially edited by Alexander and Dunbar, but, as one of the pioneers of psychosocial medicine in Britain, James Lorimer Halliday (1897–1983), pointed out in 1950, the range of chronic "diseases of adaptation or stress diseases" explored by Selye closely matched the psychosomatic diseases studied by Alexander and his colleagues.[34]

Although Selye tended to emphasize the manner in which the general adaptation syndrome emerged relatively unproblematically from his own experimental observations and clinical experience, it is evident that he mobilized a range of concepts circulating within scientific and medical debates about health and disease during the interwar years. Preoccupations with the limits of human adaptability to the stresses and strains of modern life, concerns about the psychological and physical impact of shock and fatigue, physiological studies of adaptive self-regulation, and clinical interest in the psychosomatic determinants of health collectively provided motivation and resources for Selye's formulation of the relationship between adaptation and disease. Much of Selye's subsequent research effort focused not on charting the impact of the mind or environment on physical health, however, but on identifying the biochemical mediators involved in adaptive reactions to stress.

Steroids and Stress

Similarities between the general adaptation syndrome and physiological studies of adaptive responses to environmental stresses should not disguise evident differences between Selye's work and those of his scientific predecessors and peers. First, Selye's sense of temporality clearly differed from earlier work on shock and emergency reactions. His notion of an alarm reaction shared much in common with Cannon's account of fight or flight responses to danger, but Selye's discussion of the subsequent stages of resistance and exhaustion introduced an element of chronicity that was generally missing from previous studies. Although Cannon had referred to the impact of prolonged emotional disturbances, it was Selye's work primarily that foregrounded the pathological consequences of continued physiological attempts to adapt to relentless environmental stresses. Second, in focusing on chronicity Selye emphasized the role of hormones released from the adrenal cortex rather than those produced by the adrenal medulla. Thus, while Cannon and others investigated the contribution of adrenaline and noradrenaline to emergency reactions, Selye's research became increasingly concerned with the physiological actions of cortical steroids and their regulation by pituitary hormones.[35]

Selye's fixation with steroids, which emerged from his early studies of adrenal pathology, is evident in the diversity of the research projects that he coordinated, first at McGill and subsequently at the University of Montreal. During the early 1940s the range of projects supervised by Selye and funded by government agencies, charitable organizations, and pharmaceutical companies included investigations of the anesthetic properties of steroids, attempts to synthesize new "steroid compounds of probable pharmacological interest," work on the prevention of exhaustion following shock, experiments aimed at clarifying the actions of steroids on growth and renal function, studies on the role of steroids in oncogenesis, and inquiries into the interrelation between sex hormones.[36] Selye also possessed a prodigious capacity to convert the fruits of his "steroid research program" into published articles.[37] Between his arrival at McGill in 1933 and his departure in 1945, Selye authored or coauthored approximately three hundred academic papers, many of which offered original insights into the mechanisms of physiological adaptation, the physiology of sex hormones, and the functional biochemistry of cortical steroid hormones.[38]

In 1943 Selye published arguably his most substantial contribution to the field of steroid biochemistry, a four-volume *Encyclopedia of Endocrinology* that was dedicated to providing a "classified index of the steroid hormones and related compounds." Noting the lack of a convenient handbook for investigators working in a rapidly expanding field, Selye indicated that the purpose of the encyclopedia was to promote research by providing a classification of steroids according to their "most important chemical, physical and pharmacological properties." Selye's approach to the 728 steroids already identified was comprehensive and orderly. Starting with the simplest hydrocarbon nucleus, norestrane, the volumes proceeded through the parent compounds and their substitution products, providing space for entries relating to the isolation of the steroids from normal and pathological tissues; details of their structure, synthesis, melting points, and optical rotation; comments on their pharmacological activities; details of any derivatives; and a list of reference numbers linking individual entries to the bibliography. Selye's introduction to the encyclopedia also revealed a sophisticated approach to the functional interrelations of steroid hormones, compatible with his formulation of the integrated endocrine control of adaptive stability. Although he admitted that the complex chemistry, as well as the wide range and often unpredictable combination of pharmacological actions, of steroid molecules tended to "give the impression of complete lack of orderliness," Selye insisted that the successful synthesis of many hormones and the results of ongoing research would continue to reveal logical functional correlations.[39]

According to Selye, steroids possessed a combination of independent and subordinate activities. Depending on the endocrine gland, whose function they primarily imitated, the independent actions of steroid hormones included folliculoid, testoid, luteoid, corticoid, gonadotropic, renotropic, antifolliculoid, and anesthetic activities. Each independent action was also associated with a number of subordinate actions generated by the hormone's effect on a variety of other target glands or metabolic processes. Reflecting his own research interests in adrenal function under stress, Selye cited the vital significance of the adrenocorticoid hormones as a prime example of this dual capacity: "Similarly among the corticoids some compounds have a particularly pronounced effect on sugar and others on salt metabolism, but all the corticoids exert a beneficial effect on life maintenance after adrenal deprivation. Hence both the sugar and the salt metabolism influencing activities are subordinate to the life-maintaining potency of the corticoids."[40]

While the main volumes of Selye's *Encyclopedia of Endocrinology* capture the state (and reveal the limits) of scientific knowledge about individual steroids, the "synoptic charts" detailing the naturally occurring steroid hormones that had been isolated from different tissues along with their pharmacological properties, as well as the bibliography, testify to the range of laboratory and clinical studies being pursued into the structure and function of steroids around the world.[41] Drawing on his expansive knowledge of the field, much of Selye's subsequent work during the 1940s focused on refining scientific understanding of the role of steroid hormones in health and disease. Arguing that hormones were produced for the "sole purpose of directing, regulating and coordinating the activities of the organism," he insisted that the objective of endocrinology was not the treatment of rare glandular diseases but the management of more common "hormonal derangements resulting from maladaptation to stress." Steroid hormones lay at the heart of the body's capacity to adapt to the stress of life: "not only sex," he wrote in 1949, "but the development and metabolism of the entire body, as well as its resistance and adaptability to exposure and disease, are influenced by the steroid hormones of the gonads, the adrenal cortex and the placenta."[42]

As his publications on endocrinology make clear, stress occupied an increasingly pivotal position in Selye's scheme of hormonal adaptation and resistance. Not only was it stress that initiated the chain of reactions leading, under certain conditions, to disease but individual glands and their hormonal secretions were understood primarily in terms of their involvement in homeostatic adjustments to stressful circumstances. From this perspective the corticoid hormones were "indispensable for the maintenance of life and especially for the acquisition of adaptation to changes in the external or internal environment of the body": patients suffering from adrenal insufficiency were advised to "take special care to avoid stress and strain," such as exposure to cold and excessive exercise. For Selye, adrenal function was subject to higher control: recent investigations had revealed "evidence that one of the most important physiologic roles of the anterior-lobe [of the pituitary gland] is concerned with adaptation to various types of non-specific stress" and that derangements of "the pituitary response to stress" constituted one of the causes of the diseases of adaptation.[43] During the postwar years Selye and his colleagues continued to explore the correlation between adrenal and pituitary function by investigating the physiological actions of adrenocorticotrophic hormone in shaping resistance to stress.[44]

Although most of Selye's work focused on the isolation of cortical and pituitary hormones and the identification of their physiological and pathological functions in animals subjected to stress, he was aware of the human implications of endocrine research, often speculating about the potential application of his work to a broad range of clinical problems. For other researchers and pharmaceutical companies, the clinical and financial benefits of chemical analysis of steroids were more directly relevant. Organotherapy with crude glandular extracts had become unfashionable, but awareness of the potential for certain steroids to reduce inflammation in patients with rheumatoid arthritis and allergies helped to mobilize funds and to coordinate research on the isolation and synthesis of active hormone preparations. One of the principal outcomes of these activities has been well covered by historians: in 1949 the American physician Philip S. Hench (1896–1965) and his colleagues announced the successful treatment of arthritis with a hormone, initially referred to as Compound E and subsequently named cortisone, that had been isolated from the adrenal cortex by the chemist Edward C. Kendall (1886–1972). In 1950 Hench, Kendall, and the Swiss chemist Tadeus Reichstein (1897–1996) were jointly awarded the Nobel Prize in Physiology or Medicine for their contributions to the discovery of the role of cortisone in the treatment of rheumatism.[45]

The focus of Hench and his colleagues on rheumatoid arthritis should perhaps have aligned their work closely with that of Selye, since rheumatism was commonly regarded, not just by Selye, as a "breakdown of the body's adaptive response to external stresses such as cold."[46] However, although the three Nobel laureates referred to the publications of many physiologists and biochemists in their Nobel lectures, none of them cited Selye, who was also nominated for a Nobel Prize that year.[47] It may well be that Selye's preoccupation with stress and adaptation in animals distanced him from other researchers who were applying biochemical analyses of steroid compounds directly to the treatment of human diseases in this period. In addition, as we shall see, resistance to his ideas about adrenopituitary control of endocrine function may have been stimulated by growing skepticism about the theoretical viability of the general adaptation syndrome. In 1951, for example, Kendall directly dismissed "the adaptation syndrome of Selye" as an explanation for the influence of cortisone on health and disease.[48]

Kendall's curt rejection of Selye's work should not be taken to suggest that Selye was peripheral to the fields of steroid chemistry and endocrinology during this period. As both internal endorsements of his reputation by colleagues at McGill and nominations for the Nobel Prize suggest, he was highly regarded by scholars around the world. According to Roger Guillemin, who had been one of Selye's research fellows and who later received the Nobel Prize for his isolation of hypothalamic-releasing factors, Selye was "one of the major ferments of modern endocrinology."[49] The Argentinean physiologist Bernardo A. Houssay (1887–1971), who was awarded the Nobel Prize in 1947 for his discovery of the role of anterior pituitary hormones in sugar metabolism, similarly suggested that Selye possessed "exceptional and probably unique conditions and abilities" that enabled him to "dominate all aspects of endocrinology with equal competence"; in addition to owning the "largest endocrinological library in the world," commanding many languages, and being a "brilliant teacher," Selye possessed "a personal knowledge of the major part of experimental endocrinology" and had contributed "important original studies, executed with skilful technique, to the development of the science."[50] In Houssay's words, Selye's *Textbook of Endocrinology* was a volume of "historic importance, since it is the most complete synthesis of endocrinological facts published up to date."[51]

Selye's research on steroids also attracted interest from other quarters. As Kendall pointed out in his Nobel lecture, the exigencies of war had played a crucial part in stimulating research into pharmacologically active steroids in the United States.[52] Military interest in cortical hormone preparations was related in part to their potential to reduce mental and physical fatigue. The ability of cortical extracts and purified steroids to counteract the lassitude associated with adrenal insufficiency or to improve health and stamina among overworked and anxious populations had been highlighted during the 1930s and early 1940s, leading to a commercial market for the manufacturers of hormonal extracts such as Adreno-Spermin, which promised to reverse glandular imbalances generated by stress.[53] As the stress of combat became apparent during World War II, allied military commanders on both sides of the Atlantic turned to laboratory studies of cortical steroids in the hope that the results would enable military physicians to identify and more effectively treat service personnel suffering from stress-induced fatigue.

Like shell shock and flying stress during World War I, cases of war neurosis among soldiers who had broken down "under the stress of active-service conditions" during World War II were explained primarily in terms of the fatigue and fear associated with prolonged engagement in hostile conditions.[54] In addition, psychosomatic symptoms among civilians subjected to intensive air raids were regarded as the product of anxieties precipitated by war: "It is to the war as a whole," wrote Aubrey Lewis (1900–75) in 1942, "with its accumulated stresses, that people have to adjust themselves, and signs of failure to do this can be taken as warning signals of neurosis."[55] As Selye pointed out in 1943, many of these studies of wartime illness supported his account of the general adaptation syndrome. The increased incidence of perforated peptic ulcers among British populations subjected to air raids, for example, could be explained in terms of an adrenocortical defense reaction, comparable to that produced in animals "by exposure to stress."[56] However, wartime studies of stress were only rarely linked directly to Selye's account of adaptation and disease. Although some military doctors described various stages of stress in a manner that echoed the features of Selye's triphasic general adaptation syndrome, they more often referred explicitly to Cannon's notion of alarm. According to the authors of a survey of anxiety states in the navy, for example, the "immediate stress of danger" provoked a "physiological adrenal-sympathetic response," comparable to Cannon's fight or flight reaction. If the pressures of combat persisted, this stage of "early stress" was followed (as in Selye's adaptation syndrome) by a phase of "established tension," which in turn led to a state of "anxiety with exhaustion."[57]

Although Selye's syndrome was often bypassed in this way, his work on adrenocortical steroids did shape military approaches to identifying and minimizing combat stress. After World War I the US Armed Forces had introduced a psychological screening program on the grounds that constitution determined resilience under stress. However, evidence that many supposedly stable recruits suffered from incapacitating fear and fatigue suggested that anyone could suffer from a breakdown depending on the duration and intensity of the stress to which they were exposed. Emotional casualties were thus regarded as inevitable products of war rather than as examples of lack of courage or malingering.[58] According to Roy R. Grinker (1900–1993) and John P. Spiegel (1911–91), who conducted an extensive investigation into the effects of stress on American air force personnel, the "stress of war tries men as no other test that they have encountered in civilized life." "Under sufficient stress," they continued, "any individual may show failure of adaptation, evidenced by neurotic symptoms."[59] Among British forces a different ethos prevailed. While their American counterparts emphasized environmental stress, British military authorities tended to prioritize constitutional factors: pilots who failed to cope with the demands of warfare and threatened operational efficiency were deemed to be deficient in character and, if found guilty of a "lack of moral fibre," could be returned to a basic grade or discharged.[60]

One of the challenges facing military authorities in relation to the selection of recruits and the identification of stress-related disorders was that psychological assessment was based primarily on subjective reporting of symptoms and behavior. Research carried out by the physiologists Gregory Pincus (1903–67) and Hudson Hoagland (1899–1982), however, suggested that an alternative strategy might be available, one that combined Selye's physiological studies of the role of the adrenal cortex in resisting stress with measurements of the urinary excretion of steroid metabolites. Drawing on Selye's work on histological changes in the adrenal cortex after exposure to stress and on evidence that the excretion of 17-ketosteroids increased during illness, Pincus and Hoagland investigated whether the output of 17-ketosteroids might serve as a marker of physiological stress in aircraft personnel. The results indicated that both urinary volume and the concentration of 17-ketosteroids increased when men were flying or subjected to fatiguing activities comparable to those encountered on long flights. Moreover, it appeared that while "poorer performers tended to exhibit the greatest ketosteroiduria and diuresis," pilots who were more resistant to stress-related fatigue tended to excrete "low amounts of 17-ketosteroids, as if the stress of daily living exerts little drain upon their adrenal cortex secretion."[61]

As Hoagland suggested, the results of these experiments offered not only a means of measuring physiological stress more accurately and identifying those who were less capable of resistance but also the possibility of developing a strategy for "preventing the stresses of flight from interfering too greatly with our homeostatic mechanisms."[62] Given that an individual's capacity to endure fatiguing ordeals appeared to be related to adrenal function, Pincus and Hoagland attempted to determine whether certain steroids increased resistance to stress. Although they emphasized that efficacy appeared to depend, at least to some extent, on individual motivation and the degree of stress, their studies indicated that pregnenolone in particular was effective in "counteracting psychomotor fatigue," as measured by urinary 17-ketosteroid excretion.[63] The work of Pincus and Hoagland was significant not only because it established a physiological marker for stress, one that did much to confirm Selye's emphasis on adrenocortical mediation of the stress response, but also because it provided an opportunity to circumvent industrial measures of fatigue that emphasized only productivity or performance.[64] Steroid chemistry thus promised a solution to the problems of occupational stress and nervous fatigue that clinicians, patients, industrial managers, and military authorities, as well as experimental physiologists, had been seeking since the late nineteenth century.

The originality of Selye's approach to the role of steroid hormones in adapting to chronic stress is arguably evidenced by the skeptical reception that it initially provoked from other scholars in the field, particularly Cannon. According to Selye, Cannon's resistance appeared to revolve around four of Selye's "basic tenets": the importance of chronic, rather than merely acute, responses; the central role of the adrenal cortex and pituitary gland; the nonspecific nature of adaptive responses; and the manner in which "the most diverse diseases can result from stress, depending upon the simultaneous influence of different conditioning agents."[65] In addition, Cannon may have been unimpressed by the crudity of some of Selye's experimental work. In 1922 Cannon had criticized studies that measured organ responses only in terms of size or that drew conclusions from the application of injuries, such as organ ablation, that could not be considered physiological.[66] Although Selye did include more sophisticated histological evidence, much of his early work on the effects of prolonged stress used organ weight as an indicator of physiological reaction. In spite of doubts about his methods and theories, however, Selye's theory of adaptation and disease and his emphasis on the role of steroid hormones in mediating stress reactions began to attract scientific and clinical attention because of its potential to address the rising tide of chronic disease that was threatening to submerge modern societies.

Stress and Disease

Just as Selye liked to explain the origins of the general adaptation syndrome in terms of a smooth transition from laboratory experiment to theory, he also tended to highlight the relatively unproblematic conceptual journey from adaptation to stress. Although he acknowledged that there were objections to his terminology from the start, he claimed a relatively clear lineage for his growing preoccupations with stress: laboratory research provided the evidential basis for the general adaptation syndrome, which was itself transformed by further research and clinical observation into a fully fledged pathology of stress. Yet Selye's notion of the general adaptation syndrome and his conversion to the language of stress received mixed responses. In spite of his considerable efforts to establish the validity of the syndrome and to justify his formulation of stress, many scientists and clinicians remained skeptical.

Conflicting reactions to Selye's account of adaptation and stress are particularly evident in responses to his Heberden oration on stress and the general adaptation syndrome, delivered in London in June 1950.[67] By this time Selye had moved from McGill University to establish the Institute of Experimental Medicine and Surgery at the University of Montreal. Selye's departure from McGill had been prompted by a number of factors, including increasingly strained relationships with senior colleagues, some of whom questioned the validity of Selye's work as well as the ethics of accepting sponsorship from the pharmaceutical sector without sufficient institutional control.[68] Internal disputes at McGill coincided with a generous offer from the University of Montreal, which at that time was not only investing in what Selye referred to as its "magnificent new campus" but also aiming to increase its recruitment of international researchers.[69] Following his arrival at the university in 1945, Selye rapidly established his institute as one of the prime locations for studying interactions between environmental circumstances, endocrine function, and health. It was from the institute, for example, that he began to publish his annual surveys of stress literature from 1950.[70]

Selye's relocation was accompanied by a significant shift in his approach to the language of disease. Prior to 1950 Selye had conceptualized pathology in terms of faulty adaptation to environmental circumstances; when he did use the term "stress," it signified merely the external trigger of adaptive responses.[71] This hierarchy of factors, in which stress operated only through adaptive processes, persisted, albeit in muted form, in his 1950 Heberden oration: "Stress acts only through the general adaptation syndrome," he insisted. But there are signs that Selye had begun to reconceptualize stress, referring to it not merely as an external trigger of internal processes but also as a physiological or pathological process itself. "In the biological sense," he argued in 1950, "stress is the interaction between damage and defence, just as in physics tension or pressure represents the interplay between a force and the resistance offered to it."[72] Perhaps recognizing the flexibility and fecundity of the concept, Selye increasingly employed the word "stress" rather than "adaptation" in both scholarly and popular accounts of his research. By 1956, when Selye published arguably his most influential study of the causes and pathogenesis of chronic disease, stress now took center place: in *The Stress of Life*, the general adaptation syndrome was only the visible manifestation of stress, which now constituted "the common denominator of all adaptive reactions in the body." More specifically, stress, rather than adaptation, signified the pivotal biological process at the heart of individual strategies for coping with modern life: "Stress," Selye insisted, "is essentially the rate of all the wear and tear caused by life."[73] To differentiate between the harmful agent and the biological response more clearly, Selye began to employ a new term, "stressor": "All agents can act as stressors, producing both stress and specific actions."[74]

Selye's formulation of the general adaptation syndrome and his linguistic shift toward stress generated heated debates in the *British Medical Journal* and the *Lancet*. A number of correspondents dismissed Selye's "bold attempt at a monistic pathology." Having pointed out that Selye's latest contribution had left him "in some mental confusion," H. N. Green, for example, doubted whether "Professor Selye's more recent ideas, even born as they are out of prodigious labours, will survive, *in their present form*, for very long." In particular, Green was critical of Selye's extrapolation from studies of the pathological effects of large doses of steroids administered to rats on the one hand to an ambitious account of the role of corticoids in human disease on the other. A. P. Meiklejohn similarly disapproved of Selye's reliance on a number of unsubstantiated speculations. In one of the most hostile reactions to Selye's Heberden oration, Ffrangcon Roberts exposed what he regarded as fatal contradictions at the heart of Selye's scientific framework for understanding disease. Uncritical acceptance of Selye's conflicting definitions of stress, Roberts argued, could lead only to an uncomfortable paradox: "Therefore stress, in addition to being itself and the result of itself, is also the cause of itself."[75] Although they often recognized the heuristic value of Selye's reflections on the pathogenesis of chronic disease, subsequent correspondents reinforced this sense of skepticism, contesting Selye's claims that his focus on individual adjustment to stressful environments was original, challenging Selye's theoretical interpretation of laboratory data, and emphasizing the need for further research. "The whole problem is full of obscurities," an editorial complained in response to a further article by Selye the following year, "and alternative explanations of Professor Selye's results are likely to persist until much more experimental work has been done to separate out specific physiological effects from those of a non-specific nature."[76]

Selye was exasperated by the tone of most of this correspondence, which he suggested had been written with "some animosity and little, if any, reference to facts," but he found considerable support from many other reviews of his work.[77] Selye's apparently "brilliant exposition of a most fascinating piece of research" in 1950 was initially well received by members of the Heberden Society, and according to one reviewer of Selye's first monograph on stress: "No-one has the right to pronounce judgment without carefully and critically reviewing the evidence, and no-one who reads this monumental contribution to the medical classics can fail to be profoundly impressed."[78] Selye's research continued to attract grants from state departments, charitable organizations, and pharmaceutical companies interested in the potential clinical applications of laboratory studies of stress, and many clinicians welcomed Selye's attempt to develop a novel theoretical framework for understanding a range of biological reactions and clinical manifestations that had previously resisted explanation. In 1952 the British surgeon David Le Vay applauded the manner in which Selye's "painstaking researches" helped to provide a "unitary conception of disease," integrating studies of the endocrine system with psychosomatic medicine and providing insights into the pathogenesis of functional disorders such as peptic ulcer, fibrositis, rheumatoid arthritis, and asthma.[79] During the postwar decades the central features of Selye's triphasic adaptation syndrome, and particularly his focus on the role of the adrenopituitary system in regulating stress responses, were not only adopted by allergists, clinical ecologists, and psychiatrists treating patients but also discussed in the context of sociobiological studies of aggression, psychoanalytical accounts of pain and suffering, investigations into cyclical variations in mammalian populations, studies in occupational and military psychology, and in nascent politicized deliberations about the pursuit of happiness and health on both sides of the Atlantic.[80]

Selye's studies of adaptation, steroids, and stress also generated support within the Rockefeller Foundation. In January 1950 a monthly report to the trustees explored recent studies of the relationship between adrenal function and disease. According to John S. L. Browne (1904–84), a British scientist who had received a Rockefeller Award at McGill and who had been best man at Selye's first wedding, the general adaptation syndrome constituted "the new pool of Bethesda," an original "philosophical point of view which alters our concept of disease":

> It presents the picture of a basic pathological process at work which when it mounts to a certain magnitude is the disease. And this idea, I may add, is completely at variance with the older views of scientific medicine. It is at variance with the ideas of compartmentalized disease, which is the central dogma of modern medical practice. Medical men who recognize the revolutionary and shattering nature of these developments realize that a great adjustment in our thinking has to be made. Here is the pool of Bethesda.[81]

As many of the chapters in this volume demonstrate, Selye's influence extended well beyond the scientific academy. From the early 1950s through to the 1980s, his research on adaptation and stress was reported in national newspapers, magazines, and clinical journals across the world. *Time* magazine, for example, ran a number of cover stories on the multiple manifestations of stress in the lives of contemporary Americans, often focusing on Selye's theories.[82] Medical advice books written for a general audience also transmitted Selye's message to the world. In 1956 *Healthy Minds and Bodies*, intending to provide British families with guidance on "all medical, marriage and motherhood problems," cited Selye's research on the bodily impact of stress to reinforce the book's promotion of preventative health care: "Professor Selye's conclusion to date is that stress is an important factor in the causing of all physical diseases, except, of course, those due to injury, infection or poisoning. This, as you can see, is a very forcible reminder that Worry Can Kill."[83] The uptake of Selye's ideas was facilitated by his deliberate attempts to advertise his work to a global audience. In addition to delivering lectures around the world, Selye published a number of best-selling books on stress and disease, many of which not only set out his scientific theories in laymen's terms but also established his own historical narrative of the discovery and demonstration of the general adaptation syndrome.[84] Although his scientific credibility was not universally endorsed by his peers, it was partly through Selye's popularizing zeal that stress came to be regarded as a cause of chronic disease in the decades following World War II.

Historicizing Selye

Retrospective assessments of the place and importance of Selye's work on adaptation and stress, like those expressed at the time, have been mixed. As researchers increasingly turned to clinical studies of human disease and to investigations of the psychological mediators of stress, such as appraisal and coping, Selye's experimental model, in which laboratory rats were stressed by starvation, extreme temperatures, and excessive exercise, appeared anachronistic and unethical. In 1970 an English physician, John Todd, for example, dismissed the general adaptation syndrome as one of "the errors of medicine." "Imperfections in this general-adaptation process," he wrote, "were thought to be a major cause of many maladies, notably much arterial disease and rheumatoid arthritis. Although many of Selye's observations were valuable, few now accept this theory." Fifteen years later, Paul Christian and Fernando Lolas were even more emphatic in their rejection of Selye's place in modern accounts of adaptation, stress, and disease. Although they acknowledged that the general adaptation syndrome had provided a valid model for understanding the effects of some stressors, they insisted that Selye's notions no longer fit the new "theoretical pathology" that supposedly provided the "conceptual foundation of medicine": "The Selyean concept, the original idea of the pituitary-adrenal humoral axis," they argued, "was abandoned and was no longer at the center of the discussion."[85]

Selye's detractors were only partially correct. While competing formulations of stress tended to marginalize Selye's biological focus, his emphasis on the neurohormonal mediators of adaptation and stress continued to inform medical and scientific publications as well as popular accounts of ill-health. For many clinicians and scientists Selye's notion of "diseases of adaptation," his analysis of the role of steroid hormones in mediating resistance to stress, and his promotion of stress as a novel language of disease remained paradigmatic.[86] In 1976 the British psychiatrist Richard Mackarness (1916–96) insisted that Selye would "come to rank with Louis Pasteur, Frederick Banting and Alexander Fleming among the immortals of medical research" for his role in clarifying the "mechanics of adaptation and the body's response to the threats to its stability." Two years later, Tom Cox, a prominent British occupational psychologist, similarly lauded Selye's contributions to modern understandings of stress: the capacity for the concept of stress to constructively bring together "fragments of information and relatively isolated ideas from a variety of different areas," he suggested, owed much to "the pioneering writing of Hans Selye." Many of Selye's students were also profoundly influenced by his vision and personality, and some of them, such as Roger Guillemin, made major contributions to the science of hormonal regulation and stress. In a tribute to Selye published three years after his death, a number of students and colleagues testified to his enduring impact on the field. According to Claude Fortier (1921–86), Selye was "one of the rare giants of contemporary biology," blessed with intuition, intellectual depth, and remarkable energy. As Guillemin pointed out in a more balanced evaluation of Selye's work, Selye "was the source of many ideas which, whether accepted or, more often, challenged; whether confirmed as such or eventually profoundly modified, were at the roots of modern neuroendocrinology."[87]

Measured historical reflection is needed to reconcile conflicting accounts of Selye's place in the modern history of stress. Scholarship should resort neither to uncritical adulation of his achievements nor to premature dismissal of his contributions to the field. Rather, it should aim to investigate fully the origins, development, and reception of his work within scientific, social, and cultural contexts. This chapter has attempted to extend the process of historical reconstruction. Whether embraced or discarded, Selye's formulation of adaptation and disease provided an important conceptual matrix for subsequent discussions of the mechanisms and manifestations of stress reactions, serving at the same time to fertilize research into the bio-psycho-social determinants and the pathophysiological pathways of chronic disease well into the twenty-first century. For this reason, careful study of Selye's changing approaches to stress offers a constructive window onto shifting debates about the impact of environmental circumstances on physiological regulation, individual health, and social harmony. Indeed, in many ways, Selye's journey from the physiology of shock and adaptation to the biochemistry of stress and the psychology of happiness exemplifies the complex history of modern stress research.

Notes

I am grateful to the Wellcome Trust for funding the research on which this article is based, to David Cantor and Ed Ramsden for their editorial support and comments, and to the participants in the conference at which this paper was first presented.

Epigraphs: J. S. L. Browne, "The New Pool of Bethesda," confidential monthly report to the trustees, January 1950, Rockefeller Foundation Archives, Rockefeller Archive Center, Sleepy Hollow, New York, 16; and John W. Todd, "Plain Words in Medicine," *Lancet*, June 13, 1964, 1287.

1. Hans Selye, "A Syndrome Produced by Diverse Nocuous Agents," *Nature* 138 (July 4, 1936): 32.

2. Hans Selye, *The Stress of My Life* (Toronto: McClelland and Stewart, 1977), 85.

3. Ibid., 71–72, 68–69; italics in the original.

4. John W. Mason, "A Historical View of the Stress Field," part 1, *Journal of Human Stress* 1 (1975): 6.

5. François-Joachim Beer, "L'histoire du concept biologique du stress," *Histoires des Sciences Medicales* 11 (1977): 135–40; Georgette Goupil, *Hans Selye: La sagesse du stress* (Quebec: Nouvelle Optique, 1981); Russell Viner, "Putting Stress in Life: Hans Selye and the Making of Stress Theory," *Social Studies of Science* 29, no. 3 (1999): 391–410.

6. See the Nomination Database for the Nobel Prize, *The Official Website of the Nobel Prize*, accessed September 17, 2013, http://nobelprize.org/nobel_prizes/medicine/nomination/nomination.php?string+Hans+Selye.

7. For a detailed discussion of Selye's work and its influence, see Mark Jackson, *The Age of Stress: Science and the Search for Stability* (Oxford: Oxford University Press, 2013).

8. Biographical studies and personal reminiscences include Beer, "L'histoire"; Goupil, *Hans Selye*; Andrée Yanacopoulo, *Hans Selye ou la cathédrale du stress* (Quebec: Le Jour, 1992); Paul Rosch, "Remembering Hans Selye and the Birth of 'Stress,'" *Health and Stress* 1 (2010): 1–14; and Istvan Berczi, "Stress and Disease: The Contributions of Hans Selye to Neuroimmune Biology," http://home.cc.umanitoba.ca/~berczii/page2.htm, accessed September 16, 2013. More critical historical evaluations of Selye's work include Viner, "Putting Stress in Life"; Cary L. Cooper and Philip Dewe, *Stress: A Brief History* (Malden, MA: Blackwell, 2004); Anne Harrington, *The Cure Within: A History of Mind-Body Medicine* (New York: Norton, 2008); Lea Haller, "Stress, Cortison und Homöostase: Künstliche Nebennierenrindenhormone und physiologisches Gleichgewicht, 1936–1960," *NTM Zeitschrift für Geschichte der Wissenschaften, Technik und Medizin* 18 (2010): 169–95; Serge Doublet, *The Stress Myth* (Sydney: Ispilon, 2000); Angela Patmore, *The Truth about Stress* (London: Atlantic Books, 2006); and Robert Kugelmann, *Stress: The Nature and History of Engineered Grief* (Westport, CT: Praeger, 1992).

9. Hans Selye and Thomas McKeown, "Studies on the Physiology of the Maternal Placenta in the Rat," *Proceedings of the Royal Society of London* 119 (1935): 1–31.

10. Selye, "Syndrome Produced," 32.

11. Hans Selye, "Studies on Adaptation," *Endocrinology* 21 (1937): 169–88; Selye, "The Significance of the Adrenals for Adaptation," *Science* 85 (1937): 247–48; Selye, "Adaptation Energy," *Nature*, suppl. no. 141 (1938): 926; Selye, "Experimental Evidence Supporting the Conception of 'Adaptation Energy,'" *American Journal of Physiology* 123 (1938): 758–65; Selye, "The Prevention of Adrenalin Lung Edema by the Alarm Reaction," *American Journal of Physiology* 122, no. 2 (1938): 347–51.

12. Selye, "Experimental Evidence."

13. Hans Selye, *The Story of the Adaptation Syndrome* (Montreal: Acta, 1952), 50–51.

14. On the citation and impact of Selye's article in the *Journal of Endocrinology*, see Eugene Garfield, "Citation Indexes for Science: A New Dimension in Documentation through Association of Ideas," *Science* 122 (1955): 108–11.

15. Hans Selye, "The General Adaptation Syndrome and the Diseases of Adaptation," *Journal of Clinical Endocrinology* 6, no. 2 (1946): 119, 131.

16. Francis G. Crookshank, "Science and Health," in *Science and Civilization*, ed. Francis S. Marvin (London: Oxford University Press, 1923), 247.

17. Ibid., 248. See also W. Langdon Brown, "The Return to Aesculapius," *Lancet* 2 (1933): 821–22; and Lord Horder, *Health and a Day* (London: Dent, 1937), 5–6.

18. John Eric Erichson, *On Railway and Other Injuries of the Nervous System* (Philadelphia: Lea, 1867). See also Ralph Harrington, "The Railway Journey and the Neuroses of Modernity," in *Pathologies of Travel*, ed. Richard Wrigley and George Revill (Amsterdam: Rodopi, 2000), 229–59; Nicholas Daly, "Railway Novels: Sensation Fiction and the Modernization of the Senses," *ELH* 66 (1999): 461–87; Daly, "Blood on the Tracks: Sensation Drama, the Railway, and the Dark Face of Modernity," *Victorian Studies* 42 (1998): 47–76; George M. Beard, *American Nervousness: Its Causes and Consequences* (New York: Putnam's Sons, 1881); Alfred Lief, ed., *The Common Sense Psychiatry of Adolf Meyer* (New York: McGraw-Hill, 1948); and Rhodri Hayward, "Medicine and the Mind," in *The Oxford Handbook of the History of Medicine*, ed. Mark Jackson (Oxford: Oxford University Press, 2011), 524–42.

19. For discussion of concerns about the "pathology of progress," see Charles E. Rosenberg, "Pathologies of Progress: The Idea of Civilization as Risk," *Bulletin of the History of Medicine* 72 (1998): 714–30.

20. Roberta Bivins, *Alternative Medicine? A History* (Oxford: Oxford University Press, 2007), 79.

21. Advertisement for Phyllosan, *Times*, January 30, 1934, 11; George W. Crile, *The Origin and Nature of the Emotions* (1915; repr., Charleston, SC: Bibliobazaar, 2006), 38; George W. Crile, *A Physical Interpretation of Shock, Exhaustion and Restoration* (London, Hodder and Stoughton, 1921).

22. Crile, *Origin and Nature*, 127–28, 121, 127–28, 100–101, 107–8, 127.

23. Anson Rabinbach, *The Human Motor: Energy, Fatigue and the Origins of Modernity* (Berkeley: University of California Press, 1992); William James, "The Energies of Men," *Science* 25 (1907): 326; *Report of the War Office Committee of Enquiry into "Shell-Shock"* (London: HMSO, 1922), 55–56.

24. James L. Birley, "Goulstonian Lectures on the Principles of Medical Science as Applied to Military Aviation," *Lancet*, May 29, 1920, 1147–51. Birley cited the psychological studies of Sigmund Freud and W. H. R. Rivers and the physiological investigations of Walter Cannon.

25. Carleton B. Chapman, "The Long Reach of Harvard's Fatigue Laboratory, 1926–47," *Perspectives in Biology and Medicine* 34 (1990): 17–33; Steven M. Horvath and Elizabeth C. Horvath, *The Harvard Fatigue Laboratory: Its History and Contributions* (Englewood Cliffs, NJ: Prentice Hall, 1973).

26. The role of nervous or psychological stability was embedded in psychoanalytical accounts of mental health and in debates about shell shock; see Sigmund Freud, *Beyond the Pleasure Principle and Other Writings*, trans. John Reddick (London: Penguin, 2003), 43–102; Nigel Walker, "Freud and Homeostasis," *British Journal for the Philosophy of Science* 7 (1956): 61–72; *War Office Committee*, 13, 95–96.

27. Walter B. Cannon, "Organization for Physiological Homeostasis," *Physiological Reviews* 9 (1929): 399–431; Cannon, *The Wisdom of the Body* (New York: Norton, 1932); Cannon, "Some Conditions Controlling Internal Secretion," *Journal of the American Medical Association* 79 (1922): 92–95; Cannon, "New Evidence for Sympathetic Control of Some Internal Secretions," *American Journal of Psychiatry* 79 (1922): 15–30.

28. Cannon, "New Evidence," 27; Cannon, "Some Conditions," 95.

29. Selye contributed to discussions of homeostasis and heterostasis in Chandler MacCuskey Brooks, Kiyomi Koizumi, and James O. Pinkston, eds., *The Life and Contributions of Walter Bradford Cannon, 1871–1945* (New York: SUNY Downstate Medical Center, 1975), 89–112.

30. Walter B. Cannon, "Stresses and Strains of Homeostasis," *American Journal of the Medical Sciences* 189 (1935): 1–14; Walter B. Cannon, "The Role of Emotion in Disease," *Annals of Internal Medicine* 9 (1936): 1453–65.

31. Mark Jackson, "The Pursuit of Happiness: The Social and Scientific Origins of Hans Selye's Natural Philosophy of Life," *History of the Human Sciences* 25 (2012): 13–29.

32. Franz Alexander, *Fundamentals of Psychoanalysis* (1949; repr., London: Allen and Unwin, 1960), 35–39; Helen Flanders Dunbar, *Mind and Body: Psychosomatic Medicine* (New York: Random House, 1947), viii, 4, 10. Alexander also used the term "stress" to describe emotional conflicts leading to organic disturbances; see "Psychological Aspects of Medicine," *Psychosomatic Medicine* 1 (1939): 7–18.

33. Dunbar, *Mind and Body*, 17–25.

34. Hans Selye and Claude Fortier, "Adaptive Reaction to Stress," *Psychosomatic Medicine* 12 (1950): 149–57; James L. Halliday, "Significance of the Discovery of the Effects of Cortisone," *Lancet* 256 (1950): 365–66. In *Stress without Distress* (New York: Signet, 1975), Selye included works by Alexander and Dunbar in the bibliography. Selye also included a chapter on the psychosomatic implications of his work in *The Stress of Life* (New York: McGraw-Hill, 1956), 260–72. The article by Selye and Fortier, "Adaptive Reaction to Stress," in *Psychosomatic Medicine*, also suggests reciprocal familiarity between Selye, Dunbar, and Alexander.

35. Hans Selye and Christiane Dosne, "The Action of Desoxycorticosterone Acetate and Progesterone on the Blood and Tissue Chlorides of Normal and Adrenalectomized Animals," *American Journal of Physiology* 132 (1941): 522–28; Claude Fortier and Hans Selye, "Adrenocorticotrophic Effect of Stress after Severance of the Hypothalamo-Hypophyseal Pathways," *American Journal of Physiology* 159 (1949): 433–39. In distinguishing between medullary and cortical hormones, Selye also developed innovative surgical techniques (to remove the adrenal medulla without damaging the cortex, for example, or to remove the pituitary gland) that were adopted by other researchers; see Selye, "Thymus and Adrenals in the Response of the Organism to Injuries and Intoxications," *British Journal of Experimental Pathology* 17 (1936): 234–48; and Gerald Evans, "The Adrenal Cortex and Endogenous Carbohydrate Formation," *American Journal of Physiology* 114 (1935): 297–308.

36. Hans Selye to F. Cyril James, May 31, 1943, file 38/30/81, RG 38, c. 6, McGill University Archives, Montreal (hereafter cited as MUA); Letters and research reports in file 2720, RG 2, c. 99, MUA. In 1943 Selye received a total of $40,310 from charitable, state, and pharmaceutical businesses, with a further $36,520 already promised for the following year; see file 38/30/81, RG 38, c. 6, MUA.

37. Hans Selye to Dr. H. A. Lambert, August 4, 1944, file 38/30/81, RG 38, c. 6, MUA.

38. Hans Selye and Christiane Dosne, "Effect of Cortin after Partial and after Complete Hepatectomy," *American Journal of Physiology* 128 (1940): 729–35. A full list of Selye's publications, including more than 1,400 articles and 22 monographs, was

compiled to support his nomination to the Canadian Medical Hall of Fame. I am grateful to Dr. Milagros Salas-Prato for a copy of the dossier.

39. Hans Selye, *Encyclopedia of Endocrinology*, vols. 1–4 (Montreal: Franks, 1943), 1:1, 7. Two volumes on the ovary were published three years later. For a similar discussion of the chemistry and physiology of steroid hormones, see Hans Selye, *Textbook of Endocrinology*, 2nd ed. (Montreal: Acta Endrocrinologica, 1949), 47–85.

40. Selye, *Encyclopedia of Endocrinology*, 1:8.

41. Ibid., 4:10–48.

42. Selye, *Textbook of Endocrinology*, 11–13, 50.

43. Ibid., 160, 199.

44. Hans Selye and Helen Stone, *On the Experimental Morphology of the Adrenal Cortex* (Springfield, IL: Charles C. Thomas, 1950), 95–99.

45. Harry M. Marks, "Cortisone, 1949: A Year in the Political Life of a Drug," *Bulletin of the History of Medicine* 66 (1992): 419–39; David Cantor, "Cortisone and the Politics of Empire: Imperialism and British Medicine, 1918–1955," *Bulletin of the History of Medicine* 67 (1993): 463–93; Nicolas Rasmussen, "Steroids in Arms: Science, Government, Industry, and the Hormones of the Adrenal Cortex in the United States, 1930–1950," *Medical History* 46, no. 3 (2002): 299–324; Jean-Paul Gaudillière, "Better Prepared Than Synthesized: Adolf Butendandt, Schering Ag and the Transformation of Sex Steroids into Drugs (1930–1946)," *Studies in History and Philosophy of Biological and Biomedical Sciences* 36 (2005): 612–44; Viviane Quirke, "Making British Cortisone: Glaxo and the Development of Corticosteroids in Britain in the 1950s–1960s," *Studies in History and Philosophy of Biological and Biomedical Sciences* 36 (2005): 645–74.

46. Cantor, "Cortisone," 466.

47. Edward C. Kendall, "The Development of Cortisone as a Therapeutic Agent," in *Nobel Lectures, Physiology or Medicine, 1942–1962* (Amsterdam: Elsevier, 1964), 270–88; Tadeus Reichstein, "Chemistry of the Adrenal Cortex Hormones," in *Nobel Lectures*, 289–308; Philip S. Hench, "The Reversibility of Certain Rheumatic and Nonrheumatic Conditions by the Use of Cortisone or of the Pituitary Adrenocorticotropic Hormone," in *Nobel Lectures*, 311–41.

48. Edward C. Kendall, "The Adrenal Cortex and Rheumatoid Arthritis," *British Medical Journal*, December 1, 1951, 1295–99.

49. Roger Guillemin, "A Personal Reminiscence of Hans Selye," *Experientia* 41 (1985): 560–61.

50. Selye's library contained approximately 150,000 reprints in 1943. See Jenny Kalsner, "The Unique Stress Library of Dr. Hans Selye," *Canadian Medical Association Journal* 129 (1983): 288–89; and Selye, *Encyclopedia of Endocrinology*, 1:1.

51. Bernardo A. Houssay, preface to Selye, *Textbook of Endocrinology*, xii–xiii.

52. Kendall, "Development of Cortisone," 271–72.

53. Rasmussen, "Steroids in Arms," 306–9. For a contemporary study of steroids and performance in animals, see Dwight J. Ingle, "Work Performance of Adrenalectomized Rats Treated with 11-Desoxycorticosterone Sodium Phosphate and 11-Desoxy-17-Hydroxycorticosterone," *American Journal of Physiology* 133 (1941): 676–78.

54. William Sargant and Eliot Slater, "Acute War Neuroses," *Lancet*, July 6, 1940, 1–2; Gilbert Debenham, William Sargant, Denis Hill, and Eliot Slater, "Treatment of War Neurosis," *Lancet*, January 25, 1941, 107–9.

55. Aubrey Lewis, "Incidence of Neurosis in England under War Conditions," *Lancet*, August 15, 1942, 183. For the context surrounding Lewis's report, see Stephen T. Casper, "The Origins of the Anglo-American Research Alliance and the Incidence of Civilian Neuroses in Second World War Britain," *Medical History* 52 (2008): 327–46. For other contemporary studies of combat stress, see David Stafford-Clark, "Aspects of War Medicine in the R.A.F.," *British Medical Journal*, January 30, 1943, 139–40; G. V. Stephenson and Kenneth Cameron, "Anxiety States in the Navy: A Clinical Survey and Impression," *British Medical Journal*, November 13, 1943, 603–7; Charles P. Symonds, "The Human Response to Flying Stress," *British Medical Journal*, December 4, 1943, 703–6; Symonds, "The Human Response to Flying Stress," *British Medical Journal*, December 11, 1943, 740–44; and David Stafford-Clark, "Morale and Flying Experience: Results of a Wartime Study," *Journal of Mental Science* 95 (1949): 10–50.

56. Hans Selye, "Perforated Peptic Ulcer during Air-Raid," *Lancet*, February 20, 1943, 252.

57. Stephenson and Cameron, "Anxiety States," 604.

58. Mark K. Wells, *Courage and Air Warfare: The Allied Aircrew Experience in the Second World War* (London: Cass, 1995), 77–81.

59. Roy R. Grinker and John P. Spiegel, *Men under Stress* (Philadelphia: Blakiston, 1945), vii.

60. Wells, *Courage and Air Warfare*, 186–208.

61. Gregory Pincus and Hudson Hoagland, "Steroid Excretion and the Stress of Flying," *Journal of Aviation Medicine* 14 (1943): 173–93. Although Pincus and Hoagland did not cite Selye in this paper, they subsequently became aware of his work after Selye contributed a chapter to a volume on hormones edited by Pincus; see Hans Selye, "Hypertension as a Disease of Adaptation," in *Recent Progress in Hormone Research*, vol. 3, ed. Gregory Pincus (New York: Academic Press, 1948), 343–61.

62. Hudson Hoagland, "Adventures in Biological Engineering," *Science* 100 (1944): 64.

63. Ibid., 67.

64. William Gomberg, "Measuring the Fatigue Factor," *Industrial and Labor Relations Review* 1 (1947): 80–93.

65. Selye, *Stress of My Life*, 73–74, 221–22. Selye also reflected on Cannon's reluctance to endorse his ideas at a conference in San Diego in 1978. I am grateful to Dr. David Fernandez, who collaborated with Selye in the 1970s and 1980s, for a recording of Selye's presentation to the conference and for copies of his correspondence with Selye.

66. Cannon, "Some Conditions," 94.

67. Hans Selye, "Stress and the General Adaptation Syndrome," *British Medical Journal*, June 17, 1950, 1383–92.

68. Letters and memoranda relating to Selye's work and the move to the University of Montreal are in RG 38 c. 6, file 30/38/80, 1933–46; RG 2, c. 99, file 2720, 1938–45; RG 2, c. 99, file 2721, 1944–45, MUA.

69. Selye, *Stress of My Life*, 100.

70. Hans Selye, *The Physiology and Pathology of Exposure to Stress: A Treatise Based on the Concepts of the General-Adaptation-Syndrome and the Diseases of Adaptation* (Montreal:

Acta, 1950); Hans Selye, *Annual Report on Stress* (Montreal: Acta, 1951); Hans Selye and Alexander Horava, *Second Annual Report on Stress* (Montreal: Acta, 1952).

71. Selye's application of stress and adaptation in this way echoed general usage. In 1945, in their study of the behavior of American air force pilots in combat situations, *Men under Stress*, Grinker and Spiegel argued that "under sufficient stress any individual may show failure of adaptation" (vii). Physiologists employed stress in a similar way to denote environmental factors that caused demonstrable changes in endocrine function; see Robert H. Williams, Herbert Jaffe, and Carol Kemp, "Effect of Severe Stress upon Thyroid Function," *American Journal of Physiology* 159 (1949): 291–97.

72. Selye, "Stress," 1392, 1384.

73. Selye, *Stress of Life* (1956), 54, viii. By the 1976 edition of the same book, stress was defined in even more fundamental terms as "the nonspecific response of the body to any demand"; see Hans Selye, *The Stress of Life* (New York: McGraw-Hill, 1976), 74.

74. Selye, "Stress," 1392.

75. H. N. Green, "Stress and the General Adaptation Syndrome," *British Medical Journal*, July 22, 1950, 215; A. P. Meiklejohn, "General Adaptation Syndrome," *British Medical Journal*, July 15, 1950, 164; Ffrangcon Roberts, "Stress and the General Adaptation Syndrome," *British Medical Journal*, July 8, 1950, 104–5.

76. G. S. W. Evans, letter, *British Medical Journal*, July 8, 1950, 105–6; "Diseases of Maladaptation," *British Medical Journal*, February 10, 1951, 285–86; Selye's article was published in the same issue; see Hans Selye, "Role of Somatotrophic Hormone in the Production of Malignant Nephrosclerosis, Periarteritis Nodosa, and Hypertensive Disease," *British Medical Journal*, February 10, 1951, 263–70. For other comments on Selye's approach, see "The General Adaptation Syndrome," *British Medical Journal*, June 17, 1950, 1410–11; A. Wesley Hill, "The General Adaptation Syndrome," *British Medical Journal*, July 22, 1950, 220; "Diseases of Adaptation," *Lancet*, June 10, 1950, 1078; George W. Pickering, "Significance of the Discovery of the Effects of Cortisone on Rheumatoid Arthritis," *Lancet*, July 15, 1950, 81–84; Ernst Jokl, "Adaptation in Physiological Processes," *Lancet*, December 2, 1950, 705–6.

77. Hans Selye, "Diseases of Maladaptation," *British Medical Journal*, March 3, 1951, 472–73.

78. "Rheumatic Diseases as Diseases of Adaptation: Professor Hans Selye's Heberden Oration," *British Medical Journal*, June 10, 1950, 1362–64; "What Is Stress?," *Lancet*, February 3, 1951, 279.

79. David Le Vay, "Hans Selye and a Unitary Conception of Disease," *British Journal for the Philosophy of Science* 3 (1952): 157–68.

80. Mark Jackson, *Allergy: The History of a Modern Malady* (London: Reaktion Books, 2006), 203–4; John J. Christian, "The Adreno-Pituitary System and Population Cycles in Mammals," *Journal of Mammology* 31 (1950): 247–59; John R. Clarke, "The General Adaptation Syndrome in the Study of Animal Populations," *British Journal for the Philosophy of Science* 3 (1953): 350–52; David Bakan, *Disease, Pain, and Sacrifice: Toward a Psychology of Suffering* (Chicago: University of Chicago Press, 1968); Edward O. Wilson, *Sociobiology: The New Synthesis* (1975; repr., Cambridge, MA: Belknap, 2000), 242–55.

81. Selye, *Stress of My Life*, illustration, 143; John S. L. Brown "The New Pool of Bethesda," confidential monthly report to the trustees, January 1950, Rockefeller Foundation Archives, Rockefeller Archive Center, Sleepy Hollow, New York, 16.

82. "Medicine: The Life of Stress," *Time* 56 (October 9, 1950): 93–94; "Medicine: Three-Letter Wonder," *Time* (April 16, 1951); "Medicine: Stress and Strain," *Time* 63 (January 18, 1954): 66; "Medicine: Chain of Strain?," *Time* (January 31, 1955); "Medicine: Life and Stress," *Time* (December 3, 1956); "Research: How to Handle Stress; Learn to Enjoy It," *Time* (November 29, 1963); Claudia Wallis, "Stress: Can We Cope?," *Time* (June 6, 1983): 49–54—all accessed July 10, 2009, http://www.time.com/time/magazine.

83. T. Traherne and Frank Preston, eds., *Healthy Minds and Bodies* (London: Waverley Book Company, 1956), 10.

84. Selye, *Story*; Selye, *Stress without Distress.*

85. John W. Todd, "The Errors of Medicine," *Lancet*, March 28, 1970, 665–70; Paul Christian and Fernando Lolas, "The Stress Concept as a Problem for a 'Theoretical Pathology,'" *Social Science and Medicine* 21 (1985): 1363–65.

86. Paul J. Rosch, "Stress and Cancer: A Disease of Adaptation?," in *Cancer, Stress and Death*, ed. Jean Tache, Hans Selye, and Stacey B. Day (New York: Plenum, 1979), 187–212; Angelo A. Alonso, "Health as Situational Adaptation: A Social Psychological Perspective," *Social Science and Medicine* 21 (1985): 1341–44.

87. Richard Mackarness, *Not All in the Mind* (London: Pan Books, 1976), 47; Tom Cox, *Stress* (London: Macmillan, 1978), 174; Claude Fortier, "A Giant of Biology," *Experientia* 41 (1985): 561–62; Guillemin, "Personal Reminiscence," 561.

Chapter Two

Stress and the American Vernacular

Popular Perceptions of Disease Causality

Elizabeth Siegel Watkins

FASEB Journal, the journal of the Federation of American Societies for Experimental Biology, is a well-known scholarly publication dedicated to the experimental biological and biomedical sciences. It publishes highly technical reports of the latest results of research on molecular and cellular physiology, immunology, and the like. It may thus have come as somewhat of a surprise to subscribers to find Paris Hilton as the subject of an editorial in the September 2007 issue. The journal's editor in chief used his monthly editorial space to trace the lineage of stress from Hans Selye to Paris Hilton. Hans Selye is, of course, the experimental scientist considered to be the father of the stress concept in physiology. Paris Hilton is, of course, the heiress-socialite whose dalliances and antics fill the pages of tabloid newspapers. She caught the attention of the editor in chief of *FASEB Journal* in May 2007 because a *Boston Globe* article reported her to be under such stress prior to her upcoming incarceration that she was unable to eat. As he quipped in the editorial, "Since her stress preceded the trauma, Paris Hilton may be the first well-documented case of 'Pre-Traumatic Stress Disorder.'"[1]

I begin with this story because it nicely encapsulates the interplay between professional and popular discourse in constructing the public understanding of the biomedical concept of stress. This chapter investigates when, how, and why stress entered the American vernacular.[2] As a case study in the popularization of science, it demonstrates that the processes involved are much more complicated than a simple unidirectional transmission and translation of expert knowledge into lay language. As Roger Cooter and Stephen Pumfrey explained in their 1994 essay on the history of science popularization, such a "top-down" diffusionist model is inadequate because it discounts any ability or agency on the part of nonscientists to generate or interpret knowledge about the natural world.[3]

I am especially interested in the flows of knowledge between esoteric and exoteric domains in the development of the stress concept. Broadly defined, the esoteric community consists of specialists who have MD or PhD degrees and work in the field of biomedicine as clinicians or researchers; the exoteric community of nonspecialists consists of everyone else. The boundaries between these domains, however, are both blurry and porous. Science journalists and physicians who write for mainstream magazines, for example, have a foot in both worlds. The notion of expertise is contestable, and it is one of the goals of this work to point out the multiplicity of actors engaged in the production and interpretation of the stress concept.

Building on Cooter and Pumfrey's suggestion to "be responsive to a greater plurality of the sites for the making and reproduction of scientific knowledge" and to "scrutiniz[e] popular prose and nonscientific texts for (or as) signs of orthodox and unorthodox scientific authority," this chapter explores the evolution of the stress concept as articulated in articles in newspapers and popular magazines.[4] These nonscientific texts show that journalists, popularizers, and other interpreters picked and chose meanings gleaned from the pages of scientific reports and medical studies and presented them in the context of prior knowledge and contemporary cultural values. At the same time scientists and physicians, in their lives outside their laboratories and clinics, read these newspapers and mainstream magazines and absorbed the colloquial denotations and connotations of biomedical concepts, which in turn informed subsequent research studies. With time, the term "stress" took on a multitude of meanings. Defined by Selye as a set of physiological responses he called the "general adaptation syndrome," stress has morphed into a catchall term for a vast range of human experience, including the aforementioned condition of Ms. Hilton.

Terminology has always been troublesome for stress researchers. Stress could mean the physical, emotional, or social challenge faced by an individual; the body's response to one or more of these stimuli; or the pathological result itself. One early critic observed that "stress in addition to being itself, was also the cause of itself, and the result of itself." He further elaborated, "attempting to define stress is like trying to nail a piece of jelly to a tree."[5] More recent detractors, such as Angela Patmore in *The Truth about Stress* and Serge Doublet in *The Stress Myth*, have taken issue with the imprecision of the concept in their critiques of stress research and the stress-management industry. I am not concerned with pinpointing precise definitions of stress; rather, the focus is on understandings of and references to stress as a cause of disease. I am interested in how illness has been differently explained within different historical frames, using the metaphor developed by historian Charles Rosenberg.[6] How stress was seen as a contributing etiological factor depended on the frame within which it was constructed and construed. I argue here that preexisting notions of mind-body relationships and disease causality in the context of contemporary cultural paradigms provided the frame for how stress was portrayed in popular periodicals and, in turn, how it became part of common parlance.

Since stress has been such a dominant component of both medical and popular conceptions of health and disease in recent decades—the president of the Institute of Medicine of the National Academy of Sciences declared that "no aspect of health and disease elicited more interest among leaders of the United States government in the late 1970s"—it is subject to the paradox of appearing to have been in existence forever and, at the same time, to be uniquely characteristic of the present era.[7] Indeed, from the late 1970s to the present, magazine and newspaper articles on stress have been strikingly consistent in the content of their coverage. This chapter concentrates on the 1950s, 1960s, and 1970s: the decades in which the stress concept took hold and then took off. And since the concept did not materialize in a vacuum, attention is also paid to prior explanations of the relationships between society, mind, body, and disease from the late nineteenth and early twentieth centuries. These notions were instrumental in setting the stage for the reception of stress at midcentury.

Hans Selye and the Appearance of Stress in Medical and Popular Literature

Although Hans Selye wrote about the general adaptation syndrome in a letter to *Nature* in July 1936, he did not actually use the word "stress" in that communication. His steady stream of publications over the ensuing decade notwithstanding, stress did not appear as a subject heading in *Index Medicus*, the catalog of biomedical science journal articles, until 1950. Most of the articles in that first listing came from the *Proceedings of the Association for Research in Nervous and Mental Diseases*, from the conference convened in December 1949 to discuss "Life Stress and Bodily Disease." As the 1950s progressed *Index Medicus* recorded more and more articles on the experimental physiology of stress in animal models, which studied outcomes such as gland activity, circulatory effects, hormone levels, and other biochemical markers.

Clinicians also expressed their growing interest in the effects of stress on their patients. In 1954 the British journal the *Practitioner* devoted two issues to the subject. The January issue featured an introductory piece by Selye, followed by articles by specialists on stress and the cardiovascular system, the gut, rheumatic disorders, children, dermatology, psychiatry, and sports. (This last one was penned by Roger Bannister, who four months later would become the first man to run a mile in under four minutes. Bannister wrote the article while he was a medical student; in 1975 he was knighted by Queen Elizabeth for his work as a neurologist.) The final two articles looked beyond the doctor's office for the prevention and management of stress: the first emphasized the important of leisure and the second, "The Church and Stress" by the bishop of Manchester, advocated "acceptance of the Christian faith." The February issue bypassed specialist physicians and sponsored a minisymposium on stress in general-practice medicine. After developing a common list of stress-related illnesses consisting of fifty-one separate disorders, the participants (six general practitioners, two each from urban, suburban, and rural areas) surveyed their practices for four months and found that one in five patient visits could be attributed, at least in part, to stress. In presenting this finding, the editors of the journal called for greater attention to "the etiology, prevention and treatment of this major cause of ill health."[8]

Journalists took notice of this new trend in biomedical and clinical research, and in 1951 stress appeared as a subject heading in the *Reader's Guide to Periodical Literature*, the index of articles published in popular magazines. Hans Selye featured prominently in these articles, thanks to the 1950 publication of his thousand-page tome, *The Physiology and Pathology of Exposure to Stress*, and his eagerness to bring his ideas to a wide audience. *Time* and *Newsweek* explained to their readers the hormonal basis of Selye's general adaptation syndrome and described the scientist's patience in waiting for his findings to gain notice and acceptance. *Time* also reported on the *Practitioner*'s special issue on stress, crediting the rapid growth of research studies on stress and disease to Selye's discovery: "Ever since Montreal's Dr. Hans Selye announced his theory of how stress causes disease through the 'general adaptation syndrome,' physicians have recognized that people can get serious illnesses simply from the 'stress' put on the system by emotional pressures, shock, physical fatigue, or even bad eating habits." *Reader's Digest*, with a circulation of ten million in 1955, published a flattering profile of Selye, which began, "The work of a Canadian researcher almost unknown to the public is opening dazzling vistas in medical science. It indicates that there may be common cause for almost all disease. . . . Dr. Hans Selye of Montreal believes the cause is chemical imbalance in the body—*caused by stress*."[9]

In 1956 Selye earned a new round of publicity with the publication of *The Stress of Life*, the book he wrote for a general audience. Magazine accounts boiled down his theory to a pithy maxim: "stress is the origin of disease."[10] In an interview with *Vogue*, Selye defined stress as "the rate of all the wear and tear caused by life" and attributed to it "nervous and emotional disturbances, high blood pressure, gastric and duodenal ulcers, [and] certain types of rheumatic, allergic, cardiovascular, and renal diseases." When asked, "Is stress merely nervous tension?" Selye responded, "No. But nervous and emotional factors are very often the cause of stress." *Newsweek* also tried to put a finer point on Selye's medical definition of stress, explaining that it was physical, as opposed to "a vague description of nervous strain or emotion tension."[11]

The authors of popular magazine articles used the terms "stress," "strain," and "tension" interchangeably. "Anxiety," "nerves," and "nervousness" were also part of the vocabulary used to describe emotional pressure. Only the articles that showcased the work of Selye emphasized his particular definition of stress and its physiological mechanism; others relied on conventional wisdom to guide readers through the correlation between emotional pressure and physical illness. An article on "Tension and the Nerves of the Nation" began with the claim that "16 million Americans—about one in every ten—find themselves beset this week by some kind of emotional pressure" and warned that "many of the more serious disorders, such as stomach ulcers, migraine attacks, arthritis, and high blood pressure may be psychosomatic, or emotional, in origin." A physician interviewed by *U.S. News and World Report* explained that tension "can cause or aggravate such things as high blood pressure, ulcers, angina pectoris, heart attacks and colitis. It produces nervousness, irritability, excessive worry, insomnia, speech disorders and psychoses." "Tension disorders," he claimed, "can be regarded as the chief killing disease." *Newsweek* reported on a similar position taken by the president of the National Commission on Mental Health, who declared that "nervous tension is 'a prime mover in all the principal causes of death.'"[12]

Much of the popular magazine writing on stress and tension in the 1950s offered recommendations on how to reduce, relieve, or cope with it. With titles such as "How to Live with Your Nerves," "Live with Your Nerves and Like It," "How to Deal with Your Tensions," "Tension. What It Is—And How You Can Relieve It," and "What You Can Do about Stress," these articles drew distinctions between normal (good) and pathological (bad) tension and offered behavioral strategies for dealing with the latter. Not only did they provide guidance to the already stressed, they also signaled to the rest of their readership that stress and tension were major problems in American society in the "Frantic Fifties."[13] Almost all this advice literature was either authored by physicians or based on interviews with physicians, which suggested to readers that these problems were worthy of medical attention. Furthermore, those that drew explicit connections between emotional stress (of the pathological variety) and physical ailments such as headaches, ulcers, and heart attacks deliberately blurred the boundaries between the psychic and the somatic. This link between the mind and the body was, of course, nothing new; rather, it was only the latest iteration of efforts to explain how the pace of modern life can make people sick.[14]

Nervousness as the Ancestor of Stress

In 1869 the American neurologist George M. Beard coined the medical term "neurasthenia" to describe a weakness of the nervous system, which he believed was the cause of a wide variety of seemingly unrelated symptoms presented by his patients. According to Beard, the phenomenon of nervous exhaustion was new and unique to nineteenth-century civilization. He singled out five factors responsible for taxing the nerves of Americans: steam power, the telegraph, the periodical press, the sciences, and the mental activity of women. Beard defined neurasthenia as a somatic pathology: social pressures acted on the mind, which in turn acted on the body to produce physical lesions.[15] Although his ideas were initially ignored by his medical peers, they gained traction among practicing physicians in the last two decades of the 1800s. As historian Barbara Sicherman has shown, neurasthenia "proved a satisfactory label to doctors and patients alike" by "legitimizing new roles for physicians and their patients."[16] Both groups appreciated a diagnosis that stopped short of insanity and the walls of the asylum, but at the same time acknowledged the mental and physical toll of the stresses and strains of modern living.

The medical term "neurasthenia" kept company with popular references to nerves and nervousness. The *Reader's Guide to Periodical Literature* indexed dozens of magazine articles from the 1890s through the 1910s under the category of "Nervous System—Diseases," with titles such as "Modern Nervousness and Its Cure," "Nervous Century," "Making Friends of One's Nerves," and "Age of Nerves." Many of these focused on women, combining two of Beard's five modern menaces (the periodical press and the mental activity of women). For example, in 1901 *Harper's Bazaar* ("A Monthly Magazine for Women") presented "Self-Help for Nervous Women," in 1908 *Ladies' Home Journal* informed its readers "How Women Can Keep from Being Nervous," and in 1910 *Woman's Home Companion* offered "Help for the Nervous Woman." From 1907 through 1910 Reverend Samuel McComb, associate director of the Class for the Moral Control of Nervous Disorders, a series of lectures given at Emmanuel Episcopal Church in Boston, published several articles in *Harper's Bazaar* and other magazines on suggestion therapy and moral reeducation to remedy the malady of nervousness. While some of his pieces counseled readers ("Nervous Poise and How to Get It"), others painted a more dire picture ("Nervousness—A National Menace").[17] The continual appearance of articles about nerves and nervousness in American monthly magazines helped to establish the notion that the challenges of modern life could cause people to feel unwell. While some sought treatment from the growing class of physicians specializing in neurology, others looked to spiritual counselors (e.g., the reverend McComb) or relied on themselves to deal with this modern affliction.

Into the swirl of popular and medical discourse about neurasthenia, nerves, and nervousness came a new concept, the "nervous breakdown." Essentially synonymous with neurasthenia in terms of both symptoms and causes, nervous breakdowns encompassed a broad array of mental and physical woes and were attributed to the hectic pace of modern life. Businessmen were especially vulnerable to the pressures of working too hard, but homemakers, children, and even the elderly were susceptible to anxieties that could lead to a breakdown. Although nervous breakdown enjoyed currency among some psychiatrists in the 1920s, it had its real heyday in the 1930s, 1940s, and 1950s as a concept popular among laypeople. Megan Barke, Rebecca Fribush, and Peter N. Stearns argue that "nervous breakdown never won a place in medical literature," because "the concept was too vague and generalized." Instead, it functioned more as a disease entity that could be self-diagnosed and self-treated. These historians describe nervous breakdown as "unmedical" in that its sufferers tended to eschew the professional services of physicians.[18] According to their analysis, nervous breakdown can be understood as a sort of populist notion that neither wanted nor needed legitimization from the professional medical community.

By contrast, when the editors of *Fortune* took up the subject of nervous breakdown, they looked to modern medicine for explanations and therapies. In a lengthy article published in the April 1935 issue and republished as an eighty-five-page book two months later, nervous breakdown was defined as "a state in which psychic (mental-emotional) factors prevent one from carrying on the business of modern living. The term 'nervous breakdown' has no medical standing and is a misnomer inasmuch as the nerves have practically nothing to do with the case." That said, the authors went on to declare nervous breakdown to be synonymous with serious neurosis. Although the former might have had "no medical standing," the latter did. Research for the article involved consultations with "a dozen or more men whose names loom largest in the fields of mental hygiene, psychiatry, psychoanalysis," and much of the article was devoted to the work of Freud, his acolytes, and his competitors.[19] Although neurosis was differentiated from psychosis (which often required long periods of hospitalization), it was, according to the *Fortune* editors, clearly a health problem to be diagnosed and treated by psychiatric specialists of the medical profession.

The article mentioned neurasthenia, but by 1935 that diagnosis was clearly past its prime. The authors deemed it "outmoded." "Psychiatrists don't expect it much," they explained, "and so they don't diagnose it so much." Anxiety states, by contrast, were described as "the 'modern' neuroses," in a prescient foreshadowing of the ubiquity of anxiety two decades later.[20] The connection between anxiety and illness was taken up in a May 1939 article in *Harper's Magazine* that was reprinted in condensed form in *Reader's Digest* a month later.[21] Author George W. Gray described how mental states could result in physical ailments and suggested a chemical basis for this relationship: "Anxiety thus becomes a biochemical factor. Through automatic stimulation of secretions it may release materials as upsetting to the system as bacteria."[22] Although Selye was not mentioned in the article, his ideas about hormonal responses to stress clearly informed Gray's perspective.

The *Fortune* editors dismissed the conception that overwork brought on nervous collapse as an "American legend." "The psychiatrist," they proclaimed, "doesn't believe in the popular idea of the high-powered executive lashing himself to such titanic efforts that he cracks under the sheer strain on his energy."[23] The professional opinion referenced in this article was at odds with conventional wisdom and with contemporary medical views outside the realm of psychiatry. Indeed, the trope of the business executive working himself to exhaustion and even further, to death, proved to be remarkably enduring in both popular culture and medical thought.

Closely allied to the perception that businessmen were subject to undue pressures on the job was the belief that the pace of modern life could cause stress-related illness. The distinguished physician William Osler, in his 1910 address to the Royal College of Physicians of London on angina pectoris, had asked "Has the high-pressure life of modern days made the disease more common?" Readers of the *New York Times* in the 1920s came across several articles on the detrimental effects of modern living. An article on Couéism, a sort of faith healing, quoted a pastor who warned, "Our hurried age is multiplying nervous troubles. . . . Experts tell us that one-half of all sickness is traceable to nervous disorders. Some functional disorders, like heart disease and even cancer, originate in indigestion brought on by worry and nervousness." William S. Sadler, a physician "of national reputation," came to the same conclusion:

> A quarter of a million persons a year die from a group of preventable conditions which I call "Americanitis." . . . The tension, the incessant drive of American life, the excited strain of the American temperament, are responsible for a marked mortality increase in the decade between 40 and 50. . . . Adaptation and natural selection have not had time to produce a race suited to the stress of a civilization which counts on the airplane and the wireless as commonplaces and intensifies its social and economic organization to keep pace with them.

Heart disease, in particular, was linked to modern stress. According to a report on a symposium held by the Congress of American Physicians and Surgeons in Washington in 1928, "The stress of modern life is more of a factor in deaths from heart complaints than ever before . . . with a resultant economic loss to the country of $1,502,000,000 a year from such deaths alone, not counting the cost of care, estimated at an additional $104,000,000."[24]

Advertisers used these dire figures to sell their goods and services. After a Metropolitan Life Insurance study reported an increase in deaths among men over forty-five and hypothesized that "much of the heart disease after the age of 45 . . . may well be the result, in some measure, of the increasing stress and strain of modern life," an ad for White Star Line cruises screamed "WATCH YOUR HUSBAND." The copy read, "More than two million Americans suffering from heart ailments! A great life insurance company reports decided increase in deaths among men over forty-five, and attributes this largely to the increasing stress and strain of modern life. For overworked executives a cruise is the ideal means of rest and relaxation." In January 1941 the Homestead resort in Hot Springs, Virginia, advertised its spa services at off-season low rates to "men at the top [who] know that success exacts a heavy physical toll of high tension and jangled nerves." And in 1949 *Collier's* ran an article (publicized with a full-page ad in the *New York Times*) called "Richest Man in the Cemetery" about men who "*succeed themselves to death.*"[25] This association between overwork and disease would grow even stronger in subsequent years among both physicians and the public, as researchers in the 1950s isolated stress as a primary cause of hypertension and then in the 1960s identified the so-called type A personality as especially susceptible to stress-related diseases.

Thus, by the time stress made its appearance in medical and popular literature (as cataloged in the *Index Medicus* and the *Reader's Guide to Periodical Literature*), Americans inside and outside the medical community were familiar with the conception that mental pressures could cause bodily diseases. Both physicians and nonphysicians had contributed to the conversation, as ideas flowed between the overlapping worlds of neurology, psychiatry, general medicine, and popular culture. Some aspects of this late nineteenth- and early twentieth-century heritage can be detected in the stress concept that emerged in the second half of the twentieth century, but changes in medical theories and cultural practices helped stress to develop into something quite different from its predecessors.

Stress, Anxiety, and Depression

Two streams of medical research and practice carried stress in divergent directions in the 1950s. First, stress was incorporated into the diagnosis of anxiety for which minor tranquilizers, or anxiolytics, were prescribed. Second, stress was further implicated as a risk factor for chronic disease, especially hypertension and other cardiovascular conditions, as cardiologists developed the profile of the type A personality. Both of these developments received coverage in the popular press, and these parallel pathways—along with their representations and reconfigurations by journalists and popularizers—shaped the forms that stress would take in the American vernacular.

First: anxiety. In a way, anxiety picked up where neurasthenia and nervous breakdown left off, as a generalized description of and explanation for a host of mental and physical symptoms. Historian David Herzberg described it as "a term to conjure with in virtually every version of postwar psychodynamic psychiatry."[26] Identified as "the 'chief characteristic' of the neuroses" in the first *Diagnostic and Statistical Manual* (*DSM*) put out by the American Psychiatric Association in 1952, anxiety was considered central to psychosomatic disorders, those physical conditions with no discernible organic cause.[27] Like its predecessors, anxiety incorporated both external and internal dimensions: anxious individuals suffered from the effects of outside stresses, and they displayed mental states that were especially susceptible to crisis. Until the mid-1950s the medical options available to the anxious were limited to psychoanalysis and other forms of psychotherapy.

The game changer came in 1955, when the FDA approved meprobamate, the first minor tranquilizer. Now physicians had a drug to prescribe for patients who presented with any of the constellation of symptoms that could be attributed to anxiety. Manufacturers promoted the new tranquilizers directly to doctors in advertisements in medical journals and indirectly to potential consumers in articles placed in popular magazines by public relations consultants. Readers of *Cosmopolitan*, for example, were introduced to meprobamate in 1955 in an article titled "A New Drug Brings Relief for the Tense and Anxious" that was written by Lawrence Galton, an employee of the Medical and Pharmaceutical Information Bureau, a public relations firm.[28] Marketed as Miltown by Wallace Laboratories and as Equanil by Wyeth, meprobamate became the best-selling drug in the United States within fourteen months.[29] It was succeeded in the early 1960s by the next generation of minor tranquilizers, the benzodiazepines, sold under the trade names Librium and Valium. These drugs quickly rose to the top of the prescription medication sales charts.[30]

As tranquilizers became the panacea for the epidemic of anxiety, advertisements for the drugs and articles about the condition displayed tremendous slippage between the terms "anxiety," "tension," and "stress." A cover piece in *Time* explained that "what passes for anxiety in the U.S. is really the stress of effort in a land of ambition, competition and challenge." One of the first medical journal ads for Miltown in 1955 promoted it for "anxiety, tension and mental stress." As Herzberg observed, "Psychoanalysts meant something quite different by 'anxiety' than psychologists did when they spoke of 'stress' or 'tension,' and popular references to 'worry' or 'nervousness' only further clouded the picture—but all made some claim to the mantle of medical or scientific authority."[31] With the advent of the minor tranquilizers, the legitimacy of the medical diagnosis was further validated by the pharmaceutical prescription. Consumers appreciated both the validation of their complaints—no matter what name was given to them—and the ease of popping pills as the solution.

Within two decades, however, America's infatuation with the tranquilizer ended. Tales of addiction, especially among middle-class women, turned popular opinion against Valium and the other anxiolytics. This turn was part of a broader panic about both licit and illicit drugs that swept American society in the 1970s.[32] Prescriptions for Valium dropped dramatically, as tranquilizers lost their wonder-drug status. But in the midst of this decline, another transition was taking place as diagnoses for anxiety began to be replaced by diagnoses for depression. In the words of psychiatrist Leslie Farber, "the Age of Anxiety became the Age of Depression."[33]

For the first two-thirds of the twentieth century, depression—known then as melancholia—was considered to be a serious mental illness, often treated by electroshock therapy.[34] A number of factors contributed to the reassessment of depression as a disease in the 1960s and early 1970s. Psychiatrists looked to get away from Freudian categories of neurosis and psychosis and the expensive and time-consuming practice of psychoanalysis, so they began to diagnose patients with mild depression instead of anxiety and to offer less time-intensive psychotherapies as treatment. These doctors regarded mild depression not as a symptom of anxiety but as an illness in itself. Although the tricyclic and monoamine oxidase inhibitor (MAOI) categories of antidepressant drugs had been discovered and approved for sale in the late 1950s, they were not often prescribed in the setting of the doctor's office, because mild depression had not yet taken over from anxiety, which was treated with the blockbuster minor tranquilizer drugs. The turning point came in 1972 when Senator Thomas Eagleton, the Democratic candidate for vice president, was forced to admit that he had been treated with electroshock therapy in the 1960s. While this confession of mental illness cost him his seat on the Democratic ticket, it also brought depression into the public eye and gave advocates the chance to lobby for recognition of milder forms of the condition.

Manufacturers of antidepressants took this opportunity to aggressively market these drugs, advertising them for the same symptoms as those for which the minor tranquilizers were prescribed. This campaign influenced physicians' assessments of patients' conditions: by 1975 diagnoses for depression had outstripped diagnoses for anxiety. The constellation of symptoms indicated for antidepressant drug therapy bore a marked similarity to those used to describe neurasthenia in the 1880s or nervous breakdown in the 1930s: tension, tiredness, insomnia, loss of appetite, decreased sex drive, lack of concentration, inability to make decisions, headaches, and digestive problems. Indeed, as Herzberg observed, depression "came to inherit and in some ways transform the nervous illness tradition in the 1970s."[35] The transformation came in the manner of treatment: unlike its forebears, depression necessitated medication.

The pharmaceuticalization of depression went hand in hand with physiological explanations of the etiology of depression. By 1980, according to historian Laura Hirshbein, depression was understood as a chemical imbalance in the brain, and this explanation "was in wide use in the American popular press."[36] Treatment of depression was portrayed as a simple equation:

depressed individuals had a deficiency of neurotransmitters, and antidepressant drugs corrected that deficiency. Once their neurotransmitter balance was equilibrated, patients would feel better. This rationale performed important intellectual work in the acceptance of depression by giving a physical basis to this mental illness. The prescription of drugs to treat depression would become even more prevalent in the late 1980s and 1990s with the advent of the next generation of antidepressants, the selective serotonin reuptake inhibitors (SSRIs) such as Prozac.

The framing of depression as a physical disease in and of itself clarified its relationship to stress: depression was one of the chronic diseases to which stress might be a contributing factor. The territories occupied by depression on one hand and stress on the other shared blurred and shifting boundaries during the 1960s and 1970s. Advertisements for antidepressants in the late 1960s, for example, could easily be interpreted as drug therapy for stress. Consider the text of an ad for Triavil, which, as Herzberg reported, "warned that personal or financial break-ups—indeed, 'any significant loss or severe blow to self-esteem'—could mean danger."[37] The notion that social pressure could lead to psychic effects that could lead to illness certainly characterized medical and popular conceptions of stress. But as the understanding of depression crystallized into a more physically defined entity (chemical imbalance in the brain), it moved into the more clearly defined space of a chronic disease that could be managed with pharmaceutical therapy. In this way depression was akin to hypertension. Both were somatic pathologies; both could be brought on by stress.

Stress, Coronaries, and Chronic Disease

Hypotheses about stress as a risk factor for hypertension and other chronic diseases hardened into axioms starting in the 1950s. Discussions about the relationship between stress, disease, and modern life continued apace in both medical and popular writing after World War II.[38] In an essay titled "In Praise of Idleness" in the *British Medical Journal* in 1949, Sir Heneage Ogilvie, surgeon to Guy's Hospital, blamed "modern life" for "conditions under which a great proportion of the inhabitants of the older and more civilized communities live, and these are the conditions that are causing them to break down and are producing a group of diseases that we may call the stress diseases." He singled out thyrotoxicosis (hyperthyroidism), duodenal ulcer, and nonrenal hypertension as "psychosomatic diseases, disturbances of the normal relation of mind and body by overpowering circumstances." I. McD. G. Stewart won the triennial Cary Coombs prize for the best essay on cardiology at the University of Bristol for his paper, "Coronary Disease and Stress," which was published in 1950 in the *Lancet*. In 1955

William P. Shepard, vice president for health and welfare at Metropolitan Life Insurance, asked in the *Journal of the American Geriatrics Society*, "Does thc Modern Pace Really Kill?" In comparing death rates between 1930 and 1955, he noted that overall mortality for white males over forty-five had declined, but that this group was now five times more likely to die from coronary artery disease or angina pectoris. Shepard believed that certain individuals were more susceptible to stress; it was the job of upper management and industrial physicians to work together to ensure the mental and physical health of business executives.[39]

Some physicians bypassed their colleagues and took their message directly to the public. A large advertisement in the *New York Times* promoted Dr. Max Warmbrand's *Add Years to Your Heart*, which promised to answer the question, "How does stress, emotion, worry effect [*sic*] us?" and to advise readers "how to keep your heart strong and healthy in this age of tension and frustration." An ad for Curt S. Wachtel MD's *Your Mind Can Make You Sick or Well* encouraged readers to purchase the book to learn "simple psychomechanisms that free you forever from 'nerves' and exhaustion . . . how to get rid of stress and strain . . . how to erect natural barriers against more than 30 diseases and ailments including hypertension, insomnia, ulcers and many others ranging from the common cold to heart disease."[40] Books like these reinforced notions of the interplay between mind and body.

Journalists closely followed the developments in the relationship between the stress of modern life and the rise in heart disease in the 1950s and early 1960s. Headlines such as "Rise in Heart Cases Seen, Stresses of Modern Living Cited at Meeting Here," "Heart Affliction Linked to Stress," "Stress of Work in U.S. Culture Cited as Cause of Heart Disease," "Go-Getters, Beware!," and "The Cost of Getting Ahead" made it clear that the emotional stress of overwork could produce physical sickness in the form of heart disease.[41]

This correlation received further support from the work of two San Francisco cardiologists, Meyer Friedman and Ray H. Rosenman. Starting in the late 1950s they turned their attention to the personalities and behavior patterns of their coronary patients. They found that men who showed "an intense, sustained drive for achievement" and were "continually involved in competition and deadlines, both at work and in their avocations" demonstrated a higher incidence of coronary artery disease; these men in group A (as compared to control groups B and C) displayed what came to be known as the type A personality.[42]

In 1974 Friedman and Rosenman wrote a popular book, *Type A Behavior and Your Heart*. In describing how they came to focus on personality as a risk factor for cardiovascular disease, they credited a layperson, the female president of the San Francisco Junior League, with pointing them in the right direction. They had been studying the diets of Junior Leaguers and their husbands, expecting to find that the women ate less fat and cholesterol than the coronary-prone men. When they puzzled over the fact that the diets were essentially identical, the Junior League president had the answer: "If you really want to know what is giving us heart attacks, I'll tell you. . . . It's stress, the stress they receive in their work, that's what's doing it." And that, according to the two doctors, is when the lightbulb clicked on over their heads.[43] This anecdote demonstrates nicely the bidirectional flow of information about stress and disease between professionals and nonprofessionals.

Friedman and Rosenman described a type A character as someone "who is *aggressively* involved in a *chronic, incessant* struggle to achieve more and more in less and less time." They took pains to distinguish this kind of stress from the kind that brought people into psychiatrists' offices. "It is not psychosis or a complex of worries or fears or phobias or obsessions, but a socially acceptable—indeed often praised—form of conflict."[44] Whereas the former signaled mental illness, still stigmatized in American society, the latter stemmed from laudable aspects of the American character. The former required pharmaceutical intervention; the latter could be addressed by force of will in rethinking one's priorities.

The type A pattern also differed from the life-stress model developed in the 1960s, which postulated that the timing of stressful life events could promote the onset of illness. In 1967 Thomas H. Holmes and Richard H. Rahe, psychiatrists at the University of Washington School of Medicine, developed the Social Readjustment Rating Scale, a list of forty-three life events that require personal, familial, occupational, or emotional adjustment. At the top of the scale was death of a spouse, with a score of one hundred life-change units (LCUs). A jail term merited sixty-three LCUs; marriage was worth fifty; retirement, forty-five; pregnancy, forty; and Christmas, twelve.[45] These researchers and others found "modest but statistically significant relationships . . . between mounting life change and the occurrence or onset of sudden cardiac death, myocardial infarctions, accidents, athletic injuries, tuberculosis, leukemia, multiple sclerosis, [and] diabetes."[46]

Both notions—that behavior patterns (daily stress) could, over time, lead to disease and that unsettling events (life stress) could trigger disease—found their way into the popular press, often intermingled and undifferentiated in the same article. *Mademoiselle* reprinted the Social Readjustment Rating Scale as a sidebar to a 1975 article on stress, which also made reference to Hans Selye's book, *The Stress of Life.* (Selye enjoyed a sort of renaissance of popularity in the 1970s, thanks to the publication of his second book for the general reader, *Stress without Distress,*[47] and to the seeming ubiquity of stress as a topic for public consumption.) *Good Housekeeping* referred to Friedman and Rosenman and Holmes and Rahe in its report on "What Stress Can Do to Mind and Body." The article described the susceptibility of the type A person to heart attack but also noted that life events could bring on illness. A sidebar listed the top ten events on the Holmes-Rahe scale and the number of life-change units each was worth. "A total score of 150 in one year means the person has a 37-percent chance of illness," the article explained. "A score of 300; an 80-percent chance."[48]

By referring to Friedman and Rosenman's type A personality and to Holmes and Rahe's Social Readjustment Rating Scale, journalists signaled that the work of these researchers gave scientific legitimacy to the experience of stress. Some writers in the 1970s attempted to explain the effects of stress in biological terms; they described the physiological reactions triggered by stressful encounters—such as increases in serum cholesterol levels, blood pressure, and the release of hormones from the pituitary and the adrenal glands—that eventually produced disease. Others were content simply to announce that clinicians and researchers were studying the phenomenon of stress, without giving the biological details; for them, and their readers, the mere mention of biomedical attention was enough to give the subject the status of scientific credibility. "It has long been a matter of common intuition that bottled-up anger can crack the bottle, [and] prolonged strain can make people sick," began one article. "This old folklore now has considerable scientific support."[49]

Although well into the 1970s fashion magazines addressed women, and business magazines addressed men, descriptions of the causes and consequences of stress were comparable in both forums. Arnold A. Hutschnecker, a physician writing in *Vogue* in 1971 on "Tension, the Everyday Threat to American Women . . . and What to Do about It," led with the following assertion: "If we try to answer the question why the American woman is prone to tension . . . we can say that the American woman is the victim of the very same driving force that makes her the most exquisite, attractive, and unique female in the world: her *competitiveness.*"

Six months later a nine-page exposé on "What Stress Can Do to You" in *Fortune* used similar language to describe the coronary-prone man: "If he is the kind of hard-driving, competitive perfectionist whom many corporations prize, and if this kind of stress pattern is chronic, the stress experts will tell you that he is a prime candidate for an early coronary."[50] While each article was firmly rooted in the gendered assumptions of the times, in which business executives were assumed to be male and a woman's world was thought to be circumscribed by home, marriage, and family, writers in the early 1970s considered both men and women to be vulnerable to the psychic and somatic effects of stress.

By the late 1970s stress had been featured on the covers of magazines from *Psychology Today* to *U.S. News and World Report.* The *New York Times Magazine* ran a lengthy article on the economic costs of stress in corporate America. *Today's Health,* the popular periodical put out by the American Medical Association and commonly found in doctors' waiting rooms, offered advice on "How to Avoid Harmful Stress" and "What to Do When Stress Signs Say

You're Killing Yourself." *Mademoiselle* warned its readers of the effects of stress on their complexions, and *Harper's Bazaar* promoted an antistress diet to help readers to relax *and* lose weight. All the articles drew explicit connections between stress and sickness. One began ominously: "Ulcers. Epilepsy. Asthma. Diabetes. Cancer. High blood pressure. Rheumatoid arthritis. Heart disease. Stress is a factor in any number of diseases."[51] Another noted the reciprocality of the relationship: "Any illness causes stress and stress makes any illness worse."[52] In the vernacular of popular periodicals, stress was commonly understood as an etiological factor in chronic disease.

An important component of these mass-market magazine articles on stress was advice about how to lessen, manage, or deal with it, much like the articles on tension and nerves in the 1950s. Many authors reminded readers that people needed some stress in their lives to stay motivated, citing Hans Selye's maxim that "stress is the salt of life."[53] That said, they acknowledged that a great number of Americans suffered from the effects of negative stress or overstress, which resulted from the pressures of work life, family life, and—echoing previous generations—the pace and problems of living in the modern world. They also noted that some individuals were able to handle the stresses they faced, while others were not. The type A personality accounted for many of those who had hypertension or heart attacks, but no such label was developed for people who succumbed to noncoronary chronic conditions allegedly brought on by stress.

Whatever the cause of the stress and whoever suffered from its effects, the advice given—usually at the end of the article or in an accompanying column—was consistently similar: relax. Readers were told that they themselves could control their response to stress by learning and adopting relaxation techniques. Some articles suggested existing methods, such as meditation, yoga, or self-hypnosis.[54] *Mademoiselle* recommended the purchase of a book called *The Relaxation Response*, by Harvard Medical School professor Herbert Benson. *Harper's Bazaar* interviewed C. Norman Shealy, a neurosurgeon turned holistic health proponent who touted a series of mental exercises he developed called "Biogenics." A sidebar to an article in *Psychology Today* on an experimental stress-management clinic for type A people informed readers, "On your own, you can start to change your Type A habits." The piece listed four approaches: learn to relax (music, deep muscle relaxation, and meditation were suggested as techniques), retrain your reactions, take control of your environment, and slow down. Readers who wanted more explicit instructions could send away for cassette tapes from the magazine's consumer service division.[55]

All these relaxation methods were based on self-help tenets. As Barbara Ehrenreich pointed out in an article in *Ms.*, "Most 'coping' advice focuses on what you can do to change *yourself*."[56] A physician-columnist for *Mademoiselle* declared, "We expect too much from physicians and place too much reliance on medication. Getting rid of stress is an inner achievement."[57] Readers of popular magazines were told that "pills . . . are *not* the answer"; instead, they were advised to "learn a drug-free relaxation method."[58] While Friedman and Rosenman, the architects of the type A diagnosis, did prescribe antihypertensive drugs for their patients with high blood pressure, they looked beyond pharmaceuticals to calm down their type A patients. In their book, *Type A Behavior and Your Heart*, they recommended behavior modification strategies to help the coronary-prone "reengineer" their lives.[59] Hospitals soon recognized the therapeutic (and economic) value of setting up stress-management clinics, but even in these medical settings the emphasis was on helping patients learn to relax. Although stress was somaticized, medicalized, and commercialized, it was not pharmaceuticalized. Nondrug modalities were the hallmark of stress therapy to reduce the risk of developing chronic disease.

Stress in the Twenty-First Century

By the 1980s "stress" had become an established term in the American vernacular, used to describe feelings of pressure and tension and to explain the source of some diseases. In late December 2007 my local newspaper, the *San Francisco Chronicle*, ran a front-page article with the headline, "Stress Makes Us Depressed, Fat, Sick—and We Do It to Ourselves," that bore a striking resemblance to articles published in newspapers and magazines several decades earlier. "Americans are so riddled with stress these days it's making them sick," author Erin Allday stated. "There's no doubt . . . that Americans are more stressed out than ever before."[60] Just like their ancestors more than a century earlier, and just like every generation in between, Americans living at the dawn of the twenty-first century believed their era to be the fastest paced, the most trying, and the most stressful. The telegraph and steam power of George M. Beard's time were replaced first by the telephone and the airplane, and then by the cell phone and the Internet, as markers of progress whose downside was the toll taken on people's minds and bodies.

In spite of the thousands of scientific articles published on stress since the mid-twentieth century, the physiological explanation given in the *San Francisco Chronicle* article could have been written by a journalist in the 1950s: "It comes down to a hormone called cortisol, which is released by the adrenal gland when people are under stress." The researchers who found that "chronic stress is unhealthy" came to the same conclusion as their predecessors. What was new were the numerous additional health problems attributed to stress-induced cortisol production. The list of stress-related diseases expanded beyond heart disease and depression to include obesity, autoimmune disorders, and lowered immunity, which left people vulnerable to viral or bacterial infections.

The remedies suggested for stress relief would have been familiar to a reader in the 1970s. Meditation, exercise, and positive thinking were all recommended as self-help ways to regain control, and professional help was advised for those whose stress levels had escalated beyond control. A primary care physician or psychiatrist could prescribe behavioral therapy or medication, both of which, Allday reminded her readers, were available to those who became depressed. Of course, people had to make the initial diagnosis themselves, that is, to decide whether to consult a health care professional or to manage on their own. With or without a visit to the doctor to confirm the diagnosis, stress had become almost wholly somaticized and was understood as an etiological factor in the development of a host of physical symptoms and diseases.

Stress became a prioritized field of biomedical research as a result, at least in part, of public interest in the subject. In July 1979 the Office of Science and Technology Policy of the Executive Office of the President asked the National Academy of Sciences' Institute of Medicine (IOM) to produce a report on research on stress in health and disease. In his foreword to the study, David A. Hamburg, the immediate past president of the IOM, noted the "discrepancy between the high level of public interest and the low priority of scientific commitment" to the effects of stress. The report contrasted the plethora of executive seminars and self-help books put out by the commercialized stress-management industry with the relative paucity of federal funding for scientific research on stress, and it argued for systematic research on stress as a risk factor for illness to provide a biomedical context for patients' anecdotal accounts, such as those who "explain that they have a peptic ulcer or high blood pressure 'because of the kids' or 'because of pressure at work.'"[61] Research on stress accelerated over the next twenty years; a rough count of PubMed articles generated with the keyword "stress" showed a fivefold increase in the number of medical and scientific publications in 2005 as compared to 1985.

Regardless of the occult ways in which stress worked to wreak havoc on the body, both biomedical specialists and members of the general public drew connections between the social, the psychic, and the somatic. Information about stress, health, and disease circulated in multiple directions between patients and physicians, scientists and nonscientists. Shaped by both professional discourse and everyday vernacular, stress followed in the footsteps of its predecessors—nerves and tension—and became an accepted, if poorly understood, component of the matrix within which illness could develop.

Notes

1. Gerald Weissmann, "The Experimental Pathology of Stress: Hans Selye to Paris Hilton," *FASEB Journal* 21 (September 2007): 2636.

2. My work builds on the excellent article by Russell Viner, "Putting Stress in Life: Hans Selye and the Making of Stress Theory," *Social Studies of Science* 29, no. 3 (1999): 391–410. Viner demonstrated that Selye found allies for his stress concept in four spheres beyond academic experimental biology: in psychosomatic medicine, the military, industry, and popular culture. Here I turn my attention to the last of these domains.

3. Roger Cooter and Stephen Pumfrey, "Separate Spheres and Public Places: Reflections on the History of Science Popularization and Science in Popular Culture," *History of Science* 32 (1994): 248–50.

4. Ibid., 254–55.

5. Paul J. Rosch, foreword to *Anthology of Stress Revisited,* by James H. Humphrey (New York: Novinka Books, 2005), viii, ix.

6. Angela Patmore, *The Truth about Stress* (London: Atlantic Books, 2006); Serge Doublet, *The Stress Myth* (Chesterfield, MO: Science and Humanities Press, 2000); Charles E. Rosenberg, "Disease in History: Frames and Framers," *Milbank Quarterly* 67, suppl. no. 1 (1989): 1–15.

7. David A. Hamburg, "Foreword: An Outlook on Stress Research and Health," in *Stress and Human Health: Analysis and Implications of Research; A Study by the Institute of Medicine/National Academy of Sciences,* ed. Glen R. Elliott and Carl Eisdorfer (New York: Springer, 1982), ix.

8. Bishop of Manchester, "The Church and Stress," *Practitioner* 172 (January 1954), 79; Sir Henry Ogilvie, William A. R. Thomson, and Joseph Garland, editorial, *Practitioner* 172 (January 1954): 124.

9. Hans Selye, *The Physiology and Pathology of Exposure to Stress: A Treatise Based on the Concepts of the General-Adaptation-Syndrome and the Diseases of Adaptation* (Montreal: Acta, 1950); Viner, "Putting Stress in Life," 399; "Medicine: The Life of Stress," *Time* 56 (October 9, 1950): 93–94; "Stress Diseases," *Newsweek* 35 (June 26, 1950): 40; "Medicine: Stress and Strain," *Time* 63 (January 18, 1954): 66; J. D. Ratcliff, "Stress: The Cause of All Disease?," *Reader's Digest* 66 (January 1955): 24; italics in the original.

10. Allene Talmey, "Remaking Your Idea of Stress," *Vogue* 129 (January 15, 1957), 55; "A New Approach to Tensions," *Newsweek* 48 (December 3, 1956): 55.

11. Talmey, "Idea of Stress," 54, 55; "New Approach," 55.

12. "Tension and the Nerves of the Nation . . . Psychiatry Eyes the Breaking Point," *Newsweek* 47 (March 5, 1956), 54, 55; "Tension. What It Is—And How You Can Relieve It," *U.S. News and World Report* 43 (November 1, 1957), 76; "Tension—Bad and Good," *Newsweek* 47 (May 14, 1956), 76.

13. Walter C. Alvarez, "How to Live with Your Nerves," *Reader's Digest* 58 (April 1951): 103–5; Alvarez, "Live with Your Nerves and Like It," *Cosmopolitan* 142 (February 1957): 40–45; George C. Stevenson, "How to Deal with Your Tensions," *Reader's Digest* 71 (November 1957): 44–47; "Tension. What It Is," 76–81; "What You Can Do about Stress," *Nation's Business* 46 (June 1958): 34–35. The "Frantic Fifties" quote comes from the editorial introduction to the *Cosmopolitan* article.

14. See Anne Harrington, *The Cure Within: A History of Mind-Body Medicine* (New York: Norton, 2008), for a full exploration of this subject.

15. Charles E. Rosenberg, introduction to George M. Beard, *American Nervousness: Its Causes and Consequences* (New York: Arno, 1972), n.p.

16. Barbara Sicherman, "The Uses of a Diagnosis: Doctors, Patients, and Neurasthenia," *Journal of the History of Medicine and Allied Sciences* 32 (January 1977): 38.

17. Dr. Bilsinger, "Modern Nervousness and Its Cure," *Popular Science Monthly* 42 (November 1892): 90–93; A. B. Nourse, "Nervous Century," *Era* 12 (September 1903): 257–59; A. S. Duryea, "Making Friends of One's Nerves," *Delineator* 73 (June 1909): 774; "Age of Nerves," *Living Age* 267 (November 19, 1910): 505–7; J. K. Mitchell, "Self-Help for Nervous Women," *Harper's Bazar* 35 (May–October 1901): 25–27; A. P. Call, "How Women Can Keep from Being Nervous," *Ladies' Home Journal* 25 (March 1908): 8; J. Williams, "Help for the Nervous Woman," *Woman's Home Companion* 37 (November 1910): 49; Samuel McComb, "Nervous Poise and How to Get It," *Harper's Bazaar* 43 (August 1908): 719–21; McComb, "Nervousness—A National Menace," *Everybody's Magazine* 22 (February 1910): 258–64.

18. Megan Barke, Rebecca Fribush, and Peter N. Stearns, "Nervous Breakdown in 20th-Century American Culture," *Journal of Social History* 33 (Spring 2000): 568, 574, 575, 566.

19. Editors of *Fortune*, *The Nervous Breakdown* (Garden City, NY: Doubleday, Doran, 1935), 7, v–vi.

20. Ibid., 17, 26.

21. George W. Gray, "Anxiety and Illness," *Harper's Magazine* 178 (May 1939): 605–16; Gray, "Anxiety and Illness," *Reader's Digest* 34 (June 1939): 77–80.

22. Gray, "Anxiety and Illness," *Reader's Digest*, 80.

23. Editors of *Fortune*, *Nervous Breakdown*, 39, 38.

24. William Osler, "The Lumleian Lectures on Angina Pectoris," *Lancet* 175 (March 12, 1910): 697; "Marchesa to Head Coue Institute Here," *New York Times*, January 8, 1923, 7; William S. Sadler, "Americanitis Is Accused of Wasting Many Lives," *New York Times*, January 7, 1925, X9; "Stress Death Rate of Heart Disease," *New York Times*, May 3, 1928, 5.

25. "Heart Toll in Youth Cut," *New York Times*, October 4, 1930, 17; White Star Line, display ad, *New York Times*, December 23, 1930, 14; Homestead, display ad, *New York Times*, January 9, 1941, 12; Howard Whitman, "Richest Man in the Cemetery," *Collier's* 124 (July 20, 1949), 17; italics in the original. The advertisement ran in the *New York Times* on July 22, 1949, 9.

26. David Herzberg, *Happy Pills in America: From Miltown to Prozac* (Baltimore: Johns Hopkins University Press, 2009), 32.

27. Quoted in ibid., 32–33.

28. Lawrence Galton, "A New Drug Brings Relief for the Tense and Anxious," *Cosmopolitan* 139 (August 1955): 82–83; Jeremy A. Greene and David Herzberg, "Hidden in Plain Sight: Marketing Prescription Drugs to Consumers in the Twentieth Century," *American Journal of Public Health* 100 (May 2010): 798.

29. Andrea Tone, *The Age of Anxiety: A History of America's Turbulent Affair with Tranquilizers* (New York: Basic Books, 2009), 161.

30. Edward Shorter, *A History of Psychiatry: From the Era of the Asylum to the Age of Prozac* (New York: Wiley and Sons, 1997), 317–19.

31. "The Anatomy of Angst," *Time*, March 31, 1961, 44–51, quoted in Herzberg, *Happy Pills in America*, 53; Miltown advertisement, *Journal of the American Medical Association* 159 (October 15, 1955), 38–39, pictured in Herzberg, *Happy Pills in America*, 28; Herzberg, *Happy Pills in America*, 54.

32. See both Herzberg, *Happy Pills in America*, and Tone, *Age of Anxiety*, for complementary analyses of the antidrug campaigns of the 1970s.

33. Farber, quoted in Herzberg, *Happy Pills in America*, 152.

34. For an excellent medical and cultural history of depression in twentieth-century America, see Laura D. Hirshbein, *American Melancholy: Constructions of Depression in the Twentieth Century* (New Brunswick, NJ: Rutgers University Press, 2009). See also Herzberg, *Happy Pills in America*, 152–69.

35. Herzberg, *Happy Pills in America*, 260, 152.

36. Hirshbein, *American Melancholy*, 62.

37. Herzberg, *Happy Pills in America*, 158.

38. There is an enormous literature on the effects of stress during wartime, starting with shell shock in World War I and continuing on to the diagnostic category of post-traumatic stress disorder (PTSD) in later conflicts. This topic is related to but beyond the scope of the present chapter.

39. Heneage Ogilvie, "In Praise of Idleness," *British Medical Journal*, April 16, 1949, 647; I. McD. G. Stewart, "Coronary Disease and Stress," *Lancet*, December 23, 1950, 867–70; William P. Shepard, "Does the Modern Pace Really Kill?," *Journal of the American Geriatrics Society* 3 (March 1955): 144.

40. Max Warmbrand, *Add Years to Your Heart*, display ad, *New York Times*, September 12, 1956, 31; Curt S. Wachtel, *Your Mind Can Make You Sick or Well*, display ad, *New York Times*, April 26, 1959, BR16.

41. "Rise in Heart Cases Seen, Stresses of Modern Living Cited at Meeting Here," *New York Times*, January 11, 1950, 22; "Heart Affliction Linked to Stress," *New York Times*, March 9, 1958, 82; "Stress of Work in U.S. Culture Cited as Cause of Heart Disease," *New York Times*, January 28, 1959, 23; "Go-Getters, Beware!" *Time* 74 (November 2, 1959), 80; "The Cost of Getting Ahead," *Time* 75 (May 16, 1960), 45.

42. Meyer Friedman and Ray H. Rosenman, "Association of Specific Overt Behavior Patterns with Blood and Cardiac Findings," *Journal of the American Medical Association* 169 (March 21, 1959), 1286. See also Elianne Riska, "The Rise and Fall of Type A Man," *Social Science and Medicine* 51 (2000): 1665–74.

43. Meyer Friedman and Ray H. Rosenman, *Type A Behavior and Your Heart* (New York: Knopf, 1974), 56.

44. Ibid., 67.

45. Thomas H. Holmes and Richard H. Rahe, "The Social Readjustment Rating Scale," *Journal of Psychosomatic Research* 11 (1967): 213–18. For an interesting historical analysis of Holmes's research in the 1950s on stress and tuberculosis, see Barron H. Lerner, "Can Stress Cause Disease? Revisiting the Tuberculosis Research of Thomas Holmes, 1949–1961," *Annals of Internal Medicine* 124 (April 1, 1996): 673–80.

46. Judith G. Rabkin and Elmer L. Struening, "Life Events, Stress, and Illness," *Science* 194 (December 1976): 1015.

47. Hans Selye, *Stress without Distress* (New York: Lippincott and Crowell, 1974).

48. "Stress," *Mademoiselle* 81 (April 1975): 138; M. L. S., "What Stress Can Do to Mind and Body," *Good Housekeeping* 188 (February 1979): 248–49.

49. Walter McQuade, "What Stress Can Do to You," *Fortune* 85 (January 1972): 102.

50. Arnold A. Hutschnecker, "Tension, the Everyday Threat to American Women . . . and What to Do about It," *Vogue* 151 (June 1971): 120; McQuade, "What Stress Can Do," 103.

51. David C. Glass, "Stress, Competition and Heart Attacks," *Psychology Today* 10 (December 1976): 54–57, 134; "Secrets of Coping with Stress," *U.S. News and*

World Report 82 (March 21, 1977): 51–53; Kathy Slobogin, "Stress," *New York Times*, November 20, 1977, SM 49–50, 96; J. D. Ratcliff, "How to Avoid Harmful Stress," *Today's Health* 48 (July 1970): 42–44; Kenneth Lamott, "What to Do When Stress Says You're Killing Yourself," *Today's Health* 53 (January 1975): 3–33, 59–60; "The Link between Your Emotions and Health," *Harper's Bazaar* 110 (February 1977): 131.

52. Karen Lovett Andes, "What Stress Can Do to Your Body," *Mademoiselle* 85 (October 1979): 80.

53. Hans Selye, quoted in Ratcliff, "How to Avoid Harmful Stress," 43.

54. M. L. S., "Mind and Body," 249.

55. Andes, "Your Body," 81; "Your Emotions and Health," 166; Richard M. Suinn, "How to Break the Vicious Cycle of Stress," *Psychology Today* 10 (December 1976): 60.

56. Barbara Ehrenreich, "Is Success Dangerous to Your Health?" *Ms.* 7 (May 1979): 101.

57. Dr. Allan Frank, quoted in Andes, "Your Body," 80.

58. "Stress," 138; M. L. S., "Mind and Body," 249.

59. Friedman and Rosenman, *Type A Behavior*, 180–240.

60. Erin Allday, "Stress Makes Us Depressed, Fat, Sick—and We Do It to Ourselves," *San Francisco Chronicle*, December 10, 2007, 1.

61. Hamburg, foreword to Elliott and Eisdorfer, *Stress and Human Health*, ix, 259.

Part Two

Trauma and Acute Stress

Chapter Three

Resilience for All by the Year 20–

Allan Young

The following pages describe the historical transformation of the posttraumatic *neurosis* into a now-familiar post-traumatic *stress* disorder. My approach is ethnographic in that I have emphasized transformations in epistemologies—specifically what counts as evidence and what is either taken for granted or altogether ignored. While it is important to follow how these transformations occurred, it is not useful to stick to a unilinear chronological sequence. I begin in 1980, with the publication of *DSM-III* and the debut of post-traumatic stress disorder (PTSD). PTSD was the first (and remains the only) *standardized* and *obligatory* version of a posttraumatic syndrome in the United States. By the 1990s PTSD had become, in effect, a universally accepted version. Beneath the surface of the official list of diagnostic criteria, PTSD is a heterogeneous phenomenon. There are compelling reasons to conclude that PTSD's heterogeneity is intrinsic to its logic, and it is *only* this logic that distinguishes PTSD from other disorders. Moreover, PTSD's heterogeneity is intractable: it is generally impossible to tell the subtypes apart. This is an important problem, with clinical, forensic, social, and political implications. I argue that scientific discourse on physiological stress provides researchers with possible solutions, a way of circumventing the traumatic memories believed to drive the posttraumatic syndrome. But this conception of stress, intended to stabilize and homogenize the posttraumatic syndrome, is itself polymorphic and eventually extended to include populations unimagined in 1980.

The key that unlocks this confusing situation is an understanding of the historical character of PTSD and the posttraumatic syndromes that precede it. All psychiatric disorders are historical: they change over time as a consequence of developments in psychiatry and the sciences of the mind and the brain. The posttraumatic syndromes are historical in a further sense; they are determined by historical world events, mainly violent. The section headings are intended to orient readers as the text zigzags through history. To keep the text compact, I have ignored the period before 1919.[1]

1980

Post-traumatic stress disorder begins in 1980, as a classification included among the anxiety disorders in *DSM-III*. It is preceded in *DSM-I* by a disorder called "gross stress reaction," listed among the "transient situational personality disorders."[2] Gross stress reaction affects "more or less 'normal' persons who have experienced intolerable stress" in the form of severe physical demands or extreme emotional stress, specifically fear. It is characteristically transient and, if it persists, an alternative diagnosis must be made. Leaving aside the fear and intolerable stress, it is generally unlike PTSD.[3] In *DSM-II* (1968), it disappears and there is no replacement.

In *DSM-III* and subsequent editions, PTSD comprises two elements: an etiological event, often described as the "stressor criterion," and a syndrome. The elements are connected by a defining logic: criterion A (stressor) causes B (an intrusive traumatic memory) that is in turn responsible for criteria C (avoidance and numbing) and D (symptoms of physiological arousal). Within this logic the traumatic stressor precipitates the syndrome, but it is the traumatic memory that drives the syndrome. The syndrome can be acute, lasting less than six months, or chronic, sometimes lasting a lifetime. In cases of chronic PTSD, the onset of the syndrome can be immediate or delayed. No limit is placed on the duration of the delay, and it can last for decades. PTSD research concentrates on the chronic variety, and in this chapter I do likewise.

Publications on PTSD employ the term "stress" in two ways: for psychological stress attributed to the traumatic event and traumatic memory and for psychophysiological stress underpinning criterion D. Psychological stress from PTSD is associated with anxiety and feelings of loss, guilt, shame, and anger. In some cases the stress is secondary to a person's conscious and unconscious efforts to manage posttraumatic distress by self-dosing with alcohol and drugs. PTSD psychophysiological stress is connected with the survival response (fight, flee, freeze). While the nature of the connection is not specified, researchers commonly associate PTSD arousal symptoms—outbursts of anger, hypervigilance, and exaggerated startle response—with conscious and unconscious anticipation of trauma-motif dreams and intrusive memories and images.

1920 to 1980

PTSD's memory logic originates in Sigmund Freud's account of "traumatic neurosis" in *Beyond the Pleasure Principle* (1920). He writes that the "mental apparatus" is caught off guard by a precipitating event (traumatic shock) and fails to activate its protective shield (*Reizschutz*) in time. The shock creates a quantum of energy that floods the "psychical system" and disrupts its normally quiescent state. The syndrome is a repetition compulsion, in which the ego reexperiences the traumatic memory in dreams in an effort to gain mastery. The extreme anxiety and agitation characteristic of the dreams are described as "signal anxiety"—a warning of the impending event. In the summary histories often attached to publications on PTSD during the 1980s, Abram Kardiner, an American psychiatrist, is more often mentioned than Freud. Kardiner's *The Traumatic Neuroses of War* (1941) is based on his clinical experiences with chronic cases he treated in a US Veterans Administration hospital during the 1920s. The pages on posttraumatic syndrome adopt the logic of Freud's traumatic neurosis, a debt that is acknowledged by Kardiner in his 1959 update and summary of the original book.[4] Kardiner's most significant departure from Freud is his interpretation of patients' arousal and anxiety, which he characterizes as a "physioneurosis," signifying preparation for the flee-or-fight response rather than mastery or abreaction. Freud's traumatic neurosis is now aligned with the neurophysiology of the medical mainstream. Kardiner lists the characteristics of the posttraumatic syndrome and includes features that reemerge twenty years later in criterion D: irritability, exaggerated startle response, and "explosive aggressive reaction pattern."[5] The perspective is functional: focused on the "personality as a whole" and unconcerned with biological causes or consequences.

Kardiner's 1959 paper mentions Roy Grinker, almost in passing. Grinker was a much-published neuropsychiatrist and researcher at the start of World War II. Like Kardiner, he had traveled to Vienna to be psychoanalyzed by Freud. During the war he served as a lieutenant colonel in the US Army Medical Corps in Tunisia treating ground troops and subsequently treating aircrew operating over Europe. He published two books during the war, coauthored with John P. Spiegel, *War Neuroses in North Africa* and *Men under Stress.*[6] Kardiner describes the latter book as the "most complete account of [pathogenic] war experiences in World War II." He criticizes Grinker on two points: Grinker "does not explicitly recognize the traumatic syndrome as such," and he "insists on an explanation that takes into account the neurological paths through which the pathological reactions take place." Kardiner describes the neurological account as "gratuitous," and is unsympathetic to Grinker's effort to construct a "unified theory to integrate the perspectives of psychoanalysis, psychiatry, and clinical neurology":[7] "As one proceeds from neurology through psychiatry to psychoanalysis one can discern a gradation of increasing deviation from the basic facts of anatomy and physiology susceptible of experimental proof. From a science resting directly on the foundations of biology to the descriptive field of psychiatry concerned with classifications, one arrives at more abstract, nevertheless scientific concepts concerned with dynamic factors involving intangible forces of energy."[8] Grinker's vision of the concomitance of brain and mind derives directly from Hughlings Jackson.

This celebrated neurologist described the nervous system as comprising a hierarchy of sensory-motor "centers" acquired incrementally as evolutionary adaptations. At the bottom of the hierarchy are the oldest centers—spontaneous, inflexible, reflex-like. The older centers are inhibited and controlled by centers acquired later. When a control center is disabled (by disease, alcohol, etc.), previously inhibited centers are released to perform their evolved functions, and the effect is expressed in symptoms, syndromes, and mental states. The released functions are called "positive" symptoms; a "negative" symptom, such as paralysis, results from the loss of a function. This process in which a pathology retraces the nervous system's evolutionary path in reverse order is called "dissolution." Hughlings Jackson's clinical interest focused on epilepsy and aphasia, and his most extended observations concern these disorders. Following his death in 1911, interest in the Jacksonian brain declined, the notable exceptions being W. H. R. Rivers in Britain, Paul McLean in the United States (his "triune brain" reiterates the Jacksonian scheme), Henri Ey in France (like Grinker, also a psychoanalyst), and Sigmund Freud (notably in *The Interpretation of Dreams*).[9]

Grinker repeatedly acknowledges the influence of Hughlings Jackson on his work.[10] He cites Jackson in his effort to delineate a relation between inhibition and dissolution and Freud in repression and symptom formation: "Neurologically, release of lower levels results in a greater preponderance of visceral participation in reflex activities. Psychologically, [the effect] may be roughly stated as 'turning one's emotions against oneself,' producing disturbances of function of the internal visceral organs innervated by the autonomic nervous system. It seems clear that regression to lower levels of psychologic activity has a particular applicability to the mechanisms of organ neuroses."[11] Grinker's interest in the "dynamic expressions of interplay . . . within levels of the nervous system" centered on relations between the hypothalamus and cerebral cortex. The hypothalamus, he wrote, regulates and integrates autonomic activity and is also a reservoir for prolonged excitation, experienced as intense anxiety. Unrelieved excitation produces somatic changes: attempts at the lower level to substitute for inactivity at a higher level (consciousness). The situation eventuates in symptoms and syndromes, including tachycardia, diabetes, peptic ulcers, hypertension, and migraines.[12]

The stress paradigm, emerging during the 1950s, redefined the function of the hypothalamus by incorporating it into the familiar HPA axis (hypothalamus-pituitary-adrenals). Grinker is sympathetic to these developments—the discovery of role of the hypothalamus in corticotrophin secretion and the stress response—and he strives to reconcile this new knowledge with the Jacksonian brain: "Excessive stress responses lead to disintegration and dedifferentiation of systems, parts and their differences from each other, leading to more primitive behaviors in a reversal of the developmental processes of growth and differentiation. Thus we may speak of physiological, psychological, and social *partial* regression to what existed before, inhibited but never lost."[13] Thus the stress process begins with efforts within subsystems to adapt to a challenge, a disruption of homeostasis. The efforts are exhausting, and normally subordinate levels and functions are disinhibited. The biomarkers of stress, such as corticotropin, speak of the hierarchy of responses within the subsystems. The consequent symptoms and syndromes are a collective effect of the subsystems.[14]

In his comments on *Men under Stress*, Kardiner criticizes Grinker for not explicitly recognizing "the traumatic syndrome as such."[15] Nonetheless Grinker is familiar with what can be called the soldier's traumatic situation and describes how affected soldiers respond to narcosynthesis therapy, following injection with sodium pentothol:

> Some patients act out the traumatic parts of the battle scene. . . . It is electrifying to watch the terror exhibited in the moments of supreme danger. . . . The body becomes increasingly tense and rigid; the eyes widen, and the pupils dilate, while the skin becomes covered with perspiration. The hands move about convulsively. . . . Breathing becomes incredibly rapid and shallow. The intensity of emotion sometimes becomes more than they can bear and frequently at the height of the reaction, there is a collapse and the patient falls back in bed and remains quiet for a few minutes, usually to resume the story. . . . Some patients return over and over again to one short traumatic scene, living it through repeatedly.[16]

According to Grinker, this tendency to focus on a single etiological event masks the complexity of the posttraumatic disorder in solders at war, although it may be characteristic of civilian cases:

> War neuroses are rarely the result of a single experience but many factors including monotonously repetitive dangerous stimuli, difficult physical activity, intolerable external environmental conditions, protracted and repeated evidences of desertion by all supporting and friendly human relations, and violent disruption of close personal ties with dead and wounded comrades, are a few of these factors. . . . The ego disruption is tremendous, often leading to severe regression. . . . The illness is the stimulus for a new and serious conflict with the ego ideal incrementing anxiety, so that removal from combat may become more secondary loss than gain. . . . [The] neuroses develop after the protective factors such as morale and the widened ego spans in closely knit groups have collapsed.[17]

Grinker rejects the primacy of traumatic memory but does not deny the importance of traumatizing experiences. The underlying process is complex, a product of mind, brain, and society, and cannot be reduced to the memory logic described in *Beyond the Pleasure Principle* and, later, in *DSM-III*.

Grinker's overall project is the theory of the war neuroses embracing psychoanalysis, the Jacksonian brain, "dynamic neurology," and (in the 1950s) the physiology of stress. But by the 1960s Grinker's time had passed, and the vision of an integrated field had been fragmented in autonomous research fields, connected mainly by their interest in anxiety: an ascendant psychiatric epidemiology and a stress field now bifurcated between psychological distress (exemplified by Mardi Horowitz's *Stress Response Syndromes*, 1976) and physiological stress, centered on the autonomic nervous system and the HPA axis.[18]

Unlike circumstances during and after World War II, participants and veterans of the Korean conflict (1950–53 armistice) attracted relatively little attention from psychiatric researchers. Sixty years later we know more about the mental condition of repatriated prisoners of war, and especially the collaborators and turncoats, than about the far more numerous soldiers and marines who survived otherwise.[19] The Vietnam conflict was not so different in this regard: low rates of psychiatric symptoms were reported during most of the war. Initially, low rates were attributed to high morale, rigorous training, and a one-year tour of duty; after 1967 they were commonly traced to widespread "self-dosing" with drugs.[20]

Peter Bourne's research was a significant exception to the general lack of interest in the psychophysiological effects of combat during this period.[21] An army psychiatrist, Bourne accompanied a team of twelve Special Forces soldiers to an isolated hamlet in the Vietnamese highlands. The men were highly selected, trained, and tested, and some had previous experience in perilous operations. On arrival, the unit received reliable intelligence reports that that they were the target of a large enemy force: "A clear objective threat existed in the form of death or mutilation in combat." Bourne obtained urine samples from the men for eighteen days, including four days when the attack was imminent. The attack did not occur, but the situation can be regarded as potentially traumatic. The urine samples were frozen and levels of a corticosteroid (17-OHSC) were subsequently measured. These excretions are a measure of adrenal cortical response. Levels were consistently lower than what had been reported for analogous situations in the general population. Individually and collectively, the soldiers "demonstrated an overwhelming emphasis on self-reliance, often to the point of omnipotence." According to Bourne, these features—training, experience, personality, and so on—combined with psychological defenses that included religious beliefs and idiosyncratic rituals, accounted for the absence of a physiological stress response. An earlier study of a helicopter crew operating in the combat zone had produced similar findings.[22]

John Mason is a coauthor on both of these papers. He was already a leading stress researcher and had collaborated in studies of stress physiology in people diagnosed with major depression, patients recovering from cardiac and pulmonary surgery, parents of children with neoplastic disease, and reactions of normal individuals to filmed events.[23] The Vietnam publications can be viewed as an extension of this stressful life-event research rather than work targeting the posttraumatic syndrome. This is consonant with the portrayal of stress reactions in *DSM-I* and their absence in *DSM-II.* There is one more aspect of Bourne's research worth noting, and I return to this subject toward the end of the chapter. His findings are less about the stress response in a combat situation than the absence of the response.[24] That is to say, the soldiers' "resilience" is described in psychological terms: the physiological dimension of resilience is simply undisturbed homeostasis.

1980

DSM-III represents the apotheosis of psychiatric epidemiology. The posttraumatic syndrome is standardized and defined by a memory logic, and rival classifications are excluded. The diagnostic criteria are engineered to maximize reliability and minimize false positives and false negatives. Whether by intention or default, it is an arrangement for decomposing the context of trauma—Grinker's hierarchy of subsystems, Bourne's highland narrative—into aggregates of mobile risk factors. As represented in the *DSMs*, discourse, and research, PTSD is a homogenous phenomenon. In practice, it is a heterogeneous phenomenon.

The symptoms listed for PTSD are superficially similar to the symptoms of depression and generalized anxiety disorders.[25] PTSD is distinguishable from the other disorders because traumatic memory changes the meaning (but not the appearance) of the symptoms. Since *DSM-IIIR* (1987), it has been possible to give a comorbid diagnosis to a patient. Chronic PTSD characteristically occurs together with other disorders, most often depression, generalized anxiety disorder, panic disorder, and alcohol and chemical substance-use disorders. In some affected populations comorbid depression reaches 90 percent. In most of these cases the onset of the comorbid symptoms preceded the PTSD diagnosis by several years. A clinician might wonder, did a traumatic memory produce my patient's syndrome, or is he a depressed, anxious, and dysfunctional man who is being helped to construct a serviceable etiology?

There is a further problem. Since the 1880s clinicians treating posttraumatic patients have recognized the capacity of the human mind to mimic the A-B-C-D etiology (event → memory → syndrome). Three kinds of mimicry are mentioned in the psychiatric literature during this period. The first kind begins with a real event that is not markedly distressful when initially experienced. In retrospect, sometimes long after the original event, the experience is remembered as traumatic: distressful. The causal sequence reverses the A-B-C-D sequence. It starts with C and D and progresses (usually with expert assistance) to the discovery of a plausible A and B (event and memory). Sometimes, the recollected event is recontextualized and acquires an emotional potency and psychological salience that duplicates the A-B-C-D sequence—Freud's notion of *Nachträglichkeit.* The second kind of mimicry is represented in "factitious memory," where someone develops an intense psychological identification with a borrowed or imagined etiological event or, more commonly, identifies with a distorted representation of a real autobiographical event. Factitious memory is stigmatized as a form of self-deception, but it often tokens efforts aimed at salvaging or rebuilding the individual's sense of self. The final kind of mimicry is "malingering." By definition, a malingerer is aware of dissimulating, and there is no self-deception. In practice, the boundary between fictitious and factitious memories is porous and easily transgressed through autosuggestion.

The problem is that it is very often (perhaps generally) impossible to differentiate the "true" cases of PTSD. There are two obstacles. First, autobiographical memories are intrinsically malleable representations. Remembering is correctly understood as a process in which mnemonic traces of an experience are reassembled, updated, and reschematized. Fredric Bartlett described the process in 1932 in his famous monograph, *Remembering,* and it has been intensively investigated in the intervening years, most recently by cognitive neuroscience.[26] The reconsolidation process (retrieval) appears to be an adaptation to the future, a means of enhancing the organism's ability to respond to new situations, rather than a medium providing faithful photocopies of the past. The literature on PTSD makes an empirically groundless exception for traumatic memories, which are routinely described as "indelible."[27] The second obstacle is that there are no satisfactory alternatives to the patients' self-reports. The obvious alternative is criterion D, signs and symptoms associated with the stress response. Consequently, the stress response has acquired a salience that is not entirely explained by developments in the science of stress. In the next section, I review research and writing on criterion D during the years 1980 to 2001. The events of 9/11 introduce a new perspective on traumatic stress, returning us to Bourne's mountaintop. I will describe these developments in a moment.

1980 to 2001

Biological research on PTSD is limited to the HPA axis, the hippocampus, and the autonomic nervous system (ANS). HPA research is directed to excretions neurohormones: catecholamines (epinephrine and norepinephrine) and cortisol. Excretion of catecholamines is short-lived rather than persistent. Elevated levels in PTSD are associated with episodes of autonomic arousal and, it is said, contribute to the "indelible" quality of traumatic memories. Most PTSD neuroendocrine research is directed to measuring and comparing cortisol excretions. Findings are ambiguous: some researchers find elevated levels with PTSD; others find lower than normal levels. In either event findings represent a statistically significant difference between mean values in PTSD groups and comparison groups. The deviations from the normal are clinically meaningless in that they do not reach the thresholds associated with endocrine pathologies (Addison's disease, Cushing's disease). More to the point, they are diagnostically useless. Differences between PTSD and control groups are explained by small numbers of outliers in the PTSD group; overlap between groups often exceeds 90 percent.[28]

Despite the overlap between groups, many researchers, peer reviewers, and readers widely regard hypocortisol to be a biomarker of PTSD and to reflect an underlying PTSD biology that is overtly expressed in the few outliers but also implicit in other members of the PTSD group.[29] Findings that associate PTSD with *elevated* levels of cortisol are consistent with Hans Selye's view of the role of the HPA axis during the recovery or resistance stage.[30] In contrast, the putative hypocortisol finding is "both counterintuitive, and not uniformly reproducible."[31] The problem, Rachel Yehuda writes, began with *DSM-III*, where PTSD was pictured as a normal response to an abnormal stressor. In 1980 "normal response" signified a normal HPA-axis. But subsequent research demonstrated that only a minority of exposed individuals developed the syndrome—less than 20 percent in the case of combat veterans. The prevailing view today is that PTSD is an abnormal response to a range of awful experiences that most people take in stride. Yehuda's research locates this abnormality within an HPA-axis that has been rendered "dysfunctional" or "disordered" by a combination of epigenetics and early stressors.[32]

Studies of brain images of Vietnam veterans report statistically significant differences in hippocampus volume between Vietnam-combat veterans with PTSD, combat veterans without PTSD, and veterans without combat experience and without PTSD. The smaller hippocampus in the PTSD group is consistent with the hypercortisol thesis. Researchers previously connected chronically elevated levels of cortisol in major depression with (reversible) neuronal death and reduced volume of the hippocampus. By the late 1990s opinion among researchers favored the hypocortisol thesis. Efforts to explain the reduced size of the hippocampus moved in a different direction, seeking causal pathway unconnected to cortisol. Research published in 2002 compared multiple sets of monozygotic twins: one twin had PTSD and Vietnam combat exposure, the other twin had no PTSD and no combat. Researchers discovered no significant differences between the twins and concluded that "smaller hippocampi in PTSD represent a pre-existing, *familial vulnerability factor* rather than the neurotoxic effect of trauma exposure *per se.*"[33] The toxic PTSD thesis lingers on, however, unresolved and now attracting relatively little attention.

ANS research measures responses to experimental stimuli: heart rate, blood pressure, skin conductance, eye-blink startle response, and event-related brain potentials (electrical changes recorded on the surface of the scalp). Research findings are generally inconclusive. Heart rate response (HRR) is the exception; in contrast to cortisol research, HRR can identify differences between individuals (PTSD versus normal) as well as between groups. But the question at hand is not whether a technique distinguishes between PTSD and normal individuals, but whether it can distinguish between different kinds of traumatic memories—the A-B-C-D kind and three kinds of mimicry.

Recent experimental research conducted by Susan Clancy and Richard McNally at Harvard suggests that HRR is not up to the job. The researchers recruited for the study a sample of people who believe they have been abducted and physically violated by space aliens. None of the individuals had a diagnosable psychopathology or scored in the abnormal range in response to psychological scales. All of them reported experiencing the same sequence of events, beginning with a brief episode at the moment of awakening, when they experienced full body paralysis and meaningless hallucinations—tingling sensations, buzzing sounds, flashing lights, and vague, hovering figures. Some individuals had multiple episodes. The experiences were subjectively very frightening but are in fact neurologically normal hypnopompic hallucinations. All individuals had been anxious and sought an explanation; some worried about mental or neurological diseases. All were familiar with alien abduction stories. Several individuals consulted clinicians who hypnotized them with the goal of recovering "repressed" memories. Some individuals did "recover" abduction memories. Others could obtain "no explicit autobiographical memories of the suspected events . . . but cited a variety of signs and symptoms that they believed indicated an abduction history."[34] The researchers prepared individualized scripts based on each person's reported event and other autobiographic events. Participants listened to audiotapes of their scripts, and researchers monitored their ANS responses. A control group (no abduction, no anxiety disorder) followed a parallel procedure. The abductees' heart rate and skin conductance responses to their abduction scripts were comparable to the responses of PTSD veterans and sexual abuse survivors to their traumatic event scripts and significantly higher than the responses of the controls.[35]

The key question is whether a measure can distinguish between different kinds of traumatic memories. Of course this is *my* key question, and only my question. PTSD researchers and clinicians are unconcerned. It is easy to ignore the malleability of memory problems when diagnosis is regarded as equivalent to matching a patient's self-reported symptoms and memories with the *DSM* diagnostic criteria for PTSD. The standardized and precalibrated diagnostic instruments (protocols, scales) employed for matching self-reports to symptom lists function as black boxes. In this case the malleability of memory is someone else's problem. And if there is a problem, it is a reason for refining technology rather than inquiring into epistemology.[36]

The 9/11 Attacks and the War on Terror

Posttraumatic syndromes have attracted attention for more than a century. Symptom clusters—cardiac, epigastric, sensory-motor, psychological—wax and wane in importance, putative causal mechanisms fall in and out of fashion, and expectations of patients and clinicians alter accordingly.[37] Some of the changes reflect developments in medical theories, knowledge, and technology. These syndromes have never been the exclusive domain of psychiatry. Recent proposals to eliminate the A criterion in *DSM-V* lead nowhere because they are oblivious to the social, political, and forensic significance of identifiable traumatic stressors—the importance of establishing culpability and awarding compensation for posttraumatic entitlements for veterans, workers, motorists, and so on and for establishing eligibility for asylum-seeker status.

Every diagnostic classification has a history. But the posttraumatic syndromes are historical in an additional sense. One might describe the engagement between trauma and history as disparate "episodes" that follow a single pattern. Each historical episode begins with an event of encompassing violence and a co-occurring or consequent epidemic of posttraumatic casualties. The epidemic is always a source of controversy—concerning the numbers affected, etiology, impairment, differential diagnosis, culpability and obligation, economic and social costs, and intervention and prevention strategies. Resources are mobilized for managing casualties and claimants and for conducting research. In a word, an assemblage emerges, colored by national medical traditions, institutional cultures, and popular attitudes. The posttraumatic syndromes—shell shock, PTSD, mild traumatic brain injury (TBI), Gulf War Syndrome, second-generation Holocaust trauma, and so on—and matching *subjectivities* (the patient's self-awareness of his situation) are products of these assemblages.

Epidemiological research following the 9/11 attacks focused on a phenomenon called "distant traumatic effects." PTSD researchers had been denied access to the victims of the attacks and their families. Some researchers complained about the "moratorium on research"; many others adapted by investigating the distant traumatic effects of the attacks—in one noteworthy instance, employing web-based technologies originally designed for market research surveys.[38] The distant effects were products of televised images and are compatible with the "witnessing events" medium included in the A criterion. Although TV images are not mentioned in the *DSMs*, 9/11 epidemiologists established a robust statistical association between exposure to these images and the onset of symptoms. They focused on two images: people jumping or falling to their deaths from the World Trade Center and people down below fleeing from debris and clouds of ashes. Watching the images in real time seemed to increase the risk for PTSD, and researchers likewise reported a dose-response relationship: more viewing equaled more symptoms.[39] Researchers compared the images with "flashbacks" and "flashbulb memories" associated with PTSD: repetitive, intrusive, and indelible.[40]

In the following months epidemiologists measured stress reactions to 9/11. Findings indicated very low rates of PTSD but a high incidence of nonspecific symptoms attributable to trauma, for example, intrusive mental images, sleep problems, difficulties concentrating, and hypervigilance. Evidence of two or more symptoms was often characterized as evidence of "partial PTSD," a term missing from the *DSMs*. Aggregated responses (i.e., populations rather than individuals) reached the A-B-C-D standard. The overall effect—combining distant trauma, partial PTSD, and aggregate reporting—can be characterized as "virtual PTSD," although this term should not detract from its potential significance, political rather than clinical.

The 9/11 attacks were widely described as a form of "psychological warfare" that was intended to generate a pervasiveness sense of helplessness and loss of confidence in the ability of the government to protect citizens. Respondents to structured protocols routinely indicated that the US public now believed that acts of terrorism might happen anywhere in the United States and at any moment. Editorials in the *New England Journal of Medicine*, the *Journal of the American Medical Association*, and other journals diagnosed the situation as a national public health crisis. This was the bad news. The good news was that the vast majority of Americans did not develop clinical PTSD. This can be explained in two ways. One way is that no explanation is required. This is how normal people respond to images of disquieting events that affect the lives of distant people. Alternatively, the *absence* signifies a novel *presence*—something called "resilience."

In 2003 representative Patrick Kennedy proposed a National Resilience Development Act. The proposal was sent to a congressional committee on terrorism and homeland security, where it seems to have been ignored. The American Psychological Association (APA) responded with greater enthusiasm. In 1999 it had initiated a public awareness and education program called Enhancing Resilience, promoting research into youth-related violence.[41] Four years later the APA redirected its attention to resilience in adults: "In an effort to tap the pulse of the post-9/11 nation, we conducted focus groups [around the country]. Participants described a distinct sense that 'the other shoe was about to drop' . . . [and said they] were interested in being able to be resilient in the face of such challenges."[42]

The APA produced a video documentary, *Aftermath: The Road to Resilience*, an online "consumer brochure" detailing steps to building resilience and a "tool kit" for community outreach by APA members. The APA also arranged for a series of "resilience forums" for journalists.[43] The APA's version of resilience started in an initiative to help children living in adverse conditions and at-risk for psychiatric and developmental problems. Research targeted unusual, *resilient* children who had succeeded despite great adversity—the super achievers. In the 1990s the term, as employed by social psychologists, was reconceived to mean "a common phenomenon that results in most cases from the operation of basic human adaptational systems." Resilience now acquires diagnostic features and metrics—self-efficacy, self-regulation, emotional stability, hardiness—that are incorporated into scales.[44] In 2003 Kathryn Connor and Jonathan Davidson, a psychiatrist and prominent trauma researcher, published a scale for investigating resilience and PTSD (the CD-RISC scale), because "no better evidence exists with respect to the importance of resilience than . . . the [proposed] National Resilience Development Act, which is designed to help Americans build greater psychological resilience in the face of terrorism."[45] Events are stressful because they threaten bio-psycho-social homeostasis. Resilience is the capacity to restore homeostasis: back to the status quo ante or, failing this, a descent to a lower level of homeostasis. But stressful events can also be an opportunity for achieving a higher level of homeostasis, self-actualization, and an enhanced capacity for bouncing back from adversity.[46] This possibility is foretold in a newly diagnosed condition called "posttraumatic growth."[47]

Both the National Resilience Development Act and the APA's Road to Resilience initiative took care to underline that resilience a *modifiable* trait. This is also Davidson's understanding, although there is a significant difference. The APA and Representative Kennedy want to build resilience through psychological expertise and counseling. Davidson aims to do the job with psychotropic drugs, with or without the help of cognitive behavioral therapy. Drugs can contribute to collective resilience as prophylaxis for people at risk for exposure to stressors, but drugs can also be employed for exploring the neurophysiology of resilience, with an eye on enhancement. Davidson and others divided ninety-two people with chronic PTSD into three groups, each receiving a different drug.[48] Prozac (fluoxetine) and Zoloft (setraline) are selective serotonin reuptake inhibitors (SSRI) and are commonly used for treating mood and anxiety disorders including PTSD. The third drug, Gabitril (tiagabine)—a selective GAMA reuptake inhibitor (SGRI)—is an anticonvulsant used for treating epilepsy and occasionally for treating PTSD. The researchers measured posttreatment changes in resilience scores (using the CD-RISC scale) and severity of PTSD symptoms.

CD-RISC scores improved in all three groups following treatment. Participants were inclined to rate themselves higher on items such as "able to adapt to change," "feel in control of life," "have a sense of purpose," and "can deal with what comes." On the other hand, pretreatment (baseline) resilience scores did not predict posttreatment changes in PTSD scores. Improvements in resilience promoted better outcomes—a sense of self-efficacy—but did not improve PTSD symptoms. Thus the meaning of resilience is subtly redefined: no longer a measure of resistance to pathogenesis (PTSD) but rather mastery over stress. The next job must be to find a way to sustain the improved self-reports. Does the belief that they "can handle unpleasant feelings" naturally increase participants' capacity to manage unpleasant feelings? Or must they continue taking Prozac or Zoloft? Or perhaps they should use Gabitril, since it had the strongest effect on CD-RISC scores—"a finding which suggests the possibility that GABA pathways may also play an important role in mediating resilience."[49]

Reverse Engineering

To understand the implications of these findings, one must shed antiquated ideas about normality and character. The road to the future runs from normality (an underperforming baseline) to resilience (self-efficacy, mastery over stress). To meet the future requires an act of moral imagination—to be more precise, reimagining Prozac, Zoloft, and Gabitril: "Typically, we think about and refer to drugs for depression and anxiety as 'anti' depressants and 'anti' anxiety agents. However, our data suggest . . . that these same drugs have promoting effects on positive emotions, behaviours and beliefs. We can call on increasing evidence that treatments are not only 'anti' pathology but 'pro' wellness in nature."[50]

There is a further possibility, recalling Bourne's Special Forces soldiers on a mountaintop in Vietnam: replace pharmaceuticals with heroic bodies. The rediscovery of resilience began with extraordinary people—children called the "invulnerables." In time the locus of resilience shifted, lost its heroic quality, and became "ordinary magic."[51] And then, shortly before the 9/11 attacks, PTSD researchers reclaimed the original version.[52] Only, the extraordinary people were no longer children, and the adversity and stress were no longer explained by accidents of birth and social class. The subjects for research were men who became, in a short while, the lance point in America's war against terrorism: Special Forces soldiers undergoing survival training at Fort Bragg's Special Warfare Center.

Their training was "designed to prepare soldiers to deal with situations that are beyond those in which they are routinely involved but for which they are considered at high risk, specifically, evading capture by the enemy and, when captured, surviving as prisoners of war."[53] Blood is drawn during the course, and researchers discovered high levels of neuropeptide-Y (NP-Y), when compared with ordinary soldiers. It is already known, from clinical evidence and animal studies, that NP-Y is an endogenous anxiolytic agent, buffering or reducing anxiety. Low levels of NP-Y are reported in people suffering depression and in suicide victims. "The current finding of enhanced NPY responses to acute stress individuals recognized [as] 'stress hardy' may represent a step toward improving our understanding of the various factors that contribute to stress resilience and stress vulnerability . . . [and] underscore the potential benefits of NPY agonists [stimulants] in humans."[54]

In "Voodoo Death" (1942), Walter Cannon famously described an ordinary body subjected to unremitting and inescapable fear and consumed by a runaway noradrenergic system.[55] At Fort Bragg we discover a heroic, resilient body that is happily protected from pathogenic stress by NP-Y. British SAS soldiers undergo a similar training program called R2I—"resistance to interrogation." And it provides a final twist in the history of traumatic stress, for UK and US soldiers are accused of employing their personal R2I experiences (building resilience) as templates for enhanced interrogation in the field (diminishing resilience). "When the interrogation techniques are used on British soldiers for training purposes, they are subject to a strict 48-hour time limit, and a supervisor and a psychologist are always present. It is recognized that in *inexperienced hands*, prisoners can be plunged into psychosis."[56] The theme is developed by Shane O'Mara in *Trends in Cognitive Sciences*, where he describes the "neuropsychobiological model" underlying the "enhanced and coercive interrogation techniques" employed in "war on terrorism." According to O'Mara, the Bush administration had adopted a self-defeating view of torture, based on "folk psychology" and oblivious to recent research on the neurophysiology of the HPA axis. Studies of pharmacologically induced cortisol elevations—comparable to the levels induced by water boarding, for example—have been shown to impair memory retrieval. Under torture people are talkative but do not and probably cannot provide accurate detailed information. "By contrast, mildly stressful events generally facilitate recall. The experience of capture, transport and subsequently challenging questioning would seem to be more than enough to make suspects reveal information."[57]

In the war on terror the interrogator's goal is to force someone (a putative terrorist) to retrieve and disclose memories through the application of traumatic stress. The obverse side of the terrorism coin is the efforts aimed at helping undeserving victims of traumatic stress to forestall or inhibit the involuntary reconsolidation (retrieval) of their traumatic memory. The two goals are explicitly underpinned by the same mechanism, the HPA-mediated stress process, retuned for the new century: a traumatic event stimulates elevated levels of stress-response hormones, notably norepinephrine, resulting in the consolidation of "a deeply engraved traumatic memory" manifested in intrusive thoughts and images characteristic of PTSD. The "reexperiences" stimulate the release of these stress hormones, reinforce the traumatic memory trace, and increase the likelihood of continuing series of intrusions and releases. A positive feedback loop is created through which "subclinical PTSD escalates into clinical PTSD."[58]

Propranolol is a promising solution, if taken shortly after the initial traumatic experience.[59] This beta-blocker drug inhibits the release of the stress hormones and dampens the physiological arousal that occurs when traumatized individuals are reexposed to stimuli and recall the precipitating event. When propranolol is administered after successive reexperiences (intrusive recall) of a traumatic event, a metabolic process is set in motion, interdicting further reconsolidation. At this point voluntary retrieval—consciousness of this piece of the autobiographical past—is no longer possible.[60] While this effect has yet to be demonstrated in humans, the published research has already provoked a stream of news articles and online commentaries by neuroethicists, science journalists, moral philosophers, and legal scholars. Here is an excerpt from an account in the *abcNEWS/Health* blog:

> "There are several major concerns about creating these kinds of drugs," said Felicia Cohn, a medical ethicist at University of California at Irvine's School of Medicine. "Is the act of altering memories even an appropriate medical intervention? . . . What are the effects of altering a particular person's memory but not changing the context the person is living in. We might erase a young girl's memory of a rape, but people around her will still know and inadvertently remind her," Cohn said. "It becomes a genie in the bottle question. Once a drug is available for use, it gets used appropriately and inappropriately. . . . Is it just for post-traumatic stress disorder and rape victims? Where do we draw the line? Who gets to decide what is horrific enough?"[61]

The US Department of Veterans Affairs may see propranolol and the neurophysiology of stress in a different light. In 1999 PTSD disability benefit payments were $1.7 billion. Five years later the amount rose to $4.3 billion. Most of the increase resulted from newly diagnosed Vietnam War veterans and from veterans who served in Iraq and Afghanistan. The department asked the Institute of Medicine to create a committee of experts to assess the efficacy of all therapeutic interventions for PTSD—pharmacology, psychotherapy, cognitive-behavioral therapy, and so on. (No mention was made of propranolol.) In 2008 the committee published its report: in each instance the evidence is "inadequate" to determine the efficacy of the interventions.[62]

Conclusion: Resilience for All by the Year 20–

In October 2009 the US Army initiated a service-wide skill-training program called Comprehensive Soldier Fitness. CSF is the product of Martin Seligman, former president of the American Psychological Association and creator and director of the Positive Psychology Center at the University of Pennsylvania. The Department of the Army is paying the center $31 million to facilitate the program and has allocated a further $90 million for its implementation.

> [The] program is designed to increase psychological strength and positive performance and to reduce the incidence of maladaptive responses of the entire U.S. Army. . . . There are four program elements: (a) the assessment of emotional, social, family, and spiritual fitness; (b) individualized learning modules to improve fitness in these domains; (c) formal resilience training; and (d) training of Army master resilience trainers. . . . CSF aims to move the full spectrum of responses to trauma and adversity—ranging from stress-related disorders to ordinary resilience—toward personal growth.[63]

According to General George W. Casey, current chief of staff of the US Army:

> To be clear, CSF will serve as a catalyst for changing Army culture. . . . We have trained over 2,500 master resilience trainers at the University of Pennsylvania already, and we are targeting to have them in every battalion and brigade in the Army to help design training plans and to teach our leaders how to instill resiliency in their subordinates. [The] program includes mandatory resilience training at every Army leader development school.[64]

The CSF program includes an online self-assessment to identify resiliency strengths and weaknesses. Assessment is through the Global Assessment Tool (GAT), and nearly nine hundred thousand soldiers have been used it so far. The program is intended to reassess soldiers annually and to assign targeted remedial training if scores drop below prescribed thresholds. According to Seligman, the human response to high adversity, such as combat, is normally distributed. The great majority is resilient, returns to a normal level of functioning following a brief disruption, and exhibits "posttraumatic growth." The goal is to reduce the incidence of PTSD and move the entire military population toward growth.

Seligman describes a "concrete plan" that emerged during a meeting with government notables: "The former Surgeon General of the United States, Richard Carmona, advised that civilian medicine was perversely incentivized: Of the $2 trillion the United States spends annually on health care, 75% goes into chronic disease and end-of-life care. In contrast, Army medicine is rationally incentivized—its mission is to produce health. . . . This could be a model for civilian medicine." The army surgeon general, Eric Schoomaker, suggested to the chief of staff, General Casey, that the CSF program should be removed from the taint of medicine (and the Medical Corps) and relocated in education and the fabric of everyday life. General Casey liked the idea: "The teachers of the Army are the drill sergeants, and they would become the teachers of resilience and positive psychology." Once the salutogenic effects of resilience training on soldiers and their families are demonstrated, the CSF could become a model for the civilian education of young people.[65]

Seligman was pleased with all this: "The use of resilience training and positive psychology in the Army is consciously intended as a model for civilian use . . . a model for the future of medicine generally." Enhancing emotional, social, family, and spiritual fitness among young soldiers reduces morbidity, mortality, and mental illness; improves prognosis when illness occurs; and cuts treatment costs. In the same way the program will "radically reform how civilian health care is provided." There is more. Teaching young people the skills of emotional fitness will enable them "to perform better at school and to perform better later in the workplace . . . [and perhaps they] will enjoy lives that have more positive emotion, engagement, and meaning and better relationships." And now, "these claims will be directly tested prospectively in the CSF program. . . . If it turns out that soldiers given this training perform better in their jobs, are more engaged, have more meaning in their lives, enjoy better relationships, and have more fruitful employment when they return to civilian society, this will ground a new model for our public schools. Again we will know whether this is so within the next decade."[66]

Notes

My title recalls the once-famous Alma-Ata Declaration (1978) that advocated "Health for All by the Year 2000." The International Conference on Primary Health Care directed its declaration to the WHO and its signature nations.

1. For the period prior to 1918, see Allan Young, "W. H. R. Rivers and the War Neuroses," *Journal of the History of Behavioral Sciences* 35 (1999): 359–78; and Young, *The Harmony of Illusions: Inventing Post-traumatic Stress Disorder* (Princeton, NJ: Princeton University Press, 1995.

2. American Psychiatric Association, *Diagnostic and Statistical Manual of Mental Disorders of the American Psychiatric Association* (Washington, DC, American Psychiatric Press, 1957), 1:10.

3. See, for example, Herbert C Archibald, Dorothy M. Long, Christine Miller, and Read D. Tuddenham, "Gross Stress Reaction in Combat: A 15-year Follow-up," *American Journal of Psychiatry* 119 (1965): 317–22; Herbert C. Archibald and Read D. Tuddenham, "Persistent Stress Reaction after Combat: A 20-year Follow-up." *Archives of General Psychiatry* 12 (1965): 475–81.

4. Sigmund Freud, *Beyond the Pleasure Principle* (1920; repr., London: Hogarth, 1955); Allan Young, "Our Traumatic Neurosis and Its Brain," *Science in Context* 14 (2001): 661–83; Abram Kardiner, *The Traumatic Neuroses of War* (Washington, DC: National Research Council, 1941); Kardiner, "Traumatic Neuroses of War," in *American Handbook of Psychiatry*, ed. Silvano Arieti (New York: Basic Books, 1959), 245–67.

5. Kardiner, *Traumatic Neuroses of War,* 249.

6. Roy R. Grinker and John P. Spiegel, *War Neuroses in North Africa: The Tunisian Campaign, January–May 1943* (New York: Macy Foundation, 1943); Roy R. Grinker and John P. Spiegel, *Men under Stress* (Philadelphia: Blakiston, 1945);

7. Kardiner, "Traumatic Neuroses of War," 247.

8. Roy R. Grinker, "The Interrelation of Neurology, Psychiatry, and Psychoanalysis," *Journal of the American Medical Association* 116 (1941): 2236–2241, on page 2237.

9. Allan Young, "W. H. R. Rivers and the War Neuroses," *Journal of the History of Behavioral Sciences* 35 (1999): 359–78; Young, "When Traumatic Memory Was a Problem: On the Antecedents of PTSD," in *Posttraumatic Stress Disorder: Issues and Controversies,* ed. Gerald Rosen (London: Wiley, 2004), 127–46.

10. Roy R. Grinker, "A Comparison of Psychological 'Repression' and Neurological 'Inhibition'" *Journal of Nervous and Mental Disease* 89 (1938): 765–81; Grinker. "Interrelation"; Grinker, "Psychosomatic Approach to Anxiety," *American Journal of Psychiatry* 113 (1956): 443–47.

11. Grinker, "Interrelation," 2239.

12. Ibid., 2241. See also Roy R. Grinker, "Hypothalamic Functions in Psychosomatic Interrelations," *Psychosomatic Medicine* 1 (1939): 39–45. In this Grinker compares the hypothalamus and cerebral cortex to the id and ego.

13. Roy R. Grinker, "Anxiety as a Significant Variable for a Unified Theory of Human Behavior," *Archives of General Psychiatry* 1 (1959): 537–46.

14. Grinker, "Psychosomatic Approach to Anxiety," 446.

15. Kardiner, "Traumatic Neuroses of War," Cf. Samuel Futterman and Eugene Pumpian-Mindlin, "Traumatic War Neuroses Five Years Later," *American Journal of Psychiatry* 108 (1951): 401–8.

16. Roy R. Grinker and John P. Spiegel, "Brief Psychotherapy in War Neuroses," *Psychosomatic Medicine* 6 (1944): 127. See also Grinker, "Treatment of War Neuroses," *Journal of the American Medical Association* 126 (1944): 142–45.

17. Grinker and Spiegel, "Brief Psychotherapy," 124.

18. Mardi Horowitz, *Stress Response Syndromes* (New York: Aronson, 1976).

19. For example, John C. Kluznik, Nancy Speed, Charles Van Valkenburg, and Richard Magraw, "Forty-Year Follow-Up of United States Prisoners of War, "*American Journal of Psychiatry* 143 (1986): 1443–46.

20. Young, *Harmony of Illusions.*

21. Peter G. Bourne, Robert M. Rose, and John W. Mason, "17-OHCS Levels in Combat: Special Forces 'A' Team under Threat of Attack," *Archives of General Psychiatry* 19, no. 2 (1968): 135–40.

22. Peter G. Bourne, Robert M. Rose, and John W. Mason, "Urinary 17-OHCS Levels: Data on Seven Helicopter Ambulance Medics in Combat," *Archives of General Psychiatry* 17 (July 1967): 104–10.

23. John W. Mason and Joseph V. Brady, "The Sensitivity of Psychoendocrine Systems to Social and Physical Environments," in *Psychobiological Approaches to Social Behavior,* ed. P. Herbert Leiderman and David Shapiro (Stanford, CA: Stanford University Press, 1964), 4–23; Stanford E. Friedman, John W. Mason, and David A. Hamburg, "Urinary 17-Hydroxycorticosteroid Levels in Parents of Children with Neoplastic Disease: A Study of Chronic Psychological Stress," *Psychosomatic Medicine* 25 (July–August 1963): 364–76; Douglas B. Price, Margaret Thaler, and John W.

Mason, "Pre-operative Emotional States and Adrenal Cortical Activity: Studies on Cardiac and Pulmonary Surgery Patients," *Archives of Neurology and Psychiatry* 77 (1957): 646–56.

24. Peter G. Bourne, "Military Psychiatry and the Vietnam Experience," *American Journal of Psychiatry* 127 (1970): 481–88.

25. Naomi Breslau and Glenn Davis, "Post-traumatic Stress Disorder: The Stressor Criterion," *Journal of Nervous and Mental Disease* 175 (1987): 255–64.

26. Fredrick Bartlett, *Remembering: A Study in Experimental and Social Psychology* (Cambridge: Cambridge University Press, 1932).

27. On the malleability of memory, traumatic and otherwise, see Yadin Dudai, "Predicting Not Too Much: How the Cellular Machinery of Memory Anticipates the Uncertain Future," *Philosophical Transactions of the Royal Society of London—B Biological Sciences* 364 (2009): 1255–62; Dudai, "Reconsolidation: The Advantage of Being Refocused," *Current Opinion in Neurobiology* 16 (2006): 174–78; Harmen J. Krugers, Casper C. Hoogenraad, and Laurent Groc, "Stress Hormones and AMPA Receptor Trafficking in Synaptic Plasticity and Memory," *Nature Reviews Neuroscience* 11 (2010): 675–81; Lauren French, Maryanne Garry, and Elizabeth Loftus, "False Memories: A Kind of Confabulation in Non-clinical Subjects," in *Confabulation: Views from Neuroscience, Psychiatry, Psychology, and Philosophy*, ed. William Hirstein (Oxford: Oxford University Press, 2009), 33–66; Oliver Hardt, Einar Örn Einarsson, and Karim Nader, "A Bridge over Troubled Water: Reconsolidation as a Link between Cognitive and Neuroscientific Memory Research Traditions," *Annual Review of Psychology* 61 (2010): 141–67; and Steven M. Southwick, C. Andrew Morgan III, Andreas L. Nicolaou, and Dennis S. Charney, "Consistency of Memory for Combat-Related Traumatic Events in Veterans of Operation Desert Storm," *American Journal of Psychiatry* 154 (1997): 173–77.

28. Allan Young, "How Narratives Work in Psychiatric Science: An Example from the Biological Psychiatry of PTSD," in *Narrative Research in Health and Illness*, ed. Brian Hurwitz, Trisha Greenhalgh, and Vieda Skultans (Oxford: Blackwell, 2004), 382–96.

29. Rachel Yehuda, Linda M. Bierer, Laura C. Pratchett, and Michelle Pelcovitz, "Using Biological Markers to Inform a Clinically Meaningful Treatment Response," *Annals of the New York Academy of Sciences* 1208 (2010): 158–63; Rachel Yehuda, Steven M. Southwick, Gabriel Nussbaum, Victor Wahby, Earl L. Giller, and John W. Mason, "Low Urinary Cortisol Excretion in Patients with Posttraumatic Stress Disorder," *Journal of Nervous and Mental Disease* 78 (1990): 366–68.

30. G. P. Chrousos, "Stressors, Stress, and Neuroendocrine Integration of the Adaptive Response: The 1997 Hans Selye Memorial Lecture," *Annals of the New York Academy of Sciences* 851 (1998): 311–25.

31. Rachel Yehuda, "Advances in Understanding Neuroendocrine Alterations in PTSD and Their Therapeutic Implications," *Annals of the New York Academy of Sciences* 1071 (2006): 137. See also Yehuda, "Neuroendocrinology of Trauma and Posttraumatic Stress Disorder," in *Psychological Trauma*, ed. Rachel Yehuda (Washington, DC: American Psychiatric Press, 1998), 97–132; and Yehuda, "Psychoneuroendocrinology of Post-traumatic Stress Disorder," *Psychiatric Clinics of North America* 21 (1998): 359–73.

32. Yehuda, "Understanding Neuroendocrine Alterations," 156–57.

33. Mark W. Gilbertson, Martha E. Shenton, Aleksandra Ciszewski, Kiyoto Kasai, Natasha B. Lasko, Scott P. Orr, and Roger K. Pitman, "Smaller Hippocampal Volume

Predicts Pathological Vulnerability to Psychological Trauma," *Nature Neuroscience* 5 (2002): 1245; italics added.

34. Susan Clancy, *The Trauma Myth: The Truth about the Sexual Abuse of Children—and Its Aftermath* (New York: Basic Books, 2010), 456–57.

35. Roger K. Pitman, Scott P. Orr, Dennis F. Forgue, Jacob B. de Jong, and James M. Claiborn, "Psychophysiologic Assessment of Posttraumatic Stress Disorder Imagery in Vietnam Combat Veterans," *Archives of General Psychiatry* 44 (1987): 970–75; Scott P. Orr, Natasha B. Lasko, Linda J. Metzger, Nancy J. Berry, Caryl E. Ahern, and Roger K. Pitman, "Psychophysiologic Assessment of Women with Posttraumatic Stress Disorder Resulting from Childhood Sexual Abuse," *Journal of Consulting and Clinical Psychology* 66 (1998): 906–13.

36. For efforts by PTSD researchers to retrace the history of the disorder from *DSM-III* onward, see Lawrence C. Kolb, "A Critical Survey of Hypotheses regarding Post-traumatic Stress Disorders in Light of Recent Research Findings," *Journal of Traumatic Stress* 1 (1988): 291–304; Rachel Yehuda and Alexander C. McFarlane, "Conflict between Current Knowledge about Posttraumatic Stress Disorder and Its Original Conceptual Basis," *American Journal of Psychiatry* 152 (1995): 1705–13; and Richard McNally, "Progress and Controversy in the Study of Posttraumatic Stress Disorder," *Annual Review of Psychology* 54 (2003): 229–52.

37. Edgar Jones, Robert Hodgins Vermaas, Helen McCartney, Charlotte Beech, Ian Palmer, Kenneth Hyams, and Simon Wessely, "Flashbacks and Post-traumatic Stress Disorder: The Genesis of a 20th-Century Diagnosis," *British Journal of Psychiatry* 182 (2003): 158–63; Edgar Jones, Robert Hodgins-Vermaas, Helen McCartney, Brian Everitt, Charlotte Beech, Denise Poynter, Ian Palmer, Kenneth Hyams, and Simon Wessely, "Post-combat Syndromes from the Boer War to the Gulf War: A Cluster Analysis of Their Nature and Attribution," *British Medical Journal* 324 (2002): 321–24; Edgar Jones and Simon Wessely, "Hearts, Guts and Minds: Somatization in the Military from 1900," *Journal of Psychosomatic Research* 56 (2004): 425–29; Lawrence J. Kirmayer and Allan Young, "Culture and Somatization: Clinical, Epidemiological and Ethnographic Perspectives," *Psychosomatic Medicine* 60 (1998): 420–30.

38. Rachel Yehuda, Richard Bryant, Charles Marmar, and Joseph Zohar, "Pathological Responses to Terrorism," *Neuropsychopharmacology* 30 (2005): 1793–1805, 10.

39. Roxane Cohen Silver, E. Alison Holman, Daniel N. McIntosh, Michael Poulin, and Virginia Gil-Rivas, "Nationwide Longitudinal Study of Psychological Responses to September 11," *Journal of the American Medical Association* 288 (2002): 1235–44; Roxane Cohen Silver, E. Alison Holman, Daniel N. McIntosh, Michael Poulin, Virginia Gil-Rivas, and Judith Pizarro, "Coping with a National Trauma: A Nationwide Longitudinal Study of Responses to the Terrorist Attacks of September 11," in *September 11, 2001: Mental Health in the Wake of a Terrorist Attack*, ed. Yuval Neria, Raz Gross, Randall D Marshall, and Ezra S Susser (Cambridge: Cambridge University Press, 2006), 45–70.

40. Oliver Luminet, Antonietta Curci, Elizabeth J. Marsh, Ineke Wessel, Tivu Constantin, Faruk Gencoz, and Masao Yogo, "The Cognitive, Emotional, and Social Impacts of the September 11 Attacks: Group Differences in Memory for the Reception Context of the Determinants of Flashbulb Memory," *Journal of General Psychiatry* 131 (2004): 197–224; Jones et al., "Flashbacks."

41. R. D. Fowler, "The New Enhancing Resilience Program" (letter), *APA On-line*, January 1999, http://www.apa.org/ppo/issues/p99pibernieraraons.html (no longer available).

42. Russ Newman, "The Road to Resilience," *Monitor on Psychology* 33 (2002): 62.

43. Sara Martin, "Building Resilience from the Grassroots Up," *Monitor on Psychology* 33 (2002): 52.

44. Suzanne C. Kobasa, "Stressful Life Events, Personality, and Health: An Inquiry into Hardiness," *Journal of Personality and Social Psychology* 37 (1979): 1–11; Anne S. Masten, "Ordinary Magic: Resilience Processes in Development," *American Psychologist* 56 (2001): 227–38; Michael Rutter, "Resilience in the Face of Adversity: Protective Factors and Resistance to Psychiatric Disorders," *British Journal of Psychiatry* 147 (1985): 598–611.

45. Jonathan R. T. Davidson, Victoria M. Payne, Kathryn M. Connor, Edna B. Foa, Barbara O. Rothbaum, Michael A. Hertzberg, and Richard H. Weisler, "Trauma, Resilience and Saliostasis: Effects of Treatment in Post-traumatic Stress Disorder," *International Clinical Psychopharmacology* 20 (2005): 43.

46. Kathryn M. Connor and Jonathan R. T. Davidson, "Development of a New Resilience Scale: The Connor-Davidson Resilience Scale (CD-RISC)," *Depression and Anxiety* 18 (2003): 77.

47. Richard G. Tedeschi and Lawrence G. Calhoun, "The Posttraumatic Growth Inventory: Measuring the Positive Legacy of Trauma," *Journal of Traumatic Stress* 9 (1996): 455–72.

48. Davidson et al., "Trauma, Resilience and Saliostasis."

49. Ibid., 47.

50. Ibid.

51. Masten. "Ordinary Magic."

52. Charles A. Morgan III, Sheila Wang, John Mason, Steven M. Southwick, Patrick Fox, Gary Hazlett, Dennis S. Charney, and Gary Greenfield, "Hormone Profiles in Humans Experiencing Military Survival Training," *Biological Psychiatry* 47 (2000): 891–901; Charles A. Morgan III, Sheila Wang, Steven M. Southwick, Ann Rasmusson, Gary Hazlett, Richard L. Hauger, and Dennis S. Charney, "Plasma Neuropeptide-Y Concentrations in Humans Exposed to Military Survival Training," *Biological Psychiatry* 47 (2000): 902–9. Cf. Rachel Yehuda, Sarah Brand, and Ren-Kui Yang, "Plasma NeuropeptideY Concentrations in Combat Exposed Veterans: Relationship to Trauma Exposure, Recovery from PTSD, and Coping," *Biological Psychiatry* 59 (2006): 660–63.

53. Morgan et al., "Hormone Profiles," 892.

54. Morgan et al., "Plasma Neuropeptide-Y Concentrations," 902–3, 908.

55. Walter B. Cannon, "'Voodoo' Death," *American Anthropologist* 44 (1942): 169–81; Allan Young, "Walter Cannon and the Psychophysiology of Fear," in *Greater Than the Parts: Holism in Biomedicine, 1920–1950,* ed. Christopher Lawrence and George Weisz (New York: Oxford University Press, 1998), 234–56.

56. David Leigh, "UK Forces Taught Torture Methods," *Guardian* (UK), May 8, 2004, http://www.theguardian.com/uk/2004/may/08/iraq.iraq; italics added.

57. Shane O'Mara, "Torturing the Brain: On the Folk Psychology and Folk Neurobiology Motivating 'Enhanced and Coercive Interrogation Techniques,'" *Trends in Cognitive Sciences* 13 (2009): 498.

58. Roger K. Pitman, "Post-traumatic Stress Disorder, Hormones, and Memory," *Biological Psychiatry* 26 (1989): 222.

59. Roger K. Pitman, Kathy M. Sanders, Randall M. Zusman, Anna R. Healy, Farah Cheema, Natasha B. Lasko, Larry Cahill, and Scott P. Orr, "Pilot Study of Secondary Prevention of Posttraumatic Stress Disorder with Propranolol," *Biological Psychiatry* 51 (2002): 189–42.

60. Alain Brunet, Scott P. Orr, Jacques Tremblay, Kate Robertson, Karim Nader, and Roger K. Pitman, "Effect of Post-retrieval Propranolol on Psychophysiologic Responding during Subsequent Script-Driven Traumatic Imagery in Post-traumatic Stress Disorder," *Journal of Psychiatric Research* 42 (2008): 503–6.

61. Russell Goldman, "Erasing the Pain of the Past: Scientists Are Developing Drugs That Could Eliminate Traumatic Events from Our Memories," *abcNEWS/ Health*, March 20, 2007, http://abcnews.go.com/Health/story?id=2964509&page=1.

62. Institute of Medicine, *Treatment of Posttraumatic Stress Disorder: An Assessment of the Evidence* (Washington, DC: National Academies Press, 2008).

63. Rhonda Cornum, Michael D. Matthews, and Martin E. R. Seligman, "Comprehensive Soldier Fitness: Building Resilience in a Challenging Institutional Context," *American Psychologist* 66 (2011): 4.

64. George W. Casey, "Comprehensive Soldier Fitness: A Vision for Psychological Resilience in the U.S. Army," *American Psychologist* 66 (2011): 1–3.

65. Martin E. P. Seligman and Raymond D. Fowler, "Comprehensive Soldier Fitness and the Future of Psychology," *American Psychologist* 66 (2011): 84.

66. Ibid., 85.

Chapter Four

From Primitive Fear to Civilized Stress

Sudden Unexpected Death

Otniel E. Dror

> "Voodoo Death." By this I mean the casting of a fatal spell on a person by a king or priest or voodoo doctor exerting an influence among savage and superstitious people, with the result that the person who is credulous and terrorized by the spell is said to die.
>
> Walter B. Cannon, 1934

> The sudden and unexpected death of a presumably healthy person in the midst of his accustomed activities is one of the most dramatic and disturbing events in clinical practice and everyday experience. The tragedy is heightened when autopsy examination shows an essentially normal myocardium with minimal disease of the coronary arteries and no evidence of thrombotic occlusion.
>
> Edmund D. Pellegrino, "Sudden Death"

> Since "voodoo death" can be seen as comparable to our own society's "sudden death," for which much anecdotal material is complemented by some clinical and pathophysiological assessment, we believe that "voodoo death" does refer to an empirical phenomenon whose complex dimensions are receiving more adequate description. . . . These noxious effects of belief and expectation have recently been called "nocebo."
>
> Robert A. Hahn and Arthur Kleinman, "Belief as Pathogen"

In 1942 Walter B. Cannon, head of the Department of Physiology at the Harvard Medical School, published his now-famous essay, "'Voodoo' Death." In this study Cannon elucidated the mechanisms responsible for the detrimental physiological effects of "magic" spells or "voodoo" rituals in "primitive" societies.[1] Cannon's voodoo-death essay became a model for psychosomatic effects and interrelationships.

During the interwar period, physiologists, clinicians, and anthropologists relegated voodoo deaths to the non-West and distinguished between Western and the "primitive" by defining the West as a culture that was exempt from spell-induced deaths.[2] Postwar authors took a radically different stance: they instead transformed voodoo death into one of the distinct characteristics of modern life—"sudden unexpected death" resulting from the acute stress of modernization. The voodoo-death experience came to reside in a variety of acute medical emergencies observed in everyday Western lives. The transformation of "voodoo death" into "sudden unexpected death" and of "primitive" fear into Western "stress" during the post–World War II period is the subject matter of this chapter.[3]

In presenting the genealogy of acute stress and sudden unexpected death, I offer an initial exposition of three different topics. The first pertains to the history of the "extreme." Much of the current historiography approaches extreme experiences in terms of the history and the paradigm of "trauma." This trauma paradigm often presents the history of the study of extreme experiences in terms of the history of psychology and psychiatry, a Freudian lineage and genealogy, and post-Holocaust and post-Vietnam developments.[4] There is also an important history of *physiological* modeling and the study of extreme emotions. The study of voodoo-death and sudden unexpected death uncovers aspects of this lost history of the physiology of extreme emotions.

My second general objective pertains to the historiography of twentieth-century medicine. The history of twentieth-century Western medicine focuses primarily on the shift to an epidemiology of chronic, progressive, and degenerative diseases. This shift to a Western-modern pattern of diseases construes modern life and civilization as environments of chronic exposure to low intensity assaults (with or without discontents). In presenting a case study of the acute, and in focusing on "critical situations," "emergency reactions," "shock," and "sudden death," I wish to highlight civilization in its intensity, unpredictability, discontinuity, and crisis. The medical-physiological construct of sudden unexpected death during the postwar period embodied this alternative medical cosmology.

My third objective is to highlight the histories of contemporary notions of stress, which did not draw on or emerge from Hans Selye's studies. Though many investigators and clinicians referred to the term "stress," their formulations of and approaches to stress significantly diverged from Selye's conceptions and mechanisms.

The study of acute, intense stress presented two divergent arch models of intensity and extremes. In the first, intense experiences led to intense effects. This model was construed on the emotion of intense fear, which progressively became intense stress after World War II. According to this model, intense experience—fear or stress—led to intense physiological reactions. This model underlay the logic of Hans Selye's "alarm reaction" and Walter B. Cannon's physiology of voodoo death and also offered one template for chronic low-intensity stress. Chronic low-intensity stress was the attenuated form of the acute type of stress.

In the second model of intensity, intense stress was triggered by the everyday low-intensity experiences of modern life. The trivial and contingent encounters of modern individuals with seemingly insignificant stimuli triggered an acute stress response, which then terminated in death. This second model of acute stress was embodied in the emergent nosology of "sudden unexpected death."

Both of these two models of extreme stress drew on the interwar study of surgical or traumatic shock. The study of shock provided the basic template for Cannon's interwar model of voodoo death (1942); for Hans Selye's "alarm reaction"—the basic reaction to "critical situations" and the first phase of Selye's triple-phased general adaptation syndrome (1930s–1940s); for Curt Richter's postwar model of "unexplained sudden death" (1957–58); and for George L. Engel's physiology of "syncope" (1940s).[5] Engel's physiology of syncope, which drew on the physiology of shock, was crucial for his 1960s and 1970s models of acute stress and sudden unexpected death. "Hopelessness," which became a major explanatory framework in postwar models of acute stress and death by stress—for example, in the work of Richter, Engel, and Stewart Wolf—also drew on the physiological study of shock.[6] The *physiology* of hopelessness drew on the physiology of traumatic or surgical shock.

The multiplicity of models that explained voodoo deaths and sudden unexpected deaths negotiated broader categorical distinctions. These pertained to the relationship between "civilized" and "primitive" societies and reactions, medical versus anthropological ways of knowing, physiological versus psychological models of extremes, different conceptions of causality, and the relationship between the organism and its environment. These broader contexts were enacted on the shop-floor level of the laboratory and clinic.

I begin the chapter with Cannon's interwar model of voodoo death and its interpretation as an extreme fear reaction. This extreme form of fear, which led to death, was presented as an integral aspect of the everyday experiences of primitive people in primitive societies; it was absent from the West.[7] I then shift to developments after World War II and study the transformation of voodoo death (extreme fear) into sudden unexpected death (acute stress). The shift from fear to stress entailed a series of mediating models. This first part of this chapter presents the physiological rationale and the physiological modeling of extremes, along with the historical interrelationships between a variety of interconnected models of acute fear, acute stress, shock, voodoo death, and sudden unexpected death.

After presenting the shift in models, I focus on the emergent postwar model of sudden unexpected death. I compare voodoo death with the new entity of sudden unexpected death. I study some of the salient features of sudden unexpected death, paying particular attention to its "unexpectedness" and to the relationship between "civilization" and the "primitive" in the construction of acute stress. I conclude by presenting voodoo as a "pharmakon" in Western narratives of illness and healing. Throughout the chapter I adopt an analytical rather than a contextual perspective. The different social, affective, and cultural contexts that gave rise to and were embodied in the shift in models are beyond the scope of this chapter.[8]

Voodoo Death: Death from Fear

Though Walter B. Cannon's "'Voodoo' Death" essay appeared in print only in 1942, Cannon's personal papers reveal that he had struggled with the subject seven years prior to its publication. From 1934 Cannon had developed an expansive network of correspondents with whom he engaged in a massive fact-collecting project relating to voodoo death. He approached voodoo death—a phenomenon that was "so extraordinary and so foreign to the experience of civilized people," and which took hold only "among human beings so primitive, so superstitious, so ignorant"—by adopting a two-tiered approach. First, he authenticated the reality of this "incredible" mode of death by presenting numerous reports in which the casting of a spell, the consumption of fruits that "had been taken from a tabooed place," or "bone pointing" had led to the rapid death of the victim. These reports were collected from the published literature and from Cannon's extensive personal correspondence. Then, he suggested a physiological model and rationale for the power of "sorcery," "witchcraft," or an "enchanted" spear.[9]

Two ingredients substantiated a voodoo type of death. The first was the absolute certainty that the cause of death was *immaterial*—excluding physical, chemical, or biological impacts; poisons; or other means of inflicting death. The second was the postmortem examination, which "revealed nothing that could in any way account for the fatal outcome."[10] The veracity of voodoo death depended on the discovery of dead *pathogen-free* bodies, on the "total absence of demonstrable lesions," on an autopsy that "failed to reveal any etiology for the death," and on "the paradox of a dead patient and no cause of death."[11] It was the concurrent absence of physical causes for, and physical signs in, the dead body that validated a voodoo death.[12]

After authenticating the reality of voodoo-death phenomena, Cannon transformed the phenomena of voodoo death into the emotion of fear.

Voodoo death was "an ominous and persistent state of fear." The "persistent and profound emotional state" triggered an excessive adrenaline-sympathetic "emergency" reaction, which "induced a disastrous fall of blood pressure, ending in death."[13]

The study of death by emotion harked back to some of the major physiologists of the modern era, beginning with the foundational text of Albertus Haller, *First Lines of Physiology* (1786). As Haller explained, "terror from a present evil" increases "the strength" of the force of the heart "to so great a degree, as to cause convulsions and a strong pulse; whence it" can "kill suddenly." Nineteenth-century physiologists, like Xavier Bichat, Claude Bernard, and Angelo Mosso, also discussed the lethal effects of "extreme," "profound" and "sudden" emotions. Angelo Mosso, for example, studied these killer emotions in his influential book on *Fear* (1884/1896). As Mosso explained, it was necessary to "produce . . . a sudden, unexpected agitation" in order to produce death.[14] The mechanism that nineteenth-century physiologists proposed in explaining and modeling these deaths was the "coup." A profound emotional "coup" to the nervous apparatus produced sudden death.

Early twentieth-century physiologists marginalized the nineteenth-century "coup" model and mechanism of death by emotion. They also stirred clear of nineteenth-century templates and models of mind-body interactions. Victorian hysteria, suggestion, faith, hope, influence, attention, and will were absent from physiological models of extreme emotions, as were nineteenth-century ideas of railway spine and neurasthenia. The primary model of extreme emotions and ominous fear was the war experience. The physiology of the war experience was the study of traumatic shock, which in the West modeled non-Western voodoo death. Comparable to Western wars, voodoo death was a shock-like event.

Primitive Death: The Traumatic Shock of War

The study of traumatic or surgical shock developed during the late nineteenth century. The physiology of surgical or traumatic shock explored the effects of extreme physical conditions and violent impacts on the body. Physiologists attempted to elucidate the mechanisms responsible for the systemic reaction to bodily trauma. Traumatic shock was a product of direct trauma to the body: intestinal obstruction; biliary colic; peritonitis; ingested toxins; clamped vena cava or aorta; manipulated viscera of animals; large doses of histamine, adrenaline, or formaldehyde; forced muscular exercise; extreme pain or cold; burns; severe infections; radium rays; and so on. As Noble and Collip observed, "At this time a number of ways of producing direct trauma to the tissues of the rat were investigated. . . . These included prolonged ischaemia of one or two extremities; crushing of skin, muscles, or intestine; rapid freezing of limbs, skin and muscle, or intestine; scalding of skin and muscle."[15]

During the early twentieth century, researchers expanded the purview of their studies on shock beyond physical trauma and began to study the shock effects of strong emotions and pain. These early studies on emotions and physiological shock usually focused on fear and the war experience. George W. Crile, the famous Cleveland surgeon, was one of the leading researchers who studied the effects of extreme emotions on the body and the development of physiological shock.[16]

During World War I several investigators attempted to produce shock by mimicking the effects of strong emotions. These latter studies drew on new discoveries, which demonstrated "that extreme emotion or severe pain, which are factors in some cases of shock, are accompanied by an outpouring of adrenalin from the suprarenal glands."[17] Since extreme emotions produced an outpouring of adrenaline into the bloodstream, investigators inundated animals to examine whether high levels of adrenaline—which mimicked the physiology of extreme emotions—produced shock.[18]

Walter B. Cannon's 1942 "'Voodoo' Death" essay was conceived in the context of these physiological studies on shock, extreme emotions, and traumatic deaths. Since World War I Cannon had been one of the most important contributors to the study of traumatic shock.[19] In a 1934 review Cannon presented his developing thoughts regarding shock.[20] He suggested a model of shock that was practically identical to the model that he would propose in his "'Voodoo' Death" essay. This same model already appeared in his mid-1930s correspondence in respect to voodoo death.

During the 1930s, while searching for a Western-"civilized" equivalent of "primitive" voodoo death, Cannon corresponded with the warden Lewis E. Lawes and with the psychiatrist-in-charge Ralph S. Banay, both at Sing Sing Prison: "I am writing to learn whether you have had any experience with men who are to be put to death that would bear on my interests. Of course the 'social conditions' in civilized countries are not the same as in primitive savage tribes. Possibly that would make a difference." Could Ralph Banay take a few simple tests of urine sugar, surface blood count, and blood pressure measurements at various times before the execution?[21]

The establishment of a physiological model of voodoo death—in terms of traumatic shock—became a defining moment. It provided a physiological-causal mechanism for the real and material effects of emotions in the material body. This physiological mechanism was reproduced and enacted inside the laboratory.

The new model also skirted many of the difficulties and confusions that plagued psychosomatic phenomena. The undeniable materiality of death guaranteed its reality. The dead body did not malinger, simulate, or feign.

Death by emotion was an ideal natural experiment for the effects of the psychological on the physiological. This partly explains why numerous investigators and clinicians, who did *not* adopt Cannon's physiological model of death, were interested in Cannon's "'Voodoo' Death" essay.

During the period after World War II Cannon's model of voodoo death was disassembled and deconstructed. The original model of voodoo death, which emphasized the emotions of "fear" and "terror," the physiology of shock, and the primitive origins of these forms of death, was reframed into a multiplicity of diverse models and mechanisms. Voodoo death became a model for the power of "belief" and "expectation" on the body; acute and chronic "stress"; the psychosomatic effects of emotions beyond fear and terror, like "hopelessness" or "joy"; the study of experiential extremes; brain-heart interrelationships; the "nocebo" effect; "death as adaptation"; and the physiology of "uncertainty" during "critical moments" of decision making.[22] There were multiple voodoo deaths, despite the persistent allusion of physiologists and clinicians to the "same"—that is, to Walter B. Cannon's interwar—"'Voodoo' Death." The multiplication of voodoo deaths reflected the convergence of many disciplines and perspectives, including physiology, psychoanalysis, behaviorism, psychiatry, and anthropology.

Civilized Death: The Traumatic Shock of Discontent

One of the earliest postwar studies that explicitly modeled Western sudden death on voodoo death was Curt Richter's oft-cited study, "On the Phenomenon of Sudden Death in Animals and Man" (1957).[23] Richter, head of the psychobiological laboratory at Johns Hopkins University, recognized these forms of primitive deaths in his own city of Baltimore.

Richter encountered sudden unexpected death "accidentally." It was during the course of "other experiments" that his "Wild" laboratory rats suddenly and unexpectedly died. The death of his laboratory rats soon became the focus of new experiments, leading to Richter's theory of sudden unexpected "Vagus" death. Richter's anecdotal brush with sudden unexpected death harbored global implications. His rats died not from the impact of violent stimuli and the extreme physiology of shock and fear but from the civilizing, controlling, and restraining forces of the laboratory. As Richter explained, the mere and routine act of holding and restraining the rats in the experimenter's hands was directly responsible for their sudden deaths, and by analogy and extension, for the sudden and unexpected death of individuals in "primitive" societies and "in our culture": "Apparently 'boned' victims, like wild rats, are not set for fight or flight but similarly seem resigned to their fate—their situation seems to them quite hopeless. For this reason we believe that the human victims—like our rats—may well die a parasympathetic rather than a sympathico-adrenal death, as Cannon postulated."[24]

In a much less publicized 1958 article Richter further elaborated on "unexplained sudden death." He recalled how he had come to associate his own observations on the sudden death of restrained wild rats with Cannon's shock-like voodoo-death essay. It was Philip Bard, one of Cannon's former students and collaborators, who brought Cannon's paper on voodoo death to his attention. After reading Cannon's essay, Richter became interested in the broader contexts of his discrete laboratory observations on suddenly dying rats, stating, "This search has led me to many new and unexplored fields."[25]

In reading Cannon's paper, Richter focused on one particular aspect of Cannon's model. As Richter explained, Cannon had argued that the death of laboratory animals resulted from "a combination of over-stimulation of the sympathico-adrenal system and inhibition of outward expression of the emotions." In reference to the death of humans in primitive societies, Cannon had observed that "these individuals might be dying from an excessive stimulation of the sympathico-adrenal system under circumstances in which they are inhibited from giving expression to their emotions."[26] According to Richter, death was not an outcome of the hyperactivation of the physiology of action but the inhibition of action in the face of an emergency fight-or-flight response.

In "'Voodoo' Death" Cannon had alluded in only *one* sentence to this mechanism of *in*action.[27] The dire consequences of inaction during a state of emergency received a more elaborate explanation in his 1934 review on shock.[28] Here Cannon explained why the absence of movement and of action during significant sympathetic activity contributed to the development of shock. Inaction eliminated the pumping movements of the muscles. This pumping movement was necessary to return the blood from the muscles back to the circulation. During an emergency reaction, blood flow to the muscles was greatly augmented in preparation for a fight-or-flight response. The absence of the pumping action of the muscles together with the augmented blood flow to the muscles led to the pooling of blood in the muscles. This pooling of blood decreased the effective blood volume of the total circulation and led to shock. The traumatic shock of soldiers during war was often an outcome of this combination. The injured soldier was activated for a fight-or-flight response but was often physically incapacitated by his injury and could not move and fight.

This physiological mechanism of pooled blood, physical incapacity, and shock was "considered" by Richter "also as a reaction at a much higher level of integration . . . a reaction of apparent hopelessness."[29] Richter's shift from Cannon's *physiology* of inaction to the *psychology* of hopelessness presented a radical reformulation in the nature of the explanatory models of death by emotion.

The daily laboratory practice of holding and controlling animals and arresting the fight-or-flight response emerged as an important explanatory concept in making sense of sudden unexpected death from acute stress. "Hopelessness," which was the psychological state of a restrained wild laboratory rat in the course of an experiment, became an important and persistent explanatory mechanism for acute stress and sudden unexpected death.

Richter's shift to psychology and his psychologizing of restraint laboratory rats drew on George L. Engel's and John Romano's 1940s studies on syncope. During the 1940s Engel and Romano conducted a series of "Studies of Syncope." In these studies they differentiated between different types of syncope and their distinct mechanisms, for example, hysterical versus "vasodepressor" syncope. In focusing on the "biologic" interpretation of vasodepressor syncope, Engel and Romano presented a model of syncope based on Cannon's model of shock. Vasodepressor syncope was an outcome of the concurrent combination of vasodilation in muscles (the fight-or-flight response) and "inhibition"—the inability to act. Unlike Cannon, who emphasized physical immobility, Engel and Romano emphasized the psychoanalytic mechanisms that explained inhibition and inaction in the face of a preparation for a fight-or-flight response: "The danger, then, actually arises from within the unconscious portion of the mental apparatus. . . . The patient cannot escape it. . . . The preparation for flight takes place but flight is impossible and fainting may then occur.[30]

To test their psychophysiological or physiopsychological model of vasodepressor syncope, Engel and Romano exposed one of their syncope-prone patients to the threat of a venipuncture. In this particular patient the venipuncture was the stimulus that usually induced syncope. Each time that they observed that their patient's blood pressure began to drop, they instructed their patient to exercise and run. This action on the part of the patient prevented the syncope. "These observations," they concluded, "indicate that when the patient is able to express certain aggressive feelings or to become physically active, the syncopal reaction may be overcome."[31]

Richter drew on these observations and on Cannon's voodoo-death shock model in proposing his new and famous model of sudden death. By the end of the 1950s there were two major alternative models for voodoo deaths and for sudden unexpected deaths: A Vagus (parasympathetic) *inhibition* model, which conceived death as a state of hopelessness, inaction, retreat, and conservation; and a sympathetic-adrenaline overexcitement model, which conceived death as a form of hyperactivation, aggression, and fight-or-flight response. Both of these models explained how emotions—that is, nonphysically, chemically, or biologically impacting stimuli—could induce an acute form of death in healthy and robust individuals.

Post-1950s investigators fused these two pure models, in suggesting various combinations of the physiology and of the psychology of action and inaction, activation and inhibition, attack and restraint, fight-or-flight response and conservation or retreat, aggressive feelings and hopelessness, and sympathetic and parasympathetic activation.[32] These emergent models, which drew on basic elements of the mechanisms of shock and syncope, offered a spectrum of possibilities regarding acute stress and sudden unexpected death.

In parallel with these models of death, there developed a second discourse regarding psychological death in the West. This alternative discourse and approach is not the focus of the present chapter. Yet many of the authors who adopted this alternative framework also appealed to and discussed voodoo death.

As Nolan D. C. Lewis, director of the Psychiatric Institute and Hospital in New York, wrote to Cannon in 1940,

> In my own experience in pathology, I have known of two individuals, one a white woman and the other a young colored man, who set the dates for their deaths several weeks in advance, who died on the dates set and in whose bodies I was unable by means of a complete postmortem examination to discover any cause of death. . . . I was not an amateur in postmortem work at the time. . . . In spite of a thorough histological survey of the organs including the brain, lesions sufficient to cause death were not found even by a considerable stretch of the imagination.[33]

Some mobilized Freudian theory in explaining what seemed to be a self-willed death. In "The Concept of Psychic Suicide" Abraham A. Brill had adopted Freud's "death wish" in providing a psychoanalytical framework for explaining psychic death.[34] In corresponding with Cannon, Brill explained, "Somehow, some people can make up their minds to die, and just die."[35]

Others, like the Johns Hopkins's surgeon John M. T. Finney, were all too well aware of these types of willed or foretold deaths. "You can laugh," Finney explained in 1934 to an august audience of physiologists and clinicians,

> but I have seen individuals who have lost a dear friend or relative and just die. I could mention several such interesting cases, where autopsies found nothing, no physical basis whatever. You may laugh all you like. . . . If a patient looks me steadily in the eye and quietly says he is going to die, I tell him, "All right, but you won't die on me. You go to some other surgeon."[36]

During the postwar era these anecdotes, theories, and approaches, rather than Cannon's physiology of fear, terror, and shock, became instrumental for the development of models that attempted to rethink the relationships between beliefs, expectations, and the body.

Voodoo Death: Sudden Unexpected Death

Sudden unexpected death reconfigured fundamental features of voodoo death. Interwar reports of voodoo death endowed it with a "natural history" structure; presented death as highly contained by a strict set of explicit rules and taboos; framed a linear relationship between the magnitude of the cause, the intensity of emotion, and the extent of its detrimental effects; and situated causality in the social fabric of "primitive" societies. These four features of voodoo death would undergo a radical rearrangement with the shift from primitive fear and voodoo death to Western stress and sudden unexpected death.

Many interwar reports of voodoo death presented the death as an effect or outcome of a fortuitous accident. A "young Negro unknowingly eats the inviolably banned wild hen. On discovery of his 'crime' he trembles, is overcome by fear, and dies in 24 hours"; a New Zealand "maori woman eats fruit that she only later learns has come from a tabooed place. . . . By noon of the next day she is dead."[37] This basic chance element, in which death was present in ordinary and daily incidental events, was contained by an explicit system of social rules. In primitive and fear-suffused societies voodoo death was the outcome of a breach of defined rules, even if this breach was unintended and accidental.

This primary chance element was followed by a strict determinism of consequences. The accidental transgression inescapably triggered a sequence of events that led to death.[38] This sequence of cause-effect events was linear, because the effects reflected the gravity of the primary cause—the transgression. A highly significant and charged social act led to an equally extreme emotion, which led to an equally extreme physiological reaction, ending in an equally extreme shock and death. This basic framing of voodoo death situated its pathology in the social structure and fabric of the culture of the primitive. In superstitious societies, death was immanent and omnipresent and could strike anyone at any time, because primitive societies were voodoo-death societies.

These Western representations of voodoo death structured it in terms of a medical "disease." Voodoo death was a disease of primitive societies, described in terms of its "natural history." There were known causes such as bone pointing, curses, transgressions; defined effects like the physiology of shock; and discrete and knowable outcomes (which sometimes could be remedied), or death. This structure also reflected the basic laboratory template of the stimulus-response reaction. Voodoo death was a stimulus-response, hex-death phenomenon.[39]

With the shift to sudden unexpected death in "civilized" and *stress*-suffused societies, the voodoo-death framework and cosmology underwent significant changes. One of the most important and distinctive features of sudden unexpected death, which became the namesake of this form of death, was "unexpectedness." Unexpectedness presented the Western type or mode of the pervasiveness of chance and the Western pattern of the omnipresence of death. Unexpectedness also challenged the "natural history" framing of these deaths. The absence of a natural history for these deaths, of discrete and identifiable causes, and of explicit social precepts, rules, or guides for avoiding these deaths created a "panic sentiment."[40]

Sudden unexpected death presented an actuality in which random and trivial stimuli led to acute stress that terminated in death. Cause-effect relationships could not be calculated or predicted, and death itself was condensed into a discrete moment in time. The flap of a butterfly's wings—to borrow a hyperbole from a different discipline—could generate acute stress, derange the body's physiology, and kill the subject.

The triggering mechanisms of sudden unexpected death resided in everyday experiences. "Viewing particularly gory scenes on television," winning "$1,683 on a $2 bet," the "sight of blood," "hypodermic injections," ward rounds, "fantasy materials previously repressed," interviews, and the contents of our dreams literally killed suddenly and unexpectedly.[41] As Regis A. DeSilva and Bernard Lown explained in their study on stress and sudden death, "the unpredictability of its occurrence, the absence of prodromes, and the affliction of the seemingly healthy while going about their usual activities contributed to a sense of futility." Or as Thomas N. James argued in "Chance and Sudden Death": "No one much wants to think about dying, but the idea that sudden death might largely be a matter of chance is particularly unappealing. . . . What we can deduce is that sudden unexpected death may be the ultimate game of chance in life."[42] Or as George Engel observed of a patient, "[The patient died] while celebrating his doctor's verdict that his heart was sound."[43]

This aberrant causality created a "panic sentiment." Minor causes created great effects: "The causal relation [was] peculiar. . . . A little equals a lot; and thereby this 'deranged' causality can be everywhere." This deranged causality created a panic sentiment, because "we feel that the cause is everywhere," yet this very cause is "inevitably imbued with an alien force: chance."[44] Sudden unexpected death was always under the suspicion of chance.

As research on sudden unexpected death descended from its gross clinical manifestations to the level of organs and cells, the randomness of death and the omnipresence of chance were traced to, and discovered to inhere in, the fabric of the body: "Much evidence has accumulated to indicate that the mechanism of sudden death is cardiac arrhythmia" (i.e., ventricular fibrillation). One trigger for ventricular fibrillation was the ventricular premature beat: "The ventricular premature beat *though random in occurrence*, is a precise endpoint that can be readily documented and quantified. Studying the reasons for its seemingly sporadic emergence discloses the impact of psychologic factors on cardiac arrhythmias."[45]

The mechanism for Western sudden unexpected death was thus the following: psychological factors triggered in a random fashion ventricular premature beats, which in turn predisposed the heart to lethal ventricular fibrillation. Put differently, unpredictable and sporadic encounters of an individual with specific psychological triggers in the social environment, coupled with the unpredictability of the effects of these psychological states on the production of ventricular premature beats, embodied and expressed the "unexpected" in sudden unexpected death: "The factors triggering [potentially fatal] arrhythmia may appear to be innocuous stimuli to the clinical observer but in the particular patient gain their currency and strength from symbolic meaning deeply enmeshed in a prior conditioning matrix."[46] Or as Thomas James put it in emphasizing the coincidental concurrence of unpredictable and trivial stimuli in evoking a sudden unexpected death, "The simple vagal reflex that must be anticipated as a normal response to events as mundane as coughing, sneezing or laughing also could be the single other factor needed to precipitate a lethal arrhythmia."[47]

This basic and pervasive framing of sudden unexpected death challenged the comforting "natural history" structure of disease. Sudden unexpected death challenged the basic concept that all diseases can be described in terms of discrete and known causes, that these causes have discrete and known effects, and that these effects have known and calculable outcomes. It challenged the very notion that all diseases can be totally known and rationalized, prognosticated, and ultimately remedied. Sudden unexpected death challenged the basic medical modeling that makes diseases known and knowable.

The unexpectedness of sudden unexpected death went hand in hand with its presentation as a vehement moment. This presentation accentuated the discontinuity that inhered in sudden unexpected death. As Philip Fisher observes in *The Vehement Passions*, in literature a vehement experience obliterates the history of the subject—the subject's relationships no longer exist and the moment of passion, for example, rage, overcomes and erases a long history of fondness or love that existed before. Vehement passions thus create breaks: the period before is not the period after—think, for example, of "crimes of passion."[48] This discontinuity was one of the hallmarks of sudden unexpected death. Here, however, there was a dual disruption: in the history of the subject, who was alive and is now suddenly dead, and in the history of the material body, which was normal and alive and is suddenly pathological and dead.

The unexpected break in the history of the subject precluded an "illness narrative," because sudden unexpected death was diagnosed after death. Sudden unexpected death was thus a "unitary" event—as one commentator put it—killing the victim and preventing any form of communication and anamnesis.[49] Sudden unexpected death presented a void, devoid of a history of the subject and with no illness narratives to make sense of the subject and the unexpected death.

The break in the history of the body presented a remarkable image. The reaction of medicine to the image of a discontinuous body was apparent from the beginning. Since it was obvious that the unexpectedly dying body must have had an undetected pathological history that explained its death, its history must have existed in the body prior to its death. Clinicians exerted much energy to uncover these "silent" histories of the body that would make sense of the unexpectedness of death in civilized stress-suffused societies.

Two major historiographies explained sudden unexpected death. In the first, history and causation resided in the idiosyncratic life of the individual. According to this model, seemingly trivial stimuli acquired highly significant symbolic meaning during the history of the individual. The idiosyncratic behavioristic or psychological history of an individual transformed seemingly trivial events into deadly acute stress. The mechanisms that explained this potentiation of trivial events ranged from models that appealed to conditioning to object-relation theory. In these models causation was displaced from the social structure of civilization to the particular history of civilized individuals.

The second major approach reflected the tensions that inhered in respect to the presence of a "primitive" form of death in the midst of "modern" civilization. This tension was embodied in several different models. One model implicitly adopted the widespread view that civilization had created and maintained frail and weakened bodies and constitutions. These weakened bodies succumbed to relatively trivial and minor stresses. This first model positioned sudden unexpected death as an acute "disease of civilization," because it located causality in the particular attributes of civilized frail and degenerating bodies.

A second model, which presented an alternative type of civilized hypersensitivity, inhered in the syncope model, on which sudden unexpected death was partly patterned. Modern theories of syncope, which harked back to the nineteenth century, developed in the context of the sensitive white European female, who swooned in reacting to slight trifles. The modeling of unexpected sudden death on syncope implicitly assumed aspects of this template.

A third model explained the presence of the primitive in the midst of civilized societies by appealing to the vestiges of primitive psychological-physiological reactions in the modern body. This latter model located the intrusive presence of primitive death in civilized societies in the ancient heritage of the evolutionary history of the modern body. Stewart Wolf, one of the prominent leaders of psychosomatic medicine during the postwar period, presented this type of model. Wolf's specific example was the "diving reflex." The atavistic and inappropriate reactivation of the primitive diving reflex in a grown-up human body in response to trivial and modern stresses explained sudden unexpected death: "It would appear, therefore, that the diving reflex is an atavistic response . . . invoked, seemingly inappropriately, in response to emotionally charged or threatening events."[50] Wolf's model of an atavistic response in explaining sudden death drew on his earlier studies of syncope in soldiers during a venipuncture. This reaction was perplexing since these same soldiers had withstood significant emotional situations. Wolf suggested that the pierced skin of the modern venipuncture might be symbolically associated with a primitive reaction to snake bites.[51]

These varieties of models of sudden unexpected death and acute stress implicitly negotiated the categorical distinctions between civilized and primitive. As we have seen, from its earliest beginnings in Cannon's article, the distinction between civilized and primitive suffused the study of voodoo death. Richter's study of sudden death was also framed by these categories. Richter's laboratory observations regarding the differential reactions of wild versus domesticated rats undergirded his basic theory of death. Death was the suppression of the wild instinct, of the fight-or-flight response, by the civilizing and restraining forces of the laboratory.[52]

In his 1958 study Richter had, in fact, converted the death response of wild rats into a domesticated pattern and changed the epidemiology of death by transforming the wild rats into docile, civilized variants. As he explained, "removal of the amygdaloid complex which tames the wild rats has prevented the appearance of the death reaction in a few rats."[53] By removing the amygdaloid from the wild rats' brain and taming them, Richter cured his wild rats and protected them from the detrimental effects of control and restraint.

This underlying and implicit cultural framework of wild versus civilized, of discontent, and of the suppression of the fight-or-flight response had also framed Engel's and Romano's experiments on syncope. As we recall, these investigators observed that aggressive feelings or actions eliminated the inhibitory impulse and inaction and cured their subject of his syncopal attacks.

This same underlying cultural logic also explains the shift from the sympathetic to the parasympathetic branch of the autonomic nervous system in explaining sudden death. The sympathetic branch of the autonomic nervous system was the more primitive structure of the nervous system; it was responsible for the basic instinctual fight-or-flight response of an individual organism. This system was activated during fear and rage and the struggle for existence. The parasympathetic system was often positioned in opposition to the sympathetic system. It was often activated during social emotions. Primitive societies were dominated by the adrenaline, sympathetic response (voodoo death). Civilized restraining and inhibiting societies, on the other hand, activated the parasympathetic system (sudden unexpected death). This was the cultural-physiological logic that structured the acute stress response.

Postwar models of acute stress and sudden unexpected death literally embodied the tensions and negotiations between civilization and the primitive, between parasympathetic and sympathetic, and between restraint and the fight-or-flight response. While some investigators emphasized the sympathetic, primitive, and fight-or-flight response model, others emphasized the civilizing restraint and parasympathetic reaction. Most presented models that combined these basic impulses and the internal conflict between sympathetic and parasympathetic systems.[54]

Epilogue: Voodoo Pharmakon and the Omnipresence of Stress

Paul Feyerabend was basically right when he observed that "nobody knows it [voodoo], everybody uses it as a paradigm of backwardness and confusion. And yet Voodoo has a firm though still not sufficiently understood material basis, and a study of its manifestations can be used to enrich, and perhaps even to revise, our knowledge of physiology."[55] The study of voodoo death—"the casting of a fatal spell on a person . . . with the result that the person . . . is said to die"—presented a persuasive argument for the reality of inexplicable physiological processes. Voodoo death remains a contentious issue, generating new models and possibilities regarding the mind-body conundrum, the status of the dead body (i.e., the autopsy), the reality behind alternative modes of healing, the nocebo effect, and acute stress and sudden death.

Physiologists and clinicians adopted the exotic and exoticized phenomena of voodoo death in modeling Western diseases. Rather than departing from the familiar phenomena of traumatic shock and the war experience, or from the extant and extensive nineteenth-century literature on sudden death, they adopted the voodoo-death reaction of "superstitious" societies, as they put it during the interwar years, to model and study a variety of "civilized" sudden deaths in Christian Western societies.

The *Washington Post* published a review in which "Voodoo death" is featured as the more extreme version of the detrimental effects on the health of a society under constant threat of sudden unpredictable death—but this time, from terrorism. The continuous exposure to the threat of sudden and unexpected death from terrorism has a "nocebo" effect—which is, as researchers explain, the attenuated form of voodoo death.[56]

The literature I have surveyed in this chapter represents voodoo as disease, hopelessness, stress, and death. But there is an alternative vision of voodoo as a therapeutic, spiritual, and healing faith. This alternative vision also takes us, somewhat paradoxically, to terrorism: "Since 9/11," the *New York Times* declares, "An amazing number of people are finding [meaning and guidance] . . . in voodoo."[57] Voodoo is in our contemporary predicament both a model and a template for a category of diseases and of therapies. Medicine has reframed non-Western voodoo death into the diseases of Western civilization and has suggested various forms of non-Western voodoo remedies as therapies for these same Western diseases of civilization.

As Mark Jackson, Elizabeth Siegel Watkins, and others in this volume persuasively argue, the stress concept drew on a myriad of different developments and origins, including psychosomatic medicine, research on adaptation and energy, nineteenth-century neurasthenia, and more. The implicit focus of these analyses and observations is on chronic low-intensity stress—on the "diseases of adaptation," such as peptic ulcers, arthritis, hypertension, and so on.

The origins and contexts of acute unexpected stress embodied a different conceptualization and cosmology. Despite these divergences, acute unexpected sudden stress, like chronic stress, presented the omnipresence of stress and the ever-present possibility of stress. At chronic low-intensity levels, stress was imagined as a continuous prevailing and incessant presence in the very fabric of "civilized" society (and thus akin to fear in "primitive societies"); in sudden unexpected death, stress was imagined as an ever-present possibility that could materialize unexpectedly at any moment in "civilized" societies.

These divergent models of suffusion with stress evoke two distinctive and oppositional affective moods. While chronic stress presents the *comforting* natural history narrative of a predictable and knowable disease, sudden unexpected death evokes the astonishment of a "catastrophe of instantaneous or sudden death" and a panic sentiment.[58] The function of sudden unexpected death might then be to preserve at the "very heart of contemporary society an ambiguity . . . and this ambiguity is historically necessary insofar as man still must have signs . . . but also insofar as these signs must be of uncertain content."[59]

Notes

Epigraphs: Walter B. Cannon to Dr. Daniel de la Paz, Manila, Philippine Islands, June 30, 1934, folder 889, box 67, Walter Bradford Cannon Papers (H MS c40), Harvard Medical Library in the Francis A. Countway Library of Medicine, Boston, Massachusetts (hereafter cited as WBC); E. D. Pellegrino, "Sudden Death—Problem and Perspective," in *Sudden Cardiac Death,* ed. Borys Surawicz and E. D. Pellegrino (New York: Grune & Stratton, 1964), 1–4 (see also Bernard Lown, Regis A. Desilva, Peter Reich, Benjamin J. Murawski, "Psychophysiologic Factors in Sudden Cardiac Death," *American Journal of Psychiatry* 137 [Nov. 1980]: 1325–35); and Robert A. Hahn and Arthur Kleinman, "Belief as Pathogen, Belief as Medicine: 'Voodoo Death' and the 'Placebo Phenomenon' in Anthropological Perspectives," *Medical Anthropology Quarterly* 14 (August 1983): 17.

1. Walter B. Cannon, "'Voodoo' Death," *American Anthropologist* 44 (1942): 169–81.

2. Otniel E. Dror, "'Voodoo Death': Fantasy, Excitement, and the Untenable Boundaries of Biomedical Science," in *The Politics of Healing: Essays in the Twentieth-Century History of North American Alternative Medicine*, ed. Robert D. Johnston (New York: Routledge, 2004), 71–81, 328–31.

3. In her study on the military occupation of Haiti, Mary A. Renda argues that there are "several alternative spellings of Vodou (e.g., Vodoun, Vodun)." "Voodoo," she argues, "refer[s] to the exotic phantasm that sensational writers constructed through their discourses on Haiti." In this chapter, I follow the usage of the correspondents themselves. See Renda, *Taking Haiti: Military Occupation and the Culture of U.S. Imperialism, 1915–1940* (Chapel Hill: University of North Carolina Press, 2001), 317n28.

4. Ruth Leys, *Trauma: A Genealogy* (Chicago: University of Chicago Press, 2000).

5. Cannon, "'Voodoo' Death"; Curt Richter, "On the Phenomenon of Sudden Death in Animals and Man," *Psychosomatic Medicine* 19 (1957): 191–98; George L. Engel and John Romano, "Studies of Syncope: IV. Biologic Interpretation of Vasodepressor Syncope," *Psychosomatic Medicine* 9 (1947): 289. On the general adaptation syndrome, "alarm reaction," "shock," and "counter-shock," see Hans Selye, "Studies on Adaptation," *Endocrinology* 21 (1937): 169–88; Selye, "The General Adaptation Syndrome and the Diseases of Adaptation," *Journal of Clinical Endocrinology* 6, no. 2 (1946): 117–230.

6. Stewart Wolf, "Cardiovascular Reactions to Symbolic Stimuli," *Circulation*, 18 (1958): 287–92.

7. This first section draws on and modifies my previous essay on voodoo death; see Dror, "Voodoo Death."

8. For the religious, gendered, imperialistic, and adrenaline contexts, see Dror, "Voodoo Death"; and Otniel E. Dror, "A Reflection on Feelings and the History of Science," *Isis* 100 (December 2009): 848–51.

9. Cannon, "'Voodoo' Death," 169, 175.

10. Ibid., 171.

11. Walter B. Cannon to James Humbert, June 27, 1934, folder 898, box 67, WBC; H. L. Arnold, MD, Honolulu, to Cannon, July 11, 1934, folder 899, box 67, WBC. See also Cannon to De la Paz, WBC; and Helena E. Riggs to Cannon, January 18, 1939, folder 1857, box 131, WBC.

12. The demand for dead pathogen-free bodies explains the tensions that developed between ethnographers and anthropologists on the one hand and clinicians and physiologists on the other hand, in respect to voodoo deaths during the interwar years. As the renowned French ethnologist Lévy-Bruhl had written to Cannon, the ethnologists, "basing their judgment on a large number of reports . . . admit that there are instances indicating that belief . . . does actually result in death in the course of time. On the contrary, physiologists and physicians—men who have had no acquaintance with ethnological conditions—are inclined to consider the phenomenon impossible." Lévi-Bruhl—like W. Lloyd Warner, Lauriston Sharp, and Marcel Mauss—grounded his knowledge on ethnographic modes of justification. Physicians and physiologists, on the other hand, demanded much more than a trustworthy (gentlemanly) eyewitness or a reliable narrative. Hex death would remain a fantasy as long as the bodies of the dead were unavailable. But as Morton C. Kahn explained

to Walter B. Cannon, "regarding autopsies . . . the Bush Negroes do not present themselves for hospital treatment as a rule." The slow increase in available voodoo-dead bodies during the postwar period promised to disenchant voodoo-deaths and the cosmology of voodoo-death societies by offering alternative Western explanations for these deaths. Yet as bodies did become available, and as Westernization and Christianization led to the progressive decline in the incidence of "primitive" voodoo deaths, there was a tremendous increase in the *reality* of Voodoo death and in its Western doppelganger—sudden unexpected death. For Lévi-Bruhl, see Cannon, "'Voodoo' Death," 175, where Cannon cites a letter from Lévi-Bruhl. See also Marcel Mauss, "Effet physique chez l'individu de l'idée de mort suggérée par la collectivité," *Journal de Psychologie Normale et Pathologique* 23 (1926): 652–69; Morton C. Kahn to Walter B. Cannon, October 5, 1934, folder 898, box 67, WBC; R. F. Hoernle to Cannon, March 20, 1935, folder 900, box 67, WBC; and Harry D. Eastwell, "Voodoo Death and the Mechanism for Dispatch of the Dying in East Arnhem, Australia," *American Anthropologist* 84 (1982): 5–18.

13. Cannon, "'Voodoo' Death," 176, 179.

14. Albertus Haller, *First Lines of Physiology*, trans. from Latin (1786; repr., New York: Johnson Reprint, 1966), 42; Fernand Papillon, "Physiology of the Passions," *Popular Science Monthly* 4 (1874): 552–64; Angelo Mosso, *Fear*, trans. E. Lough and Frederich Kiesow, 5th ed. (London: Longmans, Green, 1896), 242.

15. Robert L. Noble and James B. Collip, "A Quantitative Method for the Production of Experimental Traumatic Shock without Haemmorrhage in Unanaesthetized Animals," *Quarterly Journal of Experimental Physiology* 31 (1941): 187.

16. George W. Crile, *The Origin and Nature of the Emotions: Miscellaneous Papers*, ed. Amy F. Rowland (London: Saunders, 1915). On Crile, see Peter C. English, *Shock, Physiological Surgery, and George Washington Crile: Medical Innovation in the Progressive Era* (Westport, CT: Greenwood, 1980).

17. Medical Research Committee, "Memorandum upon Surgical Shock and Some Allied Conditions," *British Medical Journal*, March 24, 1917, 382.

18. Throughout the chapter I use the term "adrenaline" to denote adrenin, adrenalin, and epinephrine.

19. Walter B. Cannon, *Traumatic Shock* (New York: Appleton, 1923); Norman E. Freeman, "Decrease in Blood Volume after Prolonged Hyper-activity of the Sympathetic Nervous System," *American Journal of Physiology* 103 (1932): 185–202; Norman E. Freeman, R. S. Morison, and M. E. MacKay Sawyer, "The Effect of Dehydration on Adrenal Secretion and Its Relation to Shock," *American Journal of Physiology* 104 (1933): 628–35; and Norman E. Freeman, H. Freeman, and C. C. Miller, "The Production of Shock by the Prolonged Continuous Injection of Adrenalin in Unanesthetized Dogs," *American Journal of Physiology* 131 (1941): 545–54.

20. Walter B. Cannon, "A Consideration of Possible Toxic and Nervous Factors in the Production of Traumatic Shock," *Annals of Surgery* 100 (1934): 704–13.

21. Walter B. Cannon to Lewis E. Lawes, July 1, 1941; Ralph S. Banay to Cannon, July 15, 1941; and Cannon to Dr. Ralph S. Banay, July 17, 1941. All are in folder 903, box 67, WBC.

22. On "death as adaptation," see Stewart Wolf, "Psychosocial Forces in Myocardial Infarction and Sudden Death," *Circulation*, suppl. no. 4, vols. 39 and 40 (November 1969): 80.

23. Richter, "On the Phenomenon of Sudden Death." For explicit attempts to associate between Cannon's "'Voodoo' Death" and Western phenomena prior to Richter, see Leo W. Simmons, "The Relation between the Decline of Anxiety-Inducing and Anxiety-Resolving Factors in a Deteriorating Culture and Its Relevance to Bodily Disease," in *Life Stress and Bodily Disease: Proceedings of the Association for Research in Nervous and Mental Diseases*, ed. Harold G. Wolff, Stewart G. Wolf, and Clarence C. Hare (1950; repr., New York: Hafner, 1968), 127–36; and Leo W. Simmons and Harold G. Wolff, *Social Science in Medicine* (New York: Sage Foundation, 1954), chap. 4.

24. Richter, "On the Phenomenon of Sudden Death," 197.

25. Curt Richter, "The Phenomenon of Unexplained Sudden Death in Animals and Man," in *Physiological Bases of Psychiatry*, ed. W. Horsley Gantt (Springfield, IL: Charles C. Thomas, 1958), 117.

26. Ibid., 116–17.

27. Cannon, "'Voodoo' Death," 176.

28. Cannon, "Consideration."

29. Richter, "Animals and Man," 120.

30. Engel and Romano, "Studies of Syncope." I note that Richter suggested additional mechanisms for the parasympathetic dominance, such as a "valsalva" effect or immersion in water.

31. Ibid., 292.

32. I suggest here that Engel and others' 1950s studies of an "Infant with a Gastric Fistula" were also framed and conceived in terms of this oppositional structure of two opposing and basic impulses. The concepts and terms that appear in their 1950s studies were already present in Engel's and Romano's 1940s studies on syncope. See George L. Engel, Franz Reichsman, and Harry L. Segal, "A Study of an Infant with a Gastric Fistula: I. Behavior and the Rate of Total Hydrochloric Acid Secretion," *Psychosomatic Medicine* 18 (1956): 374–98; and John Romano and George L. Engel, "Studies of Syncope: III. Differentiation between Vasodepressor and Hysterical Fainting," *Psychosomatic Medicine* 7 (1945): 3–15.

33. Nolan D. C. Lewis to Walter B. Cannon, October 24, 1940, folder 903, box 67, WBC.

34. Abraham A. Brill, "The Concept of Psychic Suicide," *International Journal of Psycho-Analysis* 20 (1939): 251. "We know from Freud that 'probably no one finds the mental energy required to kill himself unless, in the first place, in doing so, he is at the same time killing an object with whom he has identified himself, and, in the second place, is turning against himself a death wish which has been directed against someone else.' Here, however, unlike the process in melancholia, the struggle proceeded silently, endopsychically, almost as in primitives, who feeling that they are doomed, resign themselves and die at will." In 1934 Philip Bard, Cannon's former student, inquired whether, in the context of his interest in voodoo death, Cannon had heard of the Freudian "death wish." Cannon replied that he had not. See Philip Bard to Walter B. Cannon, June 10, 1934; and Cannon to Bard, June 15, 1934. Both are in folder 1525, box 110, WBC.

35. For the correspondence between Brill and Cannon, see Walter B. Cannon to Abraham A. Brill, September 2, 1941; and Brill to Cannon, September 6, 1941. Both are in folder 903, box 67, WBC.

36. John M. T. Finney, "Discussion," following a paper by George J. Heuer and William DeWitt Andrus, "The Effect of Adrenal Cortical Extract in Controlling Shock Following the Injection of Aqueous Extracts of Closed Intestinal Loops," *Annals of Surgery* 100 (1934): 747. See also Cannon to Bard, Department of Physiology, Johns Hopkins University, June 6, 1934, folder 1525, box 110, WBC: "On Monday I had a chance to talk with Finney regarding some ideas he has concerning the dangers of operating on a person who has great fear of death from operation. I told him that I am very much interested in this phenomenon, particularly in relation to the casting of a spell by the 'medicine man' in primitive tribes and the death that is said to result therefrom."

37. Richter, "On the Phenomenon of Sudden Death," 191.

38. I note in passing that the inherent determinism of "Voodoo" death narratives, once the chance "crime" is discovered, was criticized by some postwar anthropologists, who argued that Westerners assumed that victims perceive the future as foretold, or as predetermined, once the spell had been cast. But various cultural groups, like the Yolngu, according to Janice Reid and Nancy Williams, hold no such view of the future, which is always open to various possibilities and outcomes. See "'Voodoo Death' in Arnhem Land: Whose Reality?" *American Anthropologist* 86 (1984): 121–33.

39. Several interwar ethnographers suggested an alternative conception. They conceived voodoo death as a social-interpretive and negotiated process. Fear and death were distributed over a broad temporal and spatial expanse: they did not occur in any one place during any one discrete moment in time, and they did not reside exclusively in the individual. As Lauriston Sharp ("Laurie"), of the Department of Sociology and Anthropology at Cornell, explained to Cannon in 1940: "From my own observations and reading I believe that a minor pathological condition suggests to a person that he is a victim of black magic only when he believes that there are others in the group who regard him with malevolence. It is then up to the medicine man or the group to determine whether the person really is doomed. . . . Thus the presence or absence of fear . . . appears to be very largely dependent upon the social situation of the individual as interpreted by those around him and upon group suggestion." Fear and death were not unambiguous and discrete effects. They were negotiated events that did not occur in any one particular and defined moment, did not depend on a particularly defined stimulus, and did not take place in any singularly defined space. See Lauri Sharp, Department of Sociology and Anthropology, Cornell University, to Walter B. Cannon, August 10, 1940, folder 903, box 67, WBC.

40. From Roland Barthes, "Structure of the Fait-Divers," in *Critical Essays*, trans. Richard Howard (Evanston, IL: Northwestern University Press, 1972), 185–95.

41. For some examples, see Regis A. DeSilva and Bernard Lown, "Ventricular Premature Beats, Stress, and Sudden Death," *Psychosomatics* 19 (1978): 649–61; Lown et al., "Psychophysiologic Factors"; Joel E. Dimsdale, "Emotional Causes of Sudden Death," *American Journal of Psychiatry* 134, no. 12 (December 1977): 1361–66; Richard L. Verrier and Eric L. Hagestad, "Role of the Autonomic Nervous System in Sudden Death," in *Sudden Cardiac Death*, ed. Mark E. Josephson (Philadelphia: Davis, 1985), 41–63; Jonn B. Dynes, "Sudden Death," *Diseases of the Nervous System* 30, no. 1 (January 1969): 24–28; and Ian P. Stevenson, Charles H. Duncan, Stewart Wolf, Herbert

S. Ripley, and Harold G. Wolff, "Life Situations, Emotions, and Extrasystoles," *Psychosomatic Medicine* 11, no. 5 (September–October 1949): 257–72. On "fantasy materials," see Marlene Goodfriend and Edward A. Wolpert, "Death from Fright: Report of a Case and Literature Review," *Psychosomatic Medicine* 38 (1976): 348. For sudden death in cockroaches, see L. S. Ewing, "Fighting and Death from Stress in a Cockroach," *Science* 155 (February 24, 1967): 1035–36.

42. DeSilva and Lown, "Ventricular Premature Beats," 653–56; Thomas N. James, "Chance and Sudden Death," *Journal of the American College of Cardiology* 1 (1983): 164–65.

43. George L. Engel, "A Life Setting Conductive to Illness: The Giving-Up–Given-Up Complex," *Bulletin of the Menninger Clinic* 32, no. 6 (1968): 357, reprinted from *Annals of Internal Medicine* 69 (1968): 293–300.

44. The structural similarities between medical case reports of sudden unexpected death and the *fait-divers* as studied by Roland Barthes are striking (but not analyzed in this chapter). For the citations, see Barthes, "Structure of the Fait-Divers," 185–95.

45. DeSilva and Lown, "Ventricular Premature Beats," 653–56; italics added.

46. Lown et al., "Psychophysiologic Factors," 1329.

47. James, "Chance and Sudden Death," 182.

48. Philip Fisher, *The Vehement Passions* (Princeton, NJ: Princeton University Press, 2002). Fisher gives as examples "crimes of passion," *Romeo and Juliet* and many other classical texts, in which the vehement act and moment erases a long history.

49. Lown et al., "Psychophysiologic Factors," 1331.

50. Stewart Wolf, "The End of the Rope: The Role of the Brain in Cardiac Death," *Canadian Medical Association Journal* 97 (1967): 1022.

51. Wolf, "Cardiovascular Reactions to Symbolic Stimuli," 287–92.

52. Richter's interest in domestication (qua civilization) had appeared in various publications prior to his "sudden death" article. See Curt P. Richter, "Domestication of the Norway Rat and Its Implications for the Problem of Stress," in Wolff, Wolf, and Hare, *Life Stress and Bodily Disease*, 19–47.

53. Richter, "Animals and Man," 121.

54. Similar tensions were also negotiated in reports of the sudden death of the Hmong who escaped to the West; see "The Hmong: Dying of Culture Shock?," *Science* 212 (1981): 1008. See George L. Engel, "Sudden and Rapid Death during Psychological Stress: Folklore or Folk Wisdom?," *Annals of Internal Medicine* 74 (1971): 771–82; Engel, "Psychological Factors in Instantaneous Cardiac Death," *New England of Medicine* 294 (1976): 664–65; and Engel, "Psychologic Stress, Vasodepressor (Vasovagal) Syncope, and Sudden Death," *Annals of Internal Medicine* 89 (1978): 403–12.

55. Paul K. Feyerabend, *Against Method: Outline of an Anarchistic Theory of Knowledge* (London: Verso, 1975), 50.

56. Brian Reid, "The Nocebo Effect: Placebo's Evil Twin," *Washington Post*, Tuesday, April 30, 2002, HE01.

57. Ina J. Fandrich, as quoted in Stephen Kinzer, "Interest Surges in Voodoo," *New York Times*, November 30, 2003.

58. See Engel, "Psychologic Stress," 406. We can also note that for Westerners voodoo creates the "panic sentiment," but for believers voodoo takes away the "panic."

As Yvonnne Chireau has argued, "In many cases, malign Conjure was manifested by physical maladies and inexplicable adversities such as natural disasters or sudden death. As such, Conjure served as a powerful theory for explaining unanticipated instances of misfortune." See "Conjure and Christianity in the Nineteenth Century: Religious Elements in African American Magic," *Religion and American Culture* 7 (1997): 225–47.

59. Barthes, "Structure of the Fait-Divers," 194.

Part Three

War

Chapter Five

"Stress" in US Wartime Psychiatry

World War II and the Immediate Aftermath

Theodore M. Brown

Introduction: World War II as a Watershed

In the developing literature on the history of "stress," scholars over the past two decades have begun to point to World War II as a major turning point. Gerald Grob and Robert Kugelmann, for example, both writing in the early 1990s, clearly stated that the war served as a watershed for American psychiatrists. Grob claimed, "Many psychiatrists . . . came to some novel conclusions . . . [one of which was] that environmental stress associated with combat contributed to mental maladjustment. . . . That environmental factors played a major role in the etiology of mental disorders was to be reiterated by a generation of psychiatrists who served in the military during World War II and assumed positions of leadership in the postwar era." Kugelmann insisted, "Stress comes into being as a discourse and experience during the Second World War. . . . Only in the 1940s did it become an explicit topic for research. Only then did it enter the public arena and progressively get absorbed by the general public as a lesson derived from the medical and psychological sciences."[1] Since their publications other scholars have followed Grob's and Kugelmann's lead, and it is now increasingly believed that through grappling with stress American wartime psychiatrists initiated a period in which stress concepts and stress research became central in American psychiatry and popular culture.[2]

My chapter adds to this interpretive trend and also explores several new historical dimensions. First, it describes a paradigm shift among American military psychiatrists that occurred during the war and as the result of which stress became a major rather than a peripheral concern and was transformed from being a secondary precipitating factor to being a primary causal agent. Second, it explores long-term developments and immediate historical circumstances that may have contributed to the wartime paradigm shift. Third, it presents evidence to suggest that the wartime shift in the meaning of stress was carried into domestic settings by psychiatrists after the war and contributed to the rapid dissemination of the stress concept in the postwar world.

"Stress" in World War II Military Psychiatry and Its Paradigm Shift

Stress was already a concern of US military psychiatrists at the start of the war, but their approach to it changed in two important ways during the war's course. First, stress and its effects became a more insistent and central concern, with substantially increased attention and emphasis over a short period of time. Second, stress simultaneously moved from being a general contextual factor mainly relevant as a trigger for the neurotic reactions of those military personnel already "predetermined" by their defective personalities to adverse reactions, to being a primary etiological agent that could "break" even the strongest and most "normal" of men and lead to militarily significant disability. During the course of World War II stress thus moved from background to foreground and from contributing factor to primary agent in what can be seen as a paradigm shift.

This shift is highlighted in the work of two often cited, respected, and influential American psychiatrists, Abram Kardiner and Roy R. Grinker. Kardiner's principal contribution was a monograph first published in 1941, *The Traumatic Neuroses of War.*[3] This book has a complex history and a rich literature analyzing its significance.[4] Here it is used only as a benchmark for comparison to its second edition. In the 1941 edition Kardiner referred to "stress" a number of times, always in passing. These are two examples: "a large number of these cases begin in civilian life after a period of economic stress or shock, such as the news of the death of a relative, a robbery, a business failure" and "under conditions of stress he had been inclined to stammer ever since adolescence."[5] In 1947 Kardiner published a new edition of his monograph, this one in collaboration with Herbert Spiegel. They emphasize in the preface that the second edition, unlike the first, reports the results of battlefield experience acquired during World War II. Thus there were many changes in the second edition announced by the revised title, *War Stress and Neurotic Illness.* Most important were shifts in content, such as a new ten-page section on "The Stress of War," where Kardiner writes, "Army life is always an equation in which . . . [the soldier's] natural endowment and adaptability are pitted against the cumulative effect of all these stresses at any particular time. Every soldier has his breaking point irrespective of his previous history."[6]

Grinker's contribution was a pair of books with his former chief resident at Michael Reese Hospital in Chicago, John P. Spiegel, rather than two editions of what was claimed to be the same book. Their first book was *War*

Neuroses in North Africa, originally published as a typescript in 1943.[7] Called "a descriptive masterpiece, alive with shock and wonder," *War Neuroses* focused on psychiatric casualties among the ground troops who fought under horrendous conditions in Tunisia between January and May 1943.[8] Its emphases were the classification of clinical syndromes, etiology, treatment, and psychodynamic theorizing. Of special interest here is etiology because the first Grinker and Spiegel monograph is clearly committed to the paradigm that assigned causal primacy to neurotic predisposition with a secondary role for stress as a trigger. In 1943 Grinker and Spiegel wrote as follows: "The usual story is that of an individual who has had some degree of anxiety in civilian life. . . . Under the continued stress of battle . . . the anxiety overwhelms him" and "It can be stated categorically that any man who has had functional somatic complaints [i.e., psychosomatic symptoms] in civilian life will experience a recrudescence of symptoms in much more malignant form on exposure to battle conditions. . . . Schizoid characters, who have managed to get along fairly well in stable conditions of civilian life, are apt to develop paranoid reactions when involved in the intensely hostile situation of the battlefield. Obsessive-compulsive individuals tend to develop anxiety and depression when the strain of battle overwhelms this defense." It is true that Grinker and Spiegel also vividly describe how the "continued threat of injury and death, and repeated narrow escapes produce a cumulative effect" and how "constant explosions, bangs, snaps of machine guns, whines of artillery shells, rustle of mortars, drone of airplane engines, wears down resistance," but their fundamental assumption remains that prewar neurotic predisposition is the primary factor in wartime breakdown. They write, "The realities of war . . . cooperate to produce a potential war neurosis in every soldier. When *predisposition* is combined with adequate stimulus of a certain type or degree, a neurotic breakdown is precipitated."[9]

When Grinker and Spiegel published their second book, *Men under Stress,* in 1945, their paradigm had shifted. They now focused on air force personnel in aerial combat and describe in great, vivid detail the discomforts, challenges, and emotional assaults in both the physical and psychological realms. They emphasize that stress of the magnitude experienced by their patients could break *anyone,* and their primary clinical subject is "Everyman" rather than the predisposed neurotic: "Never in the history of the study of human behavior has it been so important to understand the psychological mechanisms of 'normal' individuals in situations of stress. Under sufficient stress any individual may show failure of adaptation, evidenced by neurotic symptoms. . . . The psychological mechanisms under discussion in this book are those that apply to Everyman in his struggle to master his own environment." Even if some recruits may have had predisposing neurotic personality characteristics, it is impossible to predict until the uniquely intense and horrific experience of battle whether those predispositions would actually lead to breakdown and incapacity. In fact, realizing that intense anxiety was an externally imposed, universal, and shared reality would allow some with neurotic predispositions and life histories to do better in battle situations than nonneurotics. Certainly, the selection process was not perfect and could have erred by letting vulnerable men through in many cases, but psychiatrists should not be blamed too harshly as there was no solid basis for adequate screening. There was no proxy for the realities of combat stress, and thus no one could predict how particular men would respond until the actual, relentless experience.[10] Focus henceforth must be placed on stress as a primary causal agent and what in sufficient intensity and cumulative impact it could do to anyone.

Stress in World War II Military Psychiatry: Substantiating the Paradigm Shift

The paradigm shift described in the last section can be documented more broadly in the general wartime psychiatric literature. That literature sorts chronologically into a first phase written and published before mid-1943 and a second phase written and published afterward. The first phase is concurrent with the initially reluctant, disorganized, and lackluster early mobilization of American psychiatric resources for the war effort. The second phase is concurrent with the more impressive and robust later mobilization, much of it led by enthusiastic and respected psychiatrists eager to provide wartime service both within military ranks and as civilian consultants. The first phase was dominated by the attempt to organize psychiatric expertise to screen out psychologically damaged or vulnerable individuals in the draft-selection process and to spend less effort mobilizing treatment.[11] Not surprisingly, psychiatrists in the first phase considered stress primarily as a precipitating factor for neuroses manifested in predisposed individuals.

In fact, in that first phase stress was understood much as it had been since the turn of the twentieth century, if not earlier. American psychiatrist William Alanson White had written in 1903 that increased "stresses incident to the struggle for existence" could precipitate mental illness in vulnerable individuals, and famous clinician William Osler wrote in 1910 that "stress and strain" could be a factor in the onset of physical illnesses like angina pectoris in certain sorts of people.[12] British physician Elliot Smith in a 1918 book on *Shellshock and Its Lessons* claimed that "an intelligent man of strong will . . . might be temporarily 'bowled over' by the emotional stresses of the [military] campaign, but after a few inquiries . . . and a few explanations, he is often on his feet again."[13] Millais Culpin, a British physician treating those still suffering from war neuroses in 1921, thought that the toughest and most lingering cases were those men who had broken down quickly because "the amount of stress endured before breakdown is a measure of the man's original stamina and hence of his likely response to treatment."[14]

American military psychiatrists remained faithful to these ideas at the start of World War II. For example, William C. Porter, an Army psychiatrist who played an important role in psychiatric training throughout the wartime period and who in the early 1940s was chief of the Neuropsychiatry Section at Walter Reed Hospital, published articles in *War Medicine* and elsewhere on how to select "suitable human material" for the military and how to weed out those with potential psychiatric problems that would presumably be actualized by combat or even precombat stress. Likewise, James A. Brussel and Harold R. Wolpert collaborated on a review of "The Psychoneuroses in Military Psychiatry," which built on the assumption that individuals "prone" to mental illness could and should be weeded out in the draft-selection process.[15] The two most notable contributions in the first phase were those of Norman Q. Brill, chief of Neuropsychiatry at the Station Hospital in Fort Bragg, North Carolina, from 1941 to 1944, and J. L. Henderson and Merrill Moore, both working for the Navy Department in Pasadena, California, at the time of their March 1944 publication.

Brill's article, "War Neuroses," was published in *The Military Surgeon* in April 1942. Brill's most telling observations were these:

> In a vast majority of cases of neuroses that are being admitted to the hospital at Fort Bragg, a history of long-standing nervousness can be obtained. . . . No statistics are available at present but it is rare to find an individual whose nervous trouble began after enlistment or induction into the Army. . . . [A] hypersensitive, excessively irritable, impulsive, self-centered, infantile and moody person can "take less" than a well-adjusted mature individual and will decompensate sooner when exposed to the same stresses and strains. . . . The major factor in the prevention of war neuroses is the detection and early rejection or elimination of the emotionally unstable from active combat service.[16]

Henderson and Moore's article, "The Psychoneuroses of War" based on two hundred neuropsychiatric admissions, was published in the *New England Journal of Medicine* in March 1944. Their major conclusions were these:

> In attempting to analyze predisposing conditions, the most important factor was found to be a disturbance in family background. . . . Those patients who came from homes that were broken by separation, divorce or death, or distorted by neurotic parents, were found to have personalities insufficiently developed to deal rapidly or adequately with the problems of life, particularly with the problems of war. . . . It seems that the man who has developed a so-called "war neurosis" was predetermined before he entered the Service. It might even be said that the war neuroses are "made in America" and only come to light or are labeled in combat.[17]

The second phase of the wartime stress literature began in late 1943 and expanded in 1944. By March, articles such as Paul T. McAlpine's "Hysterical Visual Defects," which identified stress as a primary trigger of neurotic disability in previously normal men, began to appear regularly in *War Medicine* and other journals. Later in 1944 a distinguished Commission on Military Neuropsychiatry, chaired by Franklin G. Ebaugh, gave the new stress paradigm considerable legitimacy and added to the paradigm's growing momentum when the commission's work was reported in December in the *Proceedings of the Association for Research in Nervous and Mental Diseases.* John C. Whitehorn, the Henry Phipps professor of psychiatry at Johns Hopkins and secretary of the Committee on Neuropsychiatry of the National Research Council, provided the commission's keynote paper, "Changing Concepts of Psychoneurosis in Relation to Military Psychiatry." Whitehorn wrote,

> Psychiatric principles were somewhat too narrowly conceived in the early war years, when limited too sharply to the business of detecting neurotic traits or patterns. Some change to a broader basis was required, but the change which actually occurred was in the direction of inventing diagnostic labels indicative of situational factors rather than personality factors. We got a crop of diagnostic or pseudo-diagnostic terms such as "flying stress," "combat fatigue," "operational fatigue," etc. Such a shift in nomenclature was in part motivated by a kindly desire to spare valiant men the implied disgrace of the psychoneurotic label, and to spare them also some of the then current administrative implications of such labels. But this tendency to change nomenclature arose also, I believe, from an intellectually-honest necessity of recognizing the importance of the situation in the triangular relationship between situation, reaction and personality.[18]

Whitehorn's emphasis on the causal importance of "the situation" and the identification of that situation primarily with exogenous "stress" was immediately endorsed by Francis J. Braceland of the navy and Roy R. Grinker of the air force. Braceland said that Whitehorn was "progressing along the right track," and Grinker wrote as follows: "If I were permitted an extremely inaccurate generalization, I should ascribe combat neuroses to the effect of extreme stress or catastrophic experiences on personalities that are relatively well adjusted in spite of character and personality deviations or latent neuroses." In their chapter on "The Management of Neuropsychiatric Casualties in the Zone of Combat" in the *Manual of Military Neuropsychiatry*, Grinker and Spiegel put the point this way:

> The psychiatrist's first discovery is that, officially, war neuroses are not considered battle casualties. Such a view is apparently based on the assumption that the war is of lesser importance in the development of such conditions than is constitution or previous or latent neurosis. This assumption is shared by many

> psychiatrists and leads to a pessimistic therapeutic attitude. The quicker psychiatrists relinquish this idea the sooner they will achieve therapeutic successes and so prove their usefulness in combat areas. *War neuroses are caused by war*; anyone, no matter how strong or stable, may develop a war neurosis under proper circumstances.[19]

Whitehorn's "triangular" model, which emphasized situational stress as a primary causal mechanism of war neuroses, and Grinker's pragmatic insistence on aggressive therapeutic intervention to undo the effects of exogenous stress on men who were normal before the traumas of combat were both profoundly influential in the later years of the war. Theirs was the new paradigm that quickly swept away the traces of the old with its emphasis on the predetermination of war neuroses that were supposedly "made in America" rather than in combat zones and on stress as merely a circumstantial trigger far less important than personality "predisposition."

That new paradigm was given central attention by Brigadier General William C. Menninger, famous civilian psychiatrist before the war and the highest-ranking psychiatrist in the military during the war. According to Menninger,

> The psychiatric experience in the remarkable human laboratory created in the Army by this war . . . provided a controlled situation in which all men were regimented and lived under the same conditions, and presumably all were motivated towards a common goal. Perhaps the most widespread and impressive experience of the military psychiatrist was the opportunity to observe the effect of extraordinary external stress in precipitating personality disorder. The existence of psychiatric determinants, such as history of maladjustment in the family or in the individual, contributed to many of the casualties that occurred. On the other hand, far more impressive in the adjustment process than the history or the personality make-up or the internal psychodynamic stresses, was the force of factors in the environment which supported or disrupted the individual. . . . [A] large number of . . . [psychiatric casualties] undoubtedly occurred in individuals with a minimal predisposition to mental illness.[20]

Possible Reasons for the Paradigm Shift

What are the possible reasons for the paradigm shift that has been outlined? No one explanation alone would seem sufficient, especially given the quick and substantial changes involved. Even less likely is the causal influence of a broad shift in sensibility about the nature and range of "normal" and "abnormal" human personalities and behaviors. While such a shift in sensibility may have been slowly and subtly taking place, it is an unlikely major contributor to the paradigm change observed. The rapidity of the change and its very specific wartime context make the typically slow-acting and diffuse sway of cultural alteration implausible as a leading cause. More plausible is a set of shorter-acting, context-specific, and quite possibly overlapping influences. A combination of such factors is the likeliest explanation for the paradigm shift in the understanding of stress on the part of American military psychiatrists between the beginning and end of World War II.

The first influence to consider was that exercised by certain British psychiatrists, particularly Eliot Slater and Eric Wittkower. Without plunging into the tangled history of British psychiatry during the first and second world wars and in the interwar period, it is nevertheless appropriate to say that Slater and Wittkower, among others, had some influence on their American colleagues during World War II.[21] Slater had a long and distinguished career as a leader in the field of psychiatric genetics but was also known for his work adumbrating the diathesis-stress model of psychological disorders, according to which a genetic predisposition (diathesis) interacts with stressful life events to trigger abnormal behavior.[22] In 1939 he was appointed clinical director of the Sutton Emergency Hospital, where over the course of the war he was responsible for the twenty thousand psychiatric casualties who passed through his unit. In a widely influential 1940 *Lancet* article on "Acute War Neuroses," he struck a note unusual for his time by claiming that "men of reasonably sound personality may break down if the strain is severe enough."[23]

Eric Wittkower also pointed clearly in the same direction. Wittkower was an émigré psychoanalyst and psychosomatic researcher from Berlin who served as a psychiatrist in the British Army from 1940 to 1945.[24] He affiliated as a psychoanalyst with the Tavistock Institute but also further developed psychosomatic research begun on medical patients in Berlin with patients in London, including one study of cardiac patients in which he found that twenty-five of seventy-two were "non-neurotic" yet developed pain symptoms with "stress or strain" as the "precipitating agent."[25] With the beginning of the war, he got deeply involved in an important Tavistock project on "The Neuroses in War." He coauthored papers with Emanuel Miller and others, contributing significantly to a major book, *The Neuroses in War*, where he recorded the following notable observations: "Severe and prolonged stress may precipitate a breakdown in almost everybody. . . . Given sufficient emotional stress, neurotic symptoms may appear in anyone. . . . The incidence of psychosomatic illness mounted with the duration of precipitating emotional stress."[26]

A specific route of entry for these British ideas into American wartime psychiatry was Algiers in North Africa, where in 1943 Grinker and Spiegel worked alongside British military psychiatrists. Shephard describes the circumstances in these terms: "Finding the staff of the American hospital in

Algiers unsympathetic, Grinker arranged to work . . . at the large British hospital, to which many American casualties were being sent. There he and Spiegel treated many of the soldiers from Kasserine Pass as well as a number of airmen."[27]

The second influence to consider is learning through experience by running head-on into anomalies in the predispositional, stress-as-a-precipitating factor paradigm. Two reports in the literature, one published by Kurt Goldstein in *Psychosomatic Medicine* and one by E. Rogers Smith in *American Journal of Psychiatry*, will suffice as examples. First Goldstein:

> Extensive personal experience in the treatment of cases of "nervous breakdown" in men in military service has indicated that the psychologic mechanism to which the condition owes its origin must be much simpler than that which is operative in the usual neurosis. . . . These considerations . . . suggested that the nervous breakdowns of the war period were largely an expression of the simple fact that many persons cannot cope with dangerous situations presented by war events. . . . We are dealing in these cases, not with real neurosis in which maladjustment of the personality is the central factor, but with direct consequences of the overwhelming conditions. . . . I have seen extremely reliable men and officers incapacitated by acute states of anxiety who never before had shown any neurotic symptoms.[28]

E. Rogers Smith's report, describing the horrors that marine troops experienced at Guadalcanal in August 1942, is even more explicit: "Never before in history has such a group of healthy, toughened, well-trained men been subjected to such conditions as the combat troops of the U.S. Marine Corps. . . . The strain and stress experienced by these men produced a group neurosis that has not been seen before and may never be seen again. . . . We feel that from this observation we might advance the hypothesis that this type of neurosis results from the prolonged combat. . . . Each man must have a breaking point, a point beyond which he cannot carry on."[29]

These reports not only illustrate learning from experience in the brutality of battle but also suggest additional factors at work. One of these was the retrospective rationalization of the increasingly obvious inadequacy of the initial draft-selection screening process. Either psychiatrists had been utterly incompetent at identifying and excluding potentially vulnerable men or they had attempted an impossible task given the magnitude of combat-stress effects and their previously unrecognized influence on *all* military personnel. The latter explanation took psychiatrists off the hook and seemed fully consistent with wartime experience. Even if after the war psychiatrists could admit that they had initially "expected too much from induction center screening and fell in with the overselling of what psychiatry could accomplish at this level," during the war it was less demoralizing to shift attention to the impossibility of the task, given the overwhelming importance of exogenous stress compared to individual neurotic predisposition.[30] Likewise, it was less demoralizing for the hundreds of thousands of enlisted men who "broke" under the stress of combat to consider them normal but subjected to utterly abnormal and impossible circumstances than to consider them weak and vulnerable. If the symptoms neuropsychiatrists like Goldstein and Smith observed in their patients (and sometimes in themselves) were the "direct consequences of the overwhelming conditions" and could have happened to anyone because "each man must have a breaking point," then everyone involved in the screening process could be exonerated and everyone in terrifying combat situations could be spared the label "defective" or "neurotically impaired."

Another likely factor in the paradigm shift was the influence of Walter B. Cannon, one of America's leading physiologists and a most respected scientific statesmen of the prewar period.[31] He had been the George Higginson professor and chair of the Harvard Department of Physiology since 1906 and had done pioneering work in several areas including the physiology of emotion. In 1897 he noticed that when his experimental animals were frightened or in some other way disturbed, peristaltic waves in the stomach sometimes ceased abruptly. After publishing his synthetic *The Mechanical Factors of Digestion* in 1911, Cannon turned his attention to a broadly conceived investigation of the physiology of the emotions, thus becoming the first major investigator to work systematically on this topic.[32] He collected evidence to show that when an animal is strongly aroused, the sympathetic division of its autonomic nervous system works in conjunction with the hormone adrenaline to mobilize the animal for an emergency response of "flight or fight." The "sympathico-adrenal system" orchestrates changes in blood supply, sugar availability, and the blood's clotting capacity in a marshaling of resources keyed to the "violent display of energy."[33] He summarized his initial findings in a pathbreaking 1915 book, *Bodily Changes in Pain, Hunger, Fear and Rage.*

In the 1920s and 1930s Cannon pursued several fruitful lines of investigation, his most important concentrating on the complexities of chemical neurotransmission and on the maintenance of "homeostasis" (a term he coined in 1926). Beginning in 1928 he turned his attention increasingly to the clinical implications of his physiological discoveries. In this work he combined his sensitivity as a physician with the rigor of his laboratory investigations to help launch the field of American psychosomatic research. Cannon often resorted to the language of "stress," as in the following examples from a 1928 paper in the *New England Journal of Medicine*: "If . . . [physicians show] indifference [to the patient's feelings] . . . is it surprising that men and women, beset by emotional stresses, turn from us and go for help to faith healers?"; and "The doctor is properly concerned with the workings of the body and their disturbances, and he should have, therefore, a natural interest in the effects of emotional stress and in the modes of relieving it."[34] And in a widely read 1935 paper in the *American Journal of Medical Sciences* on "The Stresses and Strains of Homeostasis," Cannon explored "where the limits lie beyond which stresses overwhelm . . . [the organism's] corrective factors and significantly alter the steady state of the internal environment."[35]

By the 1940s Cannon applied his insights to the phenomenon of voodoo (curse- or magic-induced) death reported by anthropologists. In a 1942 paper in the *American Anthropologist,* Cannon wrote,

> Before denying that "voodoo" death is within the realm of possibility, let us consider the general features of the specimen reports. . . . First . . . is the fixed assurance that because of certain conditions, such as being subject to bone pointing or other magic, or failing to observe sacred tribal regulations, death is sure to supervene. . . . Thereby he becomes a pariah, wholly deprived of the confidence and social support of the tribe. . . . The question which now arises is whether an ominous and persistent state of fear can end the life of a man. Fear . . . only with difficulty can be eradicated. Associated with it are profound physiological disturbances, widespread throughout the organism. . . . If these powerful emotions prevail . . . and if this state of extreme perturbation continues in uncontrolled possession of the organism for a considerable period . . . dire results may ensue. . . . Evidence of the possibility of fatal outcome from profound emotional strain was reported by Mira in recounting his experiences as a psychiatrist in the Spanish War of 1936–39. . . . The combination of lack of food and water, anxiety, very rapid pulse and respiration, associated with a shocking experience having persistent effects, would fit well with fatal conditions reported from primitive tribes. The suggestion which I offer, therefore, is that "voodoo death" may be real, and that it may be explained as due to shocking emotional stress—to obvious repressed terror.[36]

The timing (1942), contents (using an analogy to the psychological strains of warfare), and authorship (the esteemed Walter B. Cannon) of this paper about the dire consequences of "shocking emotional stress" all point to a possible influence on American wartime psychiatrists.

Yet another set of influences, these quite explicitly noted at the time, came from the considerable body of work on "experimental neuroses." This work derived ultimately from Pavlov and people who trained with him but also showed some influence of Cannon's physiology of the emotions. Central to this new field of investigation were the extensive studies undertaken by Howard Liddell at the "Behavior Farm" on the Cornell University campus in Ithaca, New York, and by Jules Masserman in the neurophysiological laboratories of the division of psychiatry at the University of Chicago.[37] Liddell was a PhD experimental psychologist well trained in conditioning experiments, and Masserman was an MD with a neurology and neurophysiology background who had also trained at the Chicago Psychoanalytic Institute with Franz Alexander and his associates. Both Liddell and Masserman were Rockefeller Foundation grantees. They turned systematically to experimental studies in which they conditioned animals to "neuroses" by subjecting them to complex and confusing signals and circumstances often conceptualized as "frustration" or "stress." Their work was followed closely by many in the early forties, not least by Grinker and by Lawrence Kubie, a psychoanalyst with a significant neurological and neurophysiological background who also played an important role in American military psychiatry during World War II.[38] Both Grinker and Kubie, it is relevant to note, were also carefully cultivated Rockefeller grantees.[39]

Grinker, in both *War Neuroses* and *Men under Stress*, stated that it may prove useful to think of war neuroses as experimental neuroses. Both experimental animals and military personnel were "normal" before being subjected to intense stress, and some human patients showed no evidence of subjective anxiety yet exhibited tachycardia, increased perspiration, and startle reaction, just as had been observed in some experimental animals.[40] The neurotic reaction in both animal and humans may be thought of as due to the establishment of some fixed pattern in the visceral nervous system that is self-perpetuating, as if "the diencephalic waves of neural energy continued beating in closed circuits of internuncial neurons, maintaining excitation for weeks or months."[41]

Kubie, in discussing the emergency treatment for acute war neuroses in 1943 and 1944 publications, reviewed deconditioning procedures, including those that Masserman had successfully employed in alleviating the symptoms of experimental neurosis in cats. He then concluded, "It would seem reasonable to expect that by leading men repeatedly through situations which mimic closely the sights, sounds, and smells of actual battle, it may be possible to desensitize them to the stress which lies ahead. Similarly, once men have broken under that stress it would seem reasonable to suppose that similar procedures could break down the links between these sights and sounds and their superimposed terror-states, and thus return the soldier to his desensitized condition."[42]

One further possible influence meriting consideration is the tension between orthodox, strictly psychoanalytically oriented psychiatrists on the one hand and their more eclectic and often biologically oriented counterparts on the other. In response to these tensions, many of the more eclectic and biologically oriented psychiatrists turned to "stress" as a way to distance themselves from doctrinaire Freudianism without abandoning dynamic concepts entirely. The tensions in the American psychiatric community had two nodes, one primarily connected with therapeutic approaches and the other largely about biological foundations.

Nathan G. Hale discussed the first of these in his book *The Rise and Crisis of Psychoanalysis in the United States*:

> In the 1940s and 1950s . . . outside critics as well as psychoanalysts themselves . . . had begun to question the efficacy of psychoanalytic treatment. . . . Critics represented not only psychiatrists but psychologists trained in academic standards of testing and research who had entered the psychiatric and psychotherapeutic fields. . . . In 1947 Lawrence Kubie . . . [wrote] that after seeing enough of the work of even his best [psychoanalytic] colleagues, "It was no longer possible to believe that a bad therapeutic result could be explained away as due either to inadequate training or to inferior analytical ability." . . . Kubie later called for greater rigor in outcome research in psychotherapy and in psychoanalysis as well. He insisted that too little was known . . . about therapy or spontaneous recovery or about the influence of the patient's life situation to make valid judgments about comparative effectiveness.[43]

Gerald Grob discussed the second node of tension, between psychoanalytic and biologically oriented psychiatrists, in *From Asylum to Community: Mental Health Policy in Modern America*:

> Although the psychodynamic school shaped and dominated the evolution of the specialty in the two decades following World War II, its hegemony had never been absolute. Admittedly relegated to a minority position, the older biological tradition persisted in one form or another. As early as 1946, a small group of organically oriented psychiatrists, neurologists, and neurophysiologists led by George Thompson, Abram Bennett, and Johannes Nielson, and including Percival Bailey, Harry Solomon, Stanley Cobb, Samuel [*sic*] Wortis, and Karl Bowman, formed the Society of Biological Psychiatry . . . [whose] members were united by a belief in the neuronal basis of psychiatry. . . . In the APA's [American Psychiatric Association] Academic Lecture in 1956, Bailey berated his psychodynamic colleagues and suggested that psychoanalysis was a religion rather than a science. . . . Towards the close of his lecture, he urged his colleagues to . . . prove, by established criteria, that their concepts have scientific validity.[44]

The basic issues raised by Hale and Grob surfaced in an enthusiastic 1946 review of Grinker and Spiegel's *Men under Stress* in the *American Journal of Psychiatry* by Abraham Myerson, who by then was a well-established and often scathing critic of psychoanalytic orthodoxy.[45] This, in part, is what Myerson said about Grinker's book:

> It is a distinguished book, both in format and in the essential brilliancy of its English. . . . There is an especially fine description of the neurology and physiology of action, motion, sensation, mood, and feeling-tone. . . . It is refreshingly true that one can read this book and find nothing of the Oedipus complex, penis envy, castration fear; and all the various formulae of oral, anal and other eroticisms are either conspicuously absent or tentatively introduced. . . . The old psychoanalysis has disappeared though now and then the integrated habit of thought of the writers comes out as, for example, when they state that the

> American soldier loves milk because of maternal linkage. . . . [Yet the] authors have worked on and for their patients not as psychoanalysts . . . but as doctors of medicine. . . . They have set in motion physical and psychological recuperative agencies. They have used drugs. They have explained, consoled, bolstered and disciplined into integrity sick men, men who have undergone grave and disorganizing stress. It is an understatement to say that this book should be in every psychiatrist's library.[46]

While praising Grinker for his achievements, Myerson simultaneously goaded him for the relics of Freudian orthodoxy that could still be found in his book. He likely believed that Grinker was ready to depart from the dogmatic psychoanalytic fold for a more fluid and eclectic psychiatry and just needed a push. Grinker, after all, had trained originally in neurology and neurophysiology and had been recruited to psychoanalysis (and a brief personal analysis in Vienna with Freud) only as part of a conscious effort by the Rockefeller Foundation's Alan Gregg to build a grand new "psychobiology" that required an amalgam of psychoanalysis with neurophysiology and neuropsychiatry, with the biological sciences in the dominant role.[47] Grinker, in fact, had felt ambivalence about Freud and orthodox psychoanalysis from the start, held on to his neurological expertise, and progressively moved into nonpsychoanalytic experimental and theoretical territory as his career unfolded.[48] "Stress" was part of his early heterodox explorations, and Myerson sensed this. Stanley Cobb, a former neurologist too who since 1934 had, with generous Rockefeller Foundation support, been psychiatrist in chief at the Massachusetts General Hospital, could be described in similar terms as Grinker regarding his early exploration of stress perspectives.[49] This turn to stress by psychiatrists uncomfortable with the therapeutic and doctrinal dogmatism of orthodox psychoanalysis was an important thread in the late 1940s and became a major theme in the psychiatric and psychosomatic literature of the 1950s.

Postwar Dissemination

After the war American psychiatrists made serious efforts to consolidate and promote wartime lessons about the primacy and centrality of stress. These efforts were part of a larger campaign to raise the status, visibility, and influence of psychiatry and to make it an important force in domestic medicine and social policy. Psychiatrists strove to guarantee that returning veterans, especially those still suffering from psychiatric disabilities, would not be stigmatized and would have the institutional and programmatic support they needed for adequate treatment of their war-generated disorders. Even more ambitiously, they also worked to generalize from their military experience and extend their expertise about stress to a wide spectrum of civilian applications. Recognizing the general importance of environmental stress, the multiple ways it affected "normal individuals," and the need to deal with it both therapeutically and preventively became critical parts of the postwar psychiatric agenda and an early phase in the popular dissemination of the new stress concept.

Near the end of their major book on war neuroses, *Men under Stress*, Grinker and Spiegel prepared the ground for psychiatry's postwar campaign:

> War has almost always been accompanied by great advances in the medical sciences. . . . Our experiences as military psychiatrists serving combat soldiers and fliers for the last two and a half years have taught us a great deal about human beings under stress. These experiences are of value not alone for their applicability to an understanding of the problems and treatments of the psychiatric casualties of war; they are equally valuable for the understanding of the psychology and psychopathology of people under the stresses of ordinary civilian life. These may not be as continuous or as catastrophic, or their effects as sudden or dramatic, yet in essence they bring into action the same forces within the individual as do the terrifying stimuli of battle. Like any advance in medicine stimulated by war, our work should be applicable to civilian psychiatry.[50]

The lead Grinker and Spiegel provided in *Men under Stress* was soon followed by other psychiatrists, most prominently by William C. Menninger, who had been the highest-ranking military psychiatrist during the war and who emerged as a major postwar leader in the field of psychiatry.[51] In 1947 Menninger was elected president of the American Psychiatric Association and in March and September of that same year published two closely related papers in the *American Journal of Psychiatry*, laying out the central importance of the new stress concepts. In "Psychiatric Experience in the War, 1941–1946," he summarized some of the major lessons learned during the war and their implications for civilian practice:

> We learned that maintenance of mental health was largely a function of leadership, which included the extremely important element of motivating the man to want to do his job and remain loyal to his associates and his unit. The absence or weakness of these supportive factors in the presence of many excessive stresses seems to account for many of the psychiatric casualties. . . . Another observation that can be made as a result of our experience is that if intensive treatment was provided early on, in an environment in which the expectations of recovery prevailed, remarkable results were obtained.[52]

In "The Role of Psychiatry in the World Today" published in September 1947, Menninger articulated further civilian applications of wartime experience:

> One of the essential roles of psychiatry must lie in the field of prevention of mental ill health. . . . Psychiatry in the war started on the basis that treatment was the sole province and responsibility of the psychiatrist. We learned by experience, however, that our greatest contribution should have been in the field of prevention. This involved putting psychiatrists into the field to live with the soldiers, thus learning their problems, attempting to modify their stresses and develop their supports. Only there could they advise leaders effectively about immediate factors that affected mental health. It would seem that psychiatry's great opportunity is to work similarly in the fields of academic education, public health, recreation, delinquency, and industry. Our lessons in preventive psychiatry from the Army emphasized three major factors in maintaining mental health. The first, and most important, was that quality of leadership was a cause of or prevented mental ill health. We learned that the development of positive rational attitudes toward the job to be done—i.e., conscious motivation—could be a great aid to the doing of that job. . . . The development of an identification with a group, which permitted a sense of pride and provided comparative security, satisfaction, and unity of purpose, was extremely important to mental health. It was apparent that these elementary lessons which applied to the maintenance of an individual's mental health in the Army, could apply in the family, the group, the community, and the nation.[53]

Menninger developed these ideas far more extensively in his book, *Psychiatry in a Troubled World* (1948), where he devoted several hundred pages to reviewing wartime psychiatric experience with stress, its manifestations, and its consequences and to drawing out the chief implications of that experience for postwar life. He covered the latter issues principally in chapters called "Everyman: Maintenance of His Mental Health," "Lessons for Civilian Psychiatry," and "Mental Hygiene in Industry and Business." This is some of what he wrote in the first of those chapters:

> The stresses and demands of Army life were greater than the average man in civilian life has to accept. For most of us, most of the time, life is a constant struggle in which we have to change continuously to meet a rapidly changing environment. . . . The struggle may be resolved on any level between complete success and complete failure. The outcome depends upon the strength and adjustability of the personality as well as upon the amount of stress the environment imposes. . . . It was not hard for . . . [military personnel during the war] to identify with and thus easily understand similar, though more acute distress, in a comrade. . . . [This] forced the recognition of the fact that at different times the personality varies in its ability to resist stress, and that different personalities react differently to the same stress. Therefore the still-integrated person did not feel he was doomed to crack up and the disintegrated personality gained support from the fact that others had difficulty. Both could find courage to seek increased ability to resist stress.[54]

In the third of his chapters, "Mental Hygiene in Industry and Business," Menninger distilled the lessons of military experience:

> One of the more important psychiatric developments in coping with the management of ineffectiveness in the Army was the establishment of the Mental Hygiene Consultation Services. . . . The psychiatrist in these clinics worked somewhat differently than in civilian life; he used short treatment procedures, tried to relieve or help the soldier handle situational stresses, treated the individual in his relationship to group missions, and advised about the manipulation of environment. . . . In a very limited fashion this has been used in industry under various guises . . . [sometimes] described as an "emotional first aid station." . . . At the Western Electric Plant . . . it was shown, without question, that if an opportunity was provided for the employee to have a sympathetic listener who was neither censorious, critical, nor even advisory, the efficiency of the worker increased noticeably. . . . There were numerous minor matters that influenced his mental health about which the soldier "griped." . . . They were minor stresses compared to those inherent in joining the Army, leaving home, being separated from loved ones for years, or facing combat. Even though they were less severe, they were factors which produced great dissatisfaction, often cumulative. . . . Every one of these stresses has comparable analogues in civilian life, particularly in industry.[55]

Menninger's efforts to popularize stress seem to have paid off, at least if one judges by reflections in the American popular media. For example, under the headline "War Study Links Body Ills to Mental Stress," the *Los Angeles Times* reported on March 31, 1947, that "mental stress was a factor in many cases of eye trouble." On June 14, 1947, the *Chicago Daily Tribune* reported that "Attempting to keep up with the Joneses amid the stress and competition of modern living is causing an adverse effect on the mental health of the American people" and is also leading to "stomach ulcers, thyroid gland trouble, and chronic diseases." On April 23, 1949, the *New York Times* reported that "Many cardiac ailments that result from high blood pressure were caused by unnecessary 'stress and strain'" and on December 4, 1949, that "The onset of osteo-arthritis in nearly all of the patients followed directly a severe emotional stress." The media surge grew even larger in the 1950s, although by this time much of it was attributable to the efforts of Montreal-based endocrinologist Hans Selye, who had captured attention as the new stress guru.[56]

Selye's brilliantly successful self-promotional efforts have been studied by Russell Viner and others, but what should now be added to those accounts is the recognition that the ground for Selye had been prepared by Roy Grinker, William Menninger, and many other American psychiatrists in the forties.[57] Indeed, it was their work in learning from and extending wartime experience to postwar domestic applications that first drew wide attention to the centrality and significance of stress, and it seems likely that it was their work that led Selye himself to the inclusion of psychological factors in his list of exogenous stressors. Selye's early publications on "A Syndrome Produced by Diverse Nocuous Agents" (1936) and "The Prevention of Adrenalin Lung Edema by the Alarm Reaction" (1938) make no reference to psychological stimuli and no use of the word "stress." By contrast, Selye's 1946 paper, "The General Adaptation Syndrome and the Diseases of Adaptation," is replete with "stress" references.[58] It is also notable that in his 1946 paper Selye refers to the work of investigators who studied stress reactions among "aviators," although he fails to cite—quite likely deliberately and disingenuously—the best-known contemporary work on the physical and psychological challenges faced by men in flight, Grinker and Spiegel's *Men under Stress.*[59]

In short, when read closely, even some of Selye's self-promotional writing aimed at establishing his priority in the stress field can be cited in support of the claim argued here that it was the clinical encounters of American military psychiatrists during World War II and their proselytizing efforts in the immediate postwar period that most significantly contributed to focusing attention on the centrality and significance of emotional stress. It was the experience of normal men in extraordinary wartime circumstances and the insights of the psychiatrists who treated them that was the real turning point in the study of stress.

Notes

1. Gerald Grob, *From Asylum to Community: Mental Health Policy in Modern America* (Princeton, NJ: Princeton University Press, 1991), 7, 17; see also 12, 18–20; Robert Kugelmann, *Stress: The Nature and History of Engineered Grief* (Westport CN: Praeger, 1992), 52; see also 54–60.

2. See, for example, Nathan G. Hale, *The Rise and Crisis of Psychoanalysis in the United States: Freud and the Americans, 1917–1985* (New York: Oxford University Press, 1995), 188, 191, 200, 202, 207, 209; Cary L. Cooper and Philip Dewe, *Stress: A Brief History* (Malden, MA: Blackwell, 2004), 24; Hans Pols, "War Neurosis, Adjustment Problems in Veterans, and an Ill Nation: The Disciplinary Project of American Psychiatry during and after World War II," *Osiris* 22 (2007): 78, 81, 89, 92.

3. Abram Kardiner, *The Traumatic Neuroses of War* (New York: Hoeber, 1941).

4. Ben Shephard, *A War of Nerves: Soldiers and Psychiatrists in the Twentieth Century* (Cambridge, MA: Harvard University Press, 2000), 154–57.

5. Kardiner, *Traumatic Neuroses of War,* 21–23.

6. Abram Kardiner and Herbert Spiegel, *War Stress and Neurotic Illness* (New York: Hoeber, 1947), 24.

7. Roy R. Grinker and John P. Spiegel, *War Neuroses in North Africa: The Tunisian Campaign, January–May 1943* (New York: Macy Foundation, 1943). A 1945 print edition, slightly revised, is called *War Neuroses* (Philadelphia: Blakiston, 1945).

8. Shephard, *War of Nerves,* 213.

9. Grinker and Spiegel, *War Neuroses,* 29–30, 133–40, 140, 141, 142; italics added.

10. Roy R. Grinker and John P. Spiegel, *Men under Stress* (Philadelphia: Blakiston, 1945); page numbers refer to the 1963 paperback edition (New York: McGraw-Hill), 15–16, 38, 56–57, 82.

11. Robert J. Bernucci and Albert J. Glass, eds., *Neuropsychiatry in World War II* (Washington, DC: Office of the Surgeon General; Department of the Army, 1966), 1:16–37, 20–22. Cf. Shephard, *War of Nerves*, 197–201.

12. White quoted in George Rosen, "Social Stress and Mental Disease from the Eighteenth Century to the Present: Some Origins of Social Psychiatry," *Milbank Memorial Fund Quarterly*, 37 (1959): 27; Osler quoted in Lawrence E. Hinkle, "The Concept of 'Stress' in the Biological and Social Sciences," *International Journal of Psychiatry in Medicine*, 5 (1974): 331.

13. G. Elliot Smith and T. H. Pear, *Shell Shock and Its Lessons* (Manchester, UK: Manchester University Press, 1918), 67.

14. Quoted in Shephard, *War of Nerves*, 151.

15. William C. Porter, "Military Psychiatry and the Selective Service," *War Medicine* 1, no. 3 (1941): 364–71; Porter, "Military Psychiatry," *War Medicine* 2, no. 4 (1942): 543–50; James A. Brussel and Harold R. Wolpert, "The Pychoneuroses in Military Psychiatry," *War Medicine* 3, no. 2 (1943): 139–54. For Porter's career, see Bernucci and Glass, *Neuropsychiatry*, 55.

16. Norman Q. Brill, "War Neuroses," *Military Surgeon* 90 (April 1942): 390ff; reprinted in *Journal of Laboratory and Clinical Medicine* 28 (1942–43): 490, 496. Page citations from reprinted version.

17. J. L. Henderson and Merrill Moore, "The Psychoneuroses of War," *New England Journal of Medicine* 230, no. 10 (March 1944): 273, 277.

18. Paul T. McAlpine, "Hysterical Visual Defects," *War Medicine* 5, no. 5 (1944): 129–32; Commission on Military Neuropsychiatry, *Research Publications of the Association for Research in Nervous and Mental Illness*, vol. 25 (Baltimore: Willliams and Wilkins, 1946); John C. Whitehorn, "Changing Concepts of Psychoneurosis in Relation to Military Psychiatry," in Commission on Military Neuropsychiatry, *Research Publications*, 1–7; discussion following by William C. Porter, Francis Braceland, and others, 7–10.

19. Francis J. Braceland, remarks in discussion following Whitehorn's paper, "Changing Concepts," 8; Roy R. Grinker, "A Dynamic Study of War Neuroses in Flyers Returned to the United States," *Military Neuropsychiatry* 25 (1946): 26–37; Roy R. Grinker, "The Management of Neuropsychiatric Casualties in the Zone of Combat," in *Manual of Military Neuropsychiatry*, ed. Harry C. Solomon and Paul I. Yakovlev (Philadelphia: Saunders, 1944), 517; italics in the original.

20. William C. Menninger, "Psychiatric Experience in the War, 1941–1946," *American Journal of Psychiatry* 103 (1946–47): 579–80.

21. For the general history of British wartime and interwar psychiatry, see Edgar Jones and Simon Wessely, *Shell Shock to PTSD: Military Psychiatry from 1900 to the Gulf War* (New York: Psychology Press, 2005), 21–109; see also Shephard, *War of Nerves*, 1–297.

22. Irving I. Gottesman, "Eliot Slater (1904–1983): An Appreciation," *Behavior Genetics* 14 (1984): 107–10.

23. Eliot Slater, "Acute War Neuroses," *Lancet* 2 (1940): 1.

24. Hector Warnes, "Eric D. Wittkower (1899–1983)," *International Review of Psycho-Analysis* 10 (1983): 471–72.

25. Eric Wittkower, "The Psychological Factor in Cardiac Pain," *Lancet*, September 18, 1937, 665–70.

26. Emanuel Miller, ed., *The Neuroses in War* (New York: Macmillan, 1940), 6, 10, 169.

27. Shephard, *War of Nerves*, 213.

28. Kurt Goldstein, "On So-Called War Neuroses," *Psychosomatic Medicine* 5 (1943): 376.

29. E. Rogers Smith, "Neuroses Resulting from Combat," *American Journal of Psychiatry* 100 (1943): 94–95. On the extraordinary horrors of Guadalcanal, see Shephard, *War of Nerves*, 223.

30. William C. Menninger, *Psychiatry in a Troubled World: Yesterday's War and Today's Challenge* (New York: Macmillan, 1948), 41.

31. Saul Benison, A. Clifford Barger, and Elin L. Wolfe, *Walter B. Cannon: The Life and Times of a Young Scientist* (Cambridge: Belknap, 1987); Elin L. Wolfe, A. Clifford Barger, and Saul Benison, *Walter B. Cannon, Science and Society* (Cambridge: Countway Library of Medicine, 2000); Chandler MacCuskey Brooks, Kiyomi Koizumi, and James O. Pinkston, eds., *The Life and Contributions of Walter Bradford Cannon, 1871–1945* (New York: SUNY Downstate Medical Center, 1975); Saul Benison and A. Clifford Barger, "Walter Bradford Cannon," in *Dictionary of Scientific Biography*, ed. Charles C. Gillispie (New York: Scribner's Sons, 1978), 15:71–77.

32. Allan Young, "Walter Cannon and the Psychophysiology of Fear," in *Greater Than the Parts: Holism in Biomedicine, 1920–1950*, ed. Christopher Lawrence and George Weisz (New York: Oxford University Press, 1998), 234–56; Otniel E. Dror, "The Affect of Experiment: The Turn to Emotions in Anglo-American Physiology, 1900–1940," *Isis* 90 (1999): 205–37.

33. Walter B. Cannon, *Bodily Changes in Pain, Hunger, Fear and Rage* (New York: Appleton, 1915).

34. Walter B. Cannon, "The Mechanism of Emotional Disturbance of Bodily Functions," *New England Journal of Medicine*, 198 (1928): 878, 884.

35. Walter B. Cannon, "The Stresses and Strains of Homeostasis," *American Journal of the Medical Sciences* 189 (1935): 7.

36. Walter B. Cannon, "'Voodoo' Death," *American Anthropologist* 44 (1942): 169–81.

37. For an overview of Liddell's work, see James D. Block, "In Memoriam: Howard S. Liddell, Ph.D., 1895–1962," *Psychosomatic Medicine* 25 (January 1, 1963): 1–2. See also Howard S. Liddell, William Thomas James, and Oscar Daniel Anderson, *The Comparative Physiology of the Conditioned Motor Reflex* (Baltimore: Johns Hopkins University Press, 1934); Howard S. Liddell, "Conditioned Reflex Method and Experimental Neurosis," in *Personality and the Behavior Disorders*, ed. Joseph McVicker Hunt (New York: Ronald, 1944), 1:389–412; and Howard S. Liddell, "The Experimental Neurosis," *Annual Review of Physiology* 9 (1947): 569–80. For Masserman, see Jules H. Masserman, *Behavior and Neurosis: An Experimental Psychoanalytic Approach to Psychobiologic Principles* (Chicago: University of Chicago Press, 1943).

38. Edward Glover, "In Honor of Lawrence Kubie," *Journal of Nervous and Mental Diseases* 149 (1969): 5–18.

39. For Grinker as a Rockefeller grantee, see Theodore M. Brown, "Alan Gregg and the Rockefeller Foundation's Support of Franz Alexander's Psychosomatic

Research," *Bulletin of the History of Medicine* 61 (1987): 167; for Kubie, see folder 7359, box 715, series 1.5, General Education Board Collection, Rockefeller Archive Center, Sleepy Hollow, New York; folders 1342–53, boxes 109–10; and folders 950–53, box 79, series 200A, RG 1.1, Rockefeller Foundation Archives.

40. Liddell, "Experimental Neurosis," 572.

41. Grinker and Spiegel, *War Neuroses*, 131.

42. Lawrence S. Kubie, "The Emergency Care and Treatment of the Acute War Neuroses," in Solomon and Yakovlev, *Manual of Military Neuropsychiatry*, 555.

43. Hale, *Rise and Crisis*, 302–6.

44. Grob, *From Asylum to Community*, 292–93.

45. H. C. S., "Abraham Myerson (1881–1948)," *New England Journal of Medicine* 239 (1948): 982–83. See also Edward Shorter, *A History of Psychiatry: From the Era of the Asylum to the Age of Prozac* (New York: Wiley and Sons, 1997), 185.

46. Abraham Myerson, review of *Men under Stress*, by Roy R. Grinker and John P. Spiegel, *American Journal of Psychiatry* 103 (1946): 138–39.

47. Brown, "Alan Gregg," 161–64.

48. Roy R. Grinker, *Fifty Years in Psychiatry: A Living History* (Springfield, IL: Charles C. Thomas, 1979), esp. chaps. 2 and 13.

49. For a good overview of Cobb's career and contributions, see Benjamin V. White, *Stanley Cobb: A Builder of the Modern Neurosciences* (Boston: Countway Library, 1984). For Cobb's exploration of stress perspectives, see Stanley Cobb, *Borderlands of Psychiatry* (Cambridge: Harvard University Press, 1943), 149; Jacob E. Finesinger and Stanley Cobb, "Psychoneuroses and Psychosomatic Disorders," in Solomon and Yakovlev, *Manual of Military Neuropsychiatry*, 128–59, esp. 143; and Stanley Cobb, *Foundations of Neuropsychiatry* (Baltimore: Williams and Wilkins, 1952), 274.

50. Grinker and Spiegel, *Men under Stress*, 427–28.

51. Grob, *From Asylum to Community*, 28–40.

52. William C. Menninger, "Psychiatric Experience in the War, 1941–1946," reprinted in Bernard Hall, ed., *A Psychiatrist for a Troubled World: Selected Papers of William C. Menninger, M.D.* (New York: Viking, 1967), 528–42, esp. 532–33, 534.

53. "The Role of Psychiatry in the World Today," reprinted in ibid., 568–81, esp. 578–79.

54. Menninger, *Troubled World*, 351–62.

55. Ibid., 495–98.

56. See, for example, "Life of Stress," *Time* 56 (October 9, 1950): 93–94; "Stress Diseases," *Newsweek* 35 (June 26, 1950): 40; "Stress: The Cause of All Disease?," *Reader's Digest* (January 1955): 24–28.

57. Russell Viner, "Putting Stress in Life: Hans Selye and the Making of Stress Theory," *Social Studies of Science* 29, no. 3 (1999): 391–410.

58. Hans Selye, "A Syndrome Produced by Diverse Nocuous Agents," *Nature* 138 (July 4, 1936): 32; Selye, "The Prevention of Adrenalin Lung Edema by the Alarm Reaction," *American Journal of Physiology* 122, no. 2 (1938): 347–51; Selye, "The General Adaptation Syndrome and the Diseases of Adaptation," *Journal of Clinical Endocrinology* 6, no. 2 (1946): 117–230. For "stress" references, see, for example, 131 and 186.

59. For Selye's "aviators" references, see "General Adaptation Syndrome," 179 and 181.

Chapter Six

The Machinery and the Morale

Physiological and Psychological Approaches to Military Stress Research in the Early Cold War Era

TULLEY LONG

During World War II the US military launched an extensive initiative aimed at fighting the debilitating phenomenon of combat stress in its ranks. Even after the war, however, as Cold War tensions threatened to erupt in Korea, the prevention of soldier breakdown due to the psychological or emotional pressures of combat continued to present an urgent problem, and the military was keen to draw on any available tool to increase the effectiveness of soldiers on the battlefield. While psychology and psychiatry had provided certain insights during World War II on how morale and leadership could help to mitigate soldier failure, the 1940s had wrought another route for investigating and solving the problem of combat stress in the form of new physiological knowledge about the role of the pituitary and adrenal hormones in responding to stress.[1] In the early 1950s stress research within the military context sought to mobilize the most recent laboratory studies on endocrine stress responses and integrate them with the knowledge gained by military psychiatrists, all in the effort to keep their soldiers in top fighting form and, ultimately, ensure American security in an uncertain time.

The present chapter seeks to explore more deeply how the physiological concept of the stress response became constitutive of combat-stress studies by analyzing three episodes from military stress research in the 1950s: the 1952 Study of Combat Stress in Korea from the Johns Hopkins University's Operations Research Office; the 1953 Symposium on Stress held at the Walter Reed Army Medical Center; and the "psychoendocrine" research of the physiologist John W. Mason and the psychologist Joseph V. Brady at Walter Reed's Division of Neuropsychiatry. Through these case studies I argue that the translation of the physiological research on stress into the military setting was prompted by the great potential that tests based on laboratory physiology had to quantify, monitor, and predict a soldier's reaction to the stress of battle. Within a military culture in which there was an existing tradition of psychological and psychiatric approaches to combat stress, however, the shortcomings of a purely physiological notion of stress, as well as the problems with researching combat stress in the field, became apparent. Ultimately, the military's need for clear practical results forced researchers to examine more closely the interrelationships between the physiological and psychological manifestations of stress.

The idea of the physiological stress response is most often associated with the scientist Hans Selye and his theory of stress as a general, nonspecific reaction of an organism to challenges in its environment. Mediated through the endocrine cascade of the pituitary gland and the adrenal cortex, Selye saw this response as manifesting in a distinctive syndrome that proceeded in three phases: a "general alarm reaction" with the appearance of certain characteristic physiological symptoms after an injury or challenge; the stage of resistance, in which the organism appears to recover or adapt to the challenge; and finally a stage of exhaustion, marked by a return of the initial symptoms and death. In their historical treatments of Selye and the development of this "general adaptation syndrome," both Russell Viner and Anne Harrington have pointed to the role of the United States military in championing Selye's ideas and expanding physiological stress research beyond the laboratory and onto the battlefield.[2] In fact, the Korean War provided an opportunity for an interdisciplinary team of scientists and doctors from the Operations Research Office (ORO) of the Johns Hopkins University to put the theories and methods of stress physiology to the test by studying the behavior and endocrine activity of soldiers in the field. The 1952 ORO combat-stress study, while demonstrating the practical difficulties of conducting stress research in the field, actively drew on Selye's theories to make sense of the data they managed to collect.

Selye, however, was not the only architect of the pituitary-adrenocortical stress response, nor were his ideas wholly and universally adopted by the scientific community and the military. Rather, scientists' understanding and formulation of the mechanisms and actions of the stress response were still in great flux in the early 1950s. Discussions between scientists at the 1953 Walter Reed Symposium on Stress illustrated the extent to which the details of the body's physiological reaction to stressful circumstances were still vague and contentious.[3] In addition, the symposium participants emphasized the continuing importance of psychological factors in determining a soldier's ability to withstand the pressures of battle. Given the tenuous state of the existing knowledge about physiological stress, the application of stress physiology to the practical issues of combat stress proved problematic and demonstrated the deficiencies of viewing stress through a purely physiological lens, driving researchers to call for incorporation of older psychological approaches to combat stress with the newer tools of stress physiology.

While the examples of the ORO study of combat stress in Korea and the 1953 Walter Reed Symposium on Stress highlight the desire for such integrative investigations and the difficulties inherent in achieving them, research succeeded in following a new course in the 1950s at the Walter Reed Army Institute of Research. Within Walter Reed's Division of Neuropsychiatry, the military motivation to solve the operational dilemma of combat stress and a uniquely collaborative institutional environment combined to produce research that cut across different disciplines and sought to integrate the mind and the body by treating the problem of stress as a problem of the whole organism. One such integrative investigation at Walter Reed, and the example on which this essay concludes, was the "psychoendocrine" research of the physiologist John W. Mason and the psychologist Joseph V. Brady. Mason and Brady's extensive experiments on conditioned rhesus monkeys demonstrated the important connections between the psychological and emotional factors and the endocrine stress response. The products of Mason and Brady's collaboration would also eventually force the reevaluation of the generalized, purely physiological stress response proposed by Selye. Instead, Mason and Brady used the tools of psychology and physiology to argue for the importance of specificity and individual variation in the way organisms, including soldiers, react to physical and mental challenges.

The Problem of Combat Stress

During the late 1940s and 1950s US military psychiatrists and officers concerned with the psychological health of their soldiers became increasingly interested in stress research along the lines of Hans Selye's work on the general adaptation syndrome. The problem of war neuroses was certainly not new to the US military, which had first offered in-field psychiatric treatment during World War I to soldiers incapacitated by the mental pressure of battle to return them quickly to duty.[4] With the onset of World War II, psychiatrists were once again called on to help reduce the incidence of crippling war neuroses, a goal initially thought to be possible through screening programs aimed to prevent recruits with a predisposition to mental illness from joining the ranks of enlisted men. By the end of 1942, with the rate of psychiatric casualties still climbing in the wake of the devastating campaigns at Guadalcanal and in Tunisia, psychiatrists were able to convince the military leadership to renew the program of short-term, in-field psychotherapy.[5] Among this group of psychiatrists were Roy G. Grinker and John P. Spiegel, whose handbook for treating psychiatric war casualties advocated the view that anxiety, fear, and even breakdown in the face of battle were normal reactions to challenging circumstances and could be mitigated through modifying the soldier's experience of the stressful environment of war by raising morale and instilling strong bonds between members of a given military unit.[6]

While military psychiatrists focused on the external factors influencing a soldier's ability to function under stressful wartime conditions, there was also war research devoted to bolstering the internal physiological defenses. Specifically, there was interest within military medicine in the biochemical research on the hormones of the adrenal cortex. Owing to their purported capacity to make an organism less vulnerable to all kinds of challenges, including hypoxia and shock, adrenocortical extracts had become the object of an intense and competitive race during the 1930s to purify, identify, and synthesize the constituent hormones. These studies eventually attracted the military's attention after rumors surfaced that the Germans were using the extracts to fortify the pilots of the Luftwaffe at high altitudes. In 1941 the Office of Scientific Research and Development convened a committee to organize an effort to synthesize the simplest adrenocortical steroid, "Compound A." Although the group successfully synthesized the hormone, the idea that this research had military applications had been all but abandoned by 1944, after the hormone had proven to be fairly ineffective in increasing stamina and resistance to various stress-causing situations.[7]

Following the war, however, several developments revived interest in the adrenal cortex and the physiological side of stress, including the publication of Hans Selye's first thorough statement of his stress theory in 1946.[8] In addition, the research group of the biochemist Edward Kendall at the Mayo Foundation, one of the central research groups involved with the early work on adrenocortical extracts and the wartime work on Compound A, continued its efforts to synthesize the hormones of the adrenal cortex and find efficacious therapeutic uses for them. Kendall's team successfully produced the much more potent adrenocortical steroid, Compound E, and dramatically used it late in 1948 to treat the debilitating symptoms of rheumatoid arthritis. Kendall received the Nobel Prize in Physiology or Medicine in 1950 for his research on Compound E, eventually christened as cortisone. This recognition helped to create momentum behind research in endocrine physiology and sparked growing public fascination with the therapeutic potential of the hormones involved in the stress reaction described by Selye.

The military medical community shared in this postwar enthusiasm, particularly in light of the Cold War threat of communism, international instability, and the advent of the Korean conflict in 1950. With such conflicts continuing through the early Cold War period, the debilitating effects of battle stress became the focus of more intensive study. An understanding of how hormone levels and physiological function influenced the battlefield performance and psychological health of men in uniform might, it was hoped, provide new avenues by which to address the still-acute problem of combat stress. Several government institutions and affiliates established programs of stress research in the early 1950s, including research programs at the Walter Reed Army Institute of Research in Washington, DC, and the Naval Medical Research Institute in Bethesda, Maryland, as well as a combat-stress study by the Operations Research Office (ORO) of the Johns Hopkins University. The examples under scrutiny in this chapter, the 1952 ORO study of combat stress, the 1953 Walter Reed Symposium on Stress, and the psychoendocrine research of Walter Reed scientists John W. Mason and Joseph V. Brady, all demonstrate a commitment within military stress research toward finding linkages between physiological and psychological phenomena involved in an organism's stress response. Such an integrative approach promised to provide a comprehensive, operational solution to the complicated problem of battle stress that incorporated the most recent work on the endocrine processes of the pituitary and adrenal glands with the knowledge gained by military psychiatrists during the war.

The Operations Research Office's 1952 Study of Combat Stress in Korea

As with previous studies of war neuroses and battle fatigue, the 1952 ORO study of combat stress in Korea, commissioned by the US Army, sought ultimately to determine what causal factors led a soldier to breakdown in combat and what steps may be taken to prevent it. Well aware of the promising developments in laboratory research on the role of the pituitary-adrenal system in the stress response, the ORO team's leader, the psychologist Stanley W. Davis, recognized the "tremendous gap in knowledge between basic research already accomplished in laboratories throughout the country and the operational problem" of improving the performance of combat soldiers on the ground.[9] Their primary aim, therefore, was to study men in actual battle conditions and describe any discrete, quantifiable changes occurring in both the soldier's physiological and psychological states under fire that might prove valuable in improving infantry effectiveness.

Under the aegis of the ORO and the armed forces, a thirteen-member team composed of physiologists, biochemists, psychologists, and psychiatrists traveled to Korea in the fall of 1952. "It was an unusual team in many respects," Stanley Davis later wrote. "Not only did it represent all of these sciences, it also represented different interested groups in that six of the people were from the Navy, two from the Army, and five from the Operations Research Office."[10] Though a mixed group of civilian and military experts, the team seemed committed to the practical goal of improving military effectiveness through a thorough study of in situ combat stress. While the military personnel had a clear motivation toward this end, the ORO's aims are perhaps less obvious. Operations research originated as a field during World War II to streamline complex wartime decisions and strategies, as well as optimize performance and use of mechanical instruments and systems.[11] The combat-stress study was conceived as part of an initiative at the ORO aimed at "improving the effectiveness of the infantry man-weapon combination." Since stress altered and reduced the functioning of that system, the ORO very much saw the issue of combat stress as "an operational or an action problem."[12] Instead of attempting to refine the performance of tank armor or improve convoy logistics, Davis's team sought to understand how, physiologically and psychologically, the stress of combat changed soldiers' abilities to carry out their roles and what steps might be taken to ensure that infantrymen operated at peak effectiveness during the heat of battle. Any measure that might be taken prior to or during the course of combat operations, including improving the methods by which soldiers were screened for their relative effectiveness in combat or determining the "optimal" duration of exposure to combat to maintain a functional fighting unit, would be considered. Long-term effects of stress were not within the purview of the study because the team's operational approach to combat stress was an interest in, as Davis put it, "the acute problem rather than the chronic one, and in prediction, not cures."[13]

As united as the ORO team seemed in its overall goals, the scientists drew on their various disciplinary backgrounds to design the study and tackle both aspects of the operational problem: the effect of combat stress on the functions of the body and on the workings of the mind. Physiologists and biochemists devoted to the former objective comprised about half of the thirteen-member team and came from both civilian institutions and from the military.[14] Acting in a consulting capacity, Fred Elmadjian, a staff physiologist from the Worcester Foundation for Experimental Biology in Massachusetts, brought his experience in adrenal cortical physiology to the ORO's Korea study. The Worcester Foundation had been founded in 1944 by the physiologists Hudson Hoagland and Gregory Pincus as a nonprofit biomedical research institution after they became disillusioned with the strictures they felt were placed on their scientific work at Clark University. At the Worcester Foundation, Pincus and Hoagland expanded on an earlier study of fatigue in pilots to build an extensive program of research on the adrenal cortical functions of normal and stressed populations, particularly the mentally ill. They also made graduate education a priority, inviting many college and graduate students into their laboratories to get a feel for experimental science and conduct doctoral research.[15] Elmadjian was one of these graduate students, joining the Worcester staff while pursuing a master's degree at Clark and later a PhD in physiology at Tufts University.

As such, the young physiologist was heavily involved during the 1940s with the foundation's research and was thus well positioned to carry out scientific work on stress physiology for the ORO.[16]

The rest of the Korea study's physiology group was composed of officers and reservists associated with the Office of Naval Research. David Minard, who held both a medical degree and a doctorate in physiology from the University of Chicago, as well as the rank of lieutenant commander in the navy, represented the Naval Medical Research Institute in Bethesda, Maryland, where he oversaw physiology research between 1946 and 1952. His research concerned the physiological stress caused by extreme temperatures, and, as part of his military work, he helped to develop the Wet Bulb Globe Temperature Index to assess a soldier's exposure to high temperature and prevent heat-related injuries.[17] Nello Pace of the University of California at Berkeley was also interested in the effect of extreme environmental situations on human physiology, though his work focused on influences of high altitude and low atmospheric oxygen. Fresh out of his doctoral work in physiology at Berkeley when World War II commenced, Pace joined the navy and helped to organize the physiology department of the Naval Medical Research Institute (NMRI). In 1946 he left the NMRI physiology program in Minard's care and returned to Berkeley, only to be recalled to duty during the Korean War to assist with the combat-stress study as leader of the Office of Naval Research (ONR) Research Unit Number One.[18] Four members of this unit accompanied Pace to Korea to provide technical assistance for the physiological and biochemical tests of the combat-stress study.[19]

While the physiology work drew on both the ORO and the military personnel, the psychology testing was administered almost wholly through the civilian staff and consultants of the ORO. Stanley W. Davis had just earned his PhD in psychology from Cornell University when he joined the ORO as an operations analyst in 1951.[20] His doctoral research concerned a method for measuring mental fatigue that determined the threshold frequency at which an individual could detect intermittent light or sound inputs rather than mentally fuse them into a perception of a constant signal. After a prolonged or intense mental task, such as the completion of complex multiplication problems without writing anything down, Davis found the threshold frequency at which his test subjects could perceive visual flickers or auditory flutters was much lower, indicating such measurements as a promising index for fatigue.[21] As part of the ORO study, Davis designed similar fusion frequency tests to measure mental fatigue due to stimulation of battle rather than arithmetic. Lincoln F. Hanson was another newly minted psychology PhD, having received his degree from Columbia University just months before the ORO team shipped out to Korea in September 1952. His specialty was the psychology of motivation, which would have fit in with reigning notions of the importance of morale and leadership in mitigating combat stress.[22]

Finally, the psychology portion of the study also drew on the experience of the seasoned psychologist Howard S. Liddell of Cornell University.[23] Fifty-seven years old at the time of the Korean study, Liddell had already established his place as "the father of American experimental psychopathology" three decades earlier when he produced experimental neuroses in sheep using Pavlovian conditioning methods.[24] Subsequent studies on the conditioning of young sheep and goats helped to elaborate the role of maternal protection in easing the effects of external stresses.[25] Liddell took an active role in the ORO study, traveling to the front to complete the psychological observations in person rather than staying at the study's staging grounds in Japan. His work on the front lines in Korea was a life-changing experience for Liddell, resulting in a conviction that behavioral scientists held a responsibility to extend their research and conclusions toward the improvement of human behavior and the well-being of society, a belief that he espoused in his writings and public lectures during the remaining decade of his life.[26]

On the ground in Korea the team planned to carry out a battery of different physiological and psychological tests on infantrymen stationed along the main line of resistance. The bulk of the study consisted of physiological assessments aimed to estimate the pituitary-adrenal activity of the soldiers through analyzing blood, urine, and saliva for constituents, including certain hormone metabolites, electrolytes, and blood cells, that were believed to be indicative of the stress response. One other physiological evaluation, intended to evaluate the action of the autonomic nervous system in maintaining homeostasis, involved monitoring blood pressure after an injection of the vasodilator Mecholyl and observing how the body responded to the resulting low blood pressure.[27] In addition to qualitative psychiatric interviews, the ORO team also sought to gain a quantitative measure of the infantrymen's psychological response to the pressures of battle. Visual and auditory tests, similar to those Davis developed in his doctoral work, were used to gauge basic sensory perception, while higher mental functions were evaluated through a slew of paper-and-pencil tests, such as Gottschaldt figures and sequence completion.[28] In addition to these more "objective psychological measures," the team also allowed time for psychiatric interviews with soldiers to obtain the "broadest possible evaluation of the individual."[29]

This ambitious array of tests, which collectively took up to three hours to complete, were intended to be administered to the "soldier-subjects" three or four times: a baseline measurement prior to combat, once more immediately following combat when the stress response would still be active, and at several points over the subsequent weeks of recovery.[30] To administer their tests to the soldiers in a timely manner, the team placed its base of operations and a biochemical laboratory in a prefabricated shell at a Mobile Army Surgical Hospital about an hour's drive from the main line of resistance.[31] In addition, the team equipped two jeeps and a trailer with rudimentary laboratory equipment and a small gasoline generator that allowed some members of the ORO team to venture with the troops to the front lines to collect blood and urine samples following combat and to perform basic tasks, such as harvesting plasma through centrifugation.[32] Only a subset of the ORO team, likely the technicians from the ONR, made the dangerous journey to the front lines.[33] The rest of the team remained behind at the MASH, waiting to analyze the unstable biological samples as soon as they arrived. All the physiological and psychological tests were designed to be completed on the ground in Korea, with the exception of several urine samples that would be sent back to professional laboratories in the United States for evaluation.[34]

The challenges of collecting reliable data in a combat zone soon made themselves apparent. A week after the researchers' arrival in Korea, enemy offensives suspended the scheduled combat operations for the patrol that the ORO team had planned to study. When another rifle company was called to participate in a major attack a week later, the researchers could run only a limited set of precombat tests on twenty-four men due the short notice of the soldiers' deployment. Once the attacking company returned from the sixteen-hour assault, transportation and communication delays rendered it impossible to collect the blood and urine samples directly after the cessation of combat, as the research plan dictated. In addition, due to a 65 percent casualty rate in the attacking company, only five soldiers who had taken the precombat tests participated in the postcombat research, and the researchers were forced to acquire the majority of the attacking company's postcombat data from individuals for which no baseline had been obtained. Similarly, although the ORO team was able to obtain postcombat data on another rifle company that defended the position won by the attacking company in the initial assault, no precombat tests were run for the defending group.[35]

Due to the ever-changing circumstances of combat, much of the ORO team's research was eventually deemed problematic or even useless. This was particularly true for the quantitative tests for the soldiers' psychological changes, which showed negligible differences in their state of mind before and after combat. While the researchers thought these null results might be due to learning effects or insufficient sensitivity in the test design, they concluded that the reason was more likely the erratic timing of the tests and insufficient control over the testing environment. "In a combat zone it is practically impossible to establish a suitable psychology laboratory," the preliminary report explained. "The better the laboratory, i.e., the more controlled the conditions, the farther back it must be from the combat area. The farther back, the greater the time lag between the occurrence of the effects and the measurement of those effects."[36] In all the tests conducted, the researchers also noted "tremendous individual variation," which undermined the ability of the team to draw general conclusions regarding the results, especially in regard to making any meaningful correlations between the psychological and psychiatric observations and the physiological data.[37]

Despite the trouble with the quantitative psychological section of the study, the fact that the original research plan had to be abandoned and refashioned to fit the new combat operations did provide for some interesting preliminary observations on the physiological and qualitative psychological changes undergone by the infantrymen. Most notably, the two rifle companies faced different intensities and durations of combat, allowing an unforeseen opportunity for comparative study of their respective stress responses. Upon returning from the field, the assault infantrymen, who experienced unceasing, intense combat for sixteen hours against a well-defended enemy on higher ground, "gave a clear clinical impression of an extremely fatigued group." Their appearance was "drawn and gaunt" with "no spontaneous expressions of amusement," and their responses to conversation were described as "depressed and dulled," "lethargic," and "unenthusiastic." Although the defending soldiers spent five whole days in the combat zone and also showed signs of fatigue, they were "considerably more alert and cheerful" than the attacking company, even laughing and volunteering to help the ORO team with sample collection.[38]

Once the urine and blood samples were analyzed, the physiological differences between the two rifle companies also became apparent. For instance, increases in 17-ketosteroids, the metabolic end product of the adrenocortical hormones, were used as indicators of adrenal cortex activity and, therefore, the stress response. Having experienced more intense combat and having suffered higher casualties than the defending company, the attacking company unsurprisingly showed increased levels of 17-ketosteroid in their urine after returning from the front. The defending company, on the other hand, showed very low 17-ketosteroid levels, even after injection with the pituitary hormone, adrenocorticotropic hormone (ACTH), that stimulates the release of adrenocorticoids. This finding implied that, during a long exposure to moderate severity of combat, the defending soldiers had exhausted their reserve of adrenocortical hormones, leaving them unable to muster a normal physiological reaction even when the researchers tried to trigger the stress response artificially with ACTH.[39] This conclusion that the activity of the adrenal cortex could be suppressed by long-term exposure to combat was further bolstered with the observation that the defending soldiers, despite their more lively demeanor following their return from battle, took about twice as long to recover than the men of the attacking company.

In interpreting these results the authors of the ORO study on combat stress leaned heavily on the recent research elucidating of the role of the pituitary-adrenal cortical axis in adapting to stress. Specifically, they adopted

Selye's theory of the general adaptation syndrome as a framework and explanatory tool and invoked its language of nonspecificity and generality from the outset. For example, in explaining the role of the adrenal cortex in the stress response, they wrote, "Although each stress, such as a burn, wound, infection, or psychic disturbance, has a description and a response specific for the stressing agent, there is one response in the organism common to all these different conditions which involves the function of the adrenal cortex. This adrenal cortical response is called the non-specific stress response of the organism."[40] Further, while the preliminary report of 1952 did not mention Selye overtly, the physiologists of the team, particularly Elmadjian, who came to the study with experience in such research at the Worcester Foundation, would have been well aware of Selye's contribution to the field.

Popular presentations of the ORO study made the team's integration of Selye's ideas into their interpretation explicit. In a 1958 *Scientific American* article, Davis noted that the initially confounding differences observed in the attacking and defending groups "can be explained neatly . . . by Hans Selye's theory on the response of animal organisms to stress."[41] Later, in a Johns Hopkins University television program about the combat-stress study, the narrators, including ORO team member David Minard and the ORO analyst Jean Taylor, also employed Selye's three stages of adaptation in their explanations. In each case the ORO team members argued that the soldiers in the attacking group were under more stress for a shorter time, manifesting elevated adrenal activity but showing a greater capacity to recover. In both presentations this reaction was read as indicative of a classic Selye alarm-stage response. The longer recovery time that the defending soldiers experienced following their prolonged exposure to moderate combat, however, signaled that they had adapted to the stress of the battlefield and entered the resistance stage of the general adaptation syndrome.[42]

While it remains unclear just how important a physiological vision of stress like that of Hans Selye was in shaping the formulation of the ORO's initial research plan, the physiologists would have been cognizant of his theory and thus able to quickly mobilize it to interpret the puzzling results of their study. Further, the practical nature of the ORO study's goals suggest that the researchers may well have found the appeal of the physiological view of stress in its potential for application. In light of the difficulties that individual variation and uncontrolled conditions had caused for their fieldwork, the generality of Selye's stress response would mean that it would be easy to apply in military settings where group reactions to challenges and pressures of battle were important. Further, the physiology of stress provided the promise of accurate, efficient biological assays that would allow military leaders to monitor the stress responses of their men while on the ground. Even though the most positive results of the ORO study arose from the 17-ketosteroid test, which unfortunately was one of the few samples that could not be analyzed on-site in Korea, other measures, such as electrolyte ratios in saliva and urine, were tagged as possibly useful indicators of adrenal cortical activity.[43] As we will see shortly, the researchers involved with the Walter Reed Symposium on Stress were not so confident in the explanatory ability of Selye's theory or the reliability of existing physiological methods of quantifying stress.

The 1953 Symposium on Stress at Walter Reed

The same month that the ORO released its preliminary report from its study of stress in Korea, the Walter Reed Army Institute of Research in Washington, DC, held a major meeting on the subject of stress. The Symposium on Stress, held March 16–18, 1953, was the third annual symposium in a series that Colonel William Stone, the commandant of the Army Medical Service Graduate School, had organized to circulate the latest scientific findings on topics of interest to military medicine.[44] As with the ORO study, the Symposium on Stress brought together a diverse group of clinicians, psychiatrists, psychologists, and physiologists to facilitate "cross-fertilization of ideas . . . between workers of very different viewpoints and approaches."[45] While the ORO study had started out as this kind of interdisciplinary project, the difficult research setting and the ensuing dearth of usable data, particularly in the psychological section of the study, resulted in an emphasis on the recent advances in stress physiology as a way to generalize and quantify the stress responses of soldiers and ultimately improve their effectiveness in combat. In fact, when a complete report of the ORO combat-stress study finally appeared in published form in 1956, it was in the University of California Publications in Physiology series under the title "Physiological Studies on Infantrymen in Combat" and included none of the psychologists from the original research in Korea as author.[46] At the same time that this apparent retooling of the ORO study toward physiological and away from psychological analysis was underway, the 1953 Walter Reed symposium raised questions regarding the generality and accuracy of a strictly physiological view of stress and pushed for continued efforts to integrate research on physiological and psychological aspects of the problem.

The list of participant names attests to the variety of attendees and specialties represented at the symposium; among them were a number of military personnel from neuropsychiatry divisions at Walter Reed and Brooke Army Hospital in San Antonio, as well as psychiatrists and physiologists from prominent medical schools around the United States, including Harold Wolff from Cornell and Curt Richter from Johns Hopkins.[47] The three days of the symposium served to divide the meeting into three general topics. On Monday, March 16, the papers dealt with the physiological mechanisms by which organisms maintain homeostasis. The Tuesday sessions featured papers that pertained to the psychological factors of stress in a general sense. The topics of these papers, however, ranged from an abstract, technical talk on stress as "psychological transactions" that mediate the relationship between an organism and its emotional environment to more anecdotal accounts of specific individuals' reactions to stress. Finally, the papers on Wednesday all involved methods of managing and mitigating stress, with a special emphasis on experience and application in military settings. Despite the diversity in content and style, the symposium papers wrestled with a number of interlocking themes and issues: the tension between environmental and constitutional causes for an individual's reaction to stressful circumstances, the desirability of a generalizable theory of stress such as Selye's versus the recognition of its deficiencies, the reality of the wide degree of variation in individual responses, and, above all, the notion that a physiological understanding of the stress response was inseparable from the psychological aspects.

To be sure, Selye and his ideas loomed large at the Walter Reed symposium, though Selye himself was unable to attend. Unlike the ORO researchers, however, the participants of the Walter Reed symposium did not hesitate in pointing out the limitations of his ideas even as they acknowledged the great influence of his work and theories. The physiologists present mentioned Selye frequently throughout the conference, drawing attention to both his specific experimental contributions to the field and the helpfulness of the conceptual framework he established. In his introductory survey of the field, John C. Whitehorn, the Henry Phipps professor of psychiatry at the Johns Hopkins University, began by specifically acknowledging Hans Selye and "the great historical importance" and "stimulating effect" of his stress research. I. Arthur Mirsky, a professor of clinical science and psychiatry at the University of Pittsburgh, placed Selye within the esteemed lineage of physiological thinkers, such as Claude Bernard and Walter Cannon, citing Selye's work as building on the theory of homeostasis.[48] Even though the symposium occasionally aired concern over the free and casual way in which the word "stress" tended to be used, some found value in the malleability of the term. As Whitehorn explained,

> Stress is a rather broad conceptual term—like a tennis racket—with which we can manage to bat about, like tennis balls, some other concepts which are concerned with the more sharply definable reaction processes. . . . We may be able to get some use out of the term stress even if it is left vague and not very clearly defined, provided we succeed in specifying fairly sharply some of the aspects of the biological reactions to stress, in which I think we are actually more deeply interested.[49]

How sharply specified were the details of the physiology of stress in 1953? While monitoring the function of the pituitary-adrenal system provided some indication of an organism's reaction to stressful circumstances, the exact mechanisms by which the stress response acted were still far from clear at the time of the Walter Reed symposium. While Selye's theory detailed the way in which an organism responds to stimuli through activation of the adrenal cortex and subsequent liberation of cortical hormones, many questions remained. What produces a systemic response to an environmental challenge in the first place? What is the mechanism (or mechanisms) by which such a challenge initiates the alarm and resistance reactions described by Selye?

At the symposium several overview talks, given by Mirsky, Whitehorn, and others, outlined the jumble of opinions among physiologists regarding these questions.[50] While it was well known by 1953 that the anterior pituitary gland released a discrete hormone, adrenocorticotropic hormone (ACTH), which acted on the adrenal cortex, the way in which a damaging agent acted on the anterior pituitary to trigger the release of ACTH and thus the endocrine cascade of the stress response was a matter of debate.[51] While Selye believed that there must be some additional factor mediating the interaction between an outside stressor and the pituitary, others suggested a feedback mechanism in which epinephrine (adrenaline) released from the adrenal medulla directly stimulates the anterior pituitary.[52] In addition, increased ACTH secretion from the pituitary could be produced through stimulation of the hypothalamus, which was believed to secrete its own neurohormone. But, what was this agent, and could there be more than one? How did it (or they) act on the pituitary, and, indeed, what stimuli spur the hypothalamus into action in the first place? According to Mirsky, the only vague consensus that could be drawn in the matter was that the ultimate stress response of an organism must be dependent on complex interactions between neural and hormonal influences.[53]

Another major area of contestation was the mechanisms behind the action of hormones in the stress response. Although physiologists realized that hormonal activity seemed to be associated with changing rates of intracellular, enzymatic processes, some researchers actively questioned the assumption that hormones acted directly on such processes. For instance, the notion of the "permissive" nature of hormone action, advocated by the physiologist Dwight J. Ingle, was particularly intriguing to the assembled doctors and scientists.[54] Where Selye had conceived of cortical hormones directly regulating the stress response, Ingle imagined the adrenal cortex playing a supporting role, with corticosteroids influencing the responsiveness of cells and tissue to the influence of stressors. In a number of studies in the 1940s and early 1950s using intact and adrenalectomized rats, Ingle showed that typical physiological responses to hormones, such as estrogen's inhibition of hair growth or epinephrine's tendency to drain muscles of glycogen, could occur only when adrenal corticoids were present to "permit" these metabolic processes to move forward. As Mirsky summarized, "corticosteroids may be essential to, but not responsible for, the metabolic responses to damaging agents" that were part of the stress response.[55]

Ingle's work was representative of wider concerns among stress researchers regarding whether the reactions and quantifiable products under study (such as concentrations of eosinophils—a type of white blood cell—or levels of various hormone metabolites) were actually constitutive and functionally active in homeostatic mechanisms or whether they were simply indicators, artifacts, or secondary consequences of those mechanisms. As Whitehorn commented in his introductory remarks, "Some of these phenomena have been used as *indicators* of reaction to stress, without our knowing what sort of function they serve."[56] A paper presented by Rachmiel Levine, a prominent physiologist at the University of Chicago and then the chair of the Department of Medicine at Chicago's Michael Reese Hospital, illustrated these concerns. Since adrenal corticoids were known to be involved in metabolism, and a state of adrenal cortical insufficiency often lead to muscle weakness, Levine reckoned that the asthenia in adrenalectomized animals must stem from changes in muscle metabolism due to the lack of corticoids. On the contrary, Levine's experiments had shown that steroid deficiency induced muscle weakness because steroids impeded circulation in the muscle tissue, rather than acting directly in muscle metabolism. The question remained for Levine "whether a 'metabolic' change seen during the course of a stress response is primarily metabolic or whether in many instances such changes are secondary and may not be due to a set of factors non-metabolic in nature."[57]

In the same vein the possibility that some phenomena were simply indicative of stress rather than playing a primary regulatory role naturally led scientists to doubt the viability of their methods of monitoring and measuring the stress response. George Thorn of the Harvard Medical School, for instance, described his attempts to measure adrenal cortical activation resulting from injection of ACTH using levels of eosinophils and urinary 17-hydroxycorticoids (the same metabolic byproduct of adrenal cortical hormones on which the ORO study had relied).[58] Thorn and his colleagues showed that decreases in eosinophil levels occurred after administration of ACTH isolated from the pituitary gland. A corollary rise in the levels of 17-hydroxycorticoids, indicating the release of cortical steroids from the adrenal cortex and the activation of the stress response, did not always take place. The experiments suggested that eosinophil counts could not be used as an exclusive measure of the stress, as many scientists had hoped.[59]

In addition, even if certain molecules were proven to be accurate correlates of the stress response and behavior, military application of such tests required that they also be simple to analyze in the field. For instance, war research described by the physiologist Hudson Hoagland of the Worcester

Foundation for Experimental Biology demonstrated a quantifiable, inverse relationship between levels of 17-ketosteroid secretion and job performance among army pilots. Despite the promise of this method as a stress-fitness test, Hoagland himself hastened to add that such "elaborate analyses are not expedient" and suggested that other measures such as urinary potassium might prove to be more "rapid and useful assays of adrenal responsivity."[60] In light of the emphasis on military application that pervaded the conference, the holes in physiologists' understanding of the stress response, as well as the uncertainty surrounding how to efficiently and accurately measure an organism's reaction to challenges in the field, presented a serious barrier to immediate and effective deployment of stress research in combat situations.

As researchers continued to work out the niceties of the stress response as Selye had described it, they sometimes arrived at conclusions that directly challenged Selye's theory of the general adaptation syndrome. Selye's theory rested on several assumptions. First, Selye assumed that the alarm reaction and the resistance stage were both adaptive responses mediated primarily by adrenal cortical secretions. But how was the nature of this adaptation to be understood? Just as adrenal hormones might not be as integral to homeostatic mechanisms in acute instances, as Selye's initial work implied, some laboratory experiments had also shown that long-term adaptation was possible in certain instances even without the adrenal glands. Levine, for instance, recounted experiments in which an adrenalectomized animal, which would quickly become exhausted if subjected to moderate "mechanical trauma" in a revolving drum, was instead exposed to such trauma in increments over the course of a week. The experiments showed that the animal could "withstand the shock which he would not otherwise be able to bear." Levine continued,

> Therefore, if in the absence of a large section of the autonomic nervous system and in the absence of the adrenal medulla and the adrenal cortex, one can under certain conditions adapt to stimuli and react to them in the same way, exhibiting the same kind of changes that one sees in the normal animal and not succumb, then the adaptation seems to be at least in large part in the peripheral tissues rather than in transmission or mediation systems. In other words, it would seem that the cell ultimately is the main adaptive system of the body.

Such thinking suggested that Selye's idea of a centralized adaptive response, orchestrated and managed by the pituitary-adrenal system, was not entirely accurate and perhaps even drew scientific attention away from the true "locus of adaptation."[61]

The second assumption of Selye's general adaptation syndrome was that an organism responds to any number of specific stimuli in a general way. Levine's overview paper also highlighted the "divergences in reaction" to various stressful situations. In considering three such situations—starvation, obesity, and cold—Levine showed that not all chronic stresses produced the full syndrome described by Selye. In the cases of starvation and obesity, both conditions led initially to increased adrenal activity, gluconeogenesis, and other "symptoms" of the general adaptation syndrome. The survival of the fasting or obese organism, however, ultimately seemed to Levine to be dependent on pituitary and pancreatic function, respectively, rather than the adrenal cortex. Similarly, an animal exposed to cold seemed to rely on the thyroid. If different specific types of stimuli could produce various suites of physiological and hormonal response, Selye's claims regarding the generality of his theory were significantly undermined. As Levine adamantly concluded his paper,

> We tend to forget the specific changes which tissues and organs in the body as a whole undergo as a result of specific stimuli, in favor of a generalization which we have termed and accepted as "the" stress reaction. . . . Such generalization has a most inviting ring. It has stimulated a good deal of valuable work, both in the experimental and in the clinical domain. However . . . has too much attention been lavished on the nonspecific generalized reactions to a variety of stimuli, at the expense of looking for specific responses which characterize the reactions to a particular stimulus, and which may serve to distinguish them?[62]

Taking a stance directly opposed to Selye's approach, Levine focused his attention on the particular and diverse responses to stress rather than on the idea of a general or nonspecific response.

Despite the concerns of Levine and others, research on the pituitary-adrenal system during the 1930s and 1940s had clearly added to the knowledge of the body's response to environmental challenges and held great potential for the US military's goals of monitoring and relieving the debilitating effects of stress on its soldiers. For the participants of the Walter Reed symposium, however, the physiological view of stress was far from a magic bullet. In addition to the various questions about the accuracy and generality of the stress response raised in the first day of the meeting, many participants, physiologists and psychologists alike, felt a strict focus on the physiology of the stress response denied the influences of psychological and behavioral factors, which as discussed earlier, had long been of great interest and importance within the military. Rather, a full understanding of combat stress required the integration of both its psychological and physiological aspects.

One of the first papers that challenged a purely physiological view of stress was presented by Curt Richter, the influential psychobiologist from Johns Hopkins University, who argued that there are also behavioral adaptations that the organism can make when it attempts to counteract a stressing agent and maintain homeostasis. Richter's animal experiments probed the question of how the organism can control its electrolyte balance or body temperature through behavioral adaptations when the glands required for such metabolic regulation were surgically removed. Richter's thyroidectomized rats would, for instance, engage in vigorous nest-building exercises to prevent loss of body heat. Beyond reinforcing the idea that stress is a whole-organism response that is not simply physiological, Richter's approach to the problem of stress addressed how organisms could positively adapt to environmental challenges. In this way he departed from the focus of Selye and others interested in the medical aspects of stress, who were more concerned with "all the bodily changes that result from the breakdown of homeostasis as a result of stress."[63]

It was also crucial to acknowledge individual variation and the importance of context and past experience. The effectiveness of an organism's behavioral or psychological response, however positive, differed greatly from individual to individual and even from situation to situation, a fact that echoed the troubled psychological studies of the ORO. As the symposium participants repeated again and again in the second and third day of the symposium, any number of factors could affect an individual soldier's response to the pressures of combat. In his address on the second day of the symposium, Colonel Albert J. Glass, chief of the Neuropsychiatric Division at Brooke Army Hospital, explained how aspects of a soldier's personality, including his level of aggressiveness, sense of conscience or self-criticism, or egocentricity, all played a role in his ability to control fear and confront danger in a battle situation, thereby resisting the pressures driving him toward breakdown. In addition to these kinds of variations, the specificity of an individual's response seemed to depend on his perception of a situation, as well as the details of his past and present experiences. Among the US Air Force fliers that the psychiatrist Douglas Bond of Western Reserve University treated during World War II, the men's ability or inability to withstand the pressures of warfare lay not only in their dispositions but also in their particular experiences in battle and their perception of the danger or risk involved. If a flier's buddy was killed or his unit had suffered a large number of losses, he would be much more likely to have an anxiety reaction due to the psychic trauma of his particular experience.[64]

Although individual personality and specific circumstance were recognized to be central factors contributing to combat stress, from an operational standpoint such issues could not be evaluated, due to the extreme difficulty of accurately measuring or predicting how a personality type might react to the charged, ever-fluctuating environment of the combat zone. Since stress responses depended in part on experience and hence on chance events, individual human behavior was ultimately not fully predictable. "Probably one of the important lessons we learned from World War II," Henry W. Brosin, a professor of psychiatry from the University of Pittsburgh, reminded his audience, "was that even after men with massive physical and psychiatric incapacity had been selected out at some early stage of training, it was not easy to predict how long or arduous a service a man could give before he failed." Bond concurred, adding that it was the hefty element of chance involved in an individual's experience that rendered impossible the notion of selecting for men who would remain functional and well adjusted. "How can we select the men who will not sit next to those who will get their heads shot off?" he queried.[65]

For military purposes, then, it was far easier to control for the other psychological properties that had been proven to help control fear of battle and combat failure. To this end many of the Walter Reed symposium's speakers emphasized the same themes and directives that Grinker and Spiegel espoused a decade earlier, such as the importance of encouraging morale and group coherence, as well as providing adequate motivation and strong leadership. Additionally, several of the psychiatrists in attendance, including Spiegel himself and Jurgen Ruesch of the University of California School of Medicine, spoke about the value of maintaining strong communication both during and following stressful situations, because free flow of information strengthens group bonds, mitigates the pressures on the individual, and ultimately improves morale.[66] By looking at patterns of stress in groups, as well as aiming to modify the psychological environment in which a soldier operated, this approach sidestepped the difficulties inherent in examining and correcting for the highly variable stress responses in individuals.

For the participants in the Walter Reed symposium, these issues of motivation and morale, while ostensibly the domain of psychology, had real consequences for the successful functioning of the soldier in the heat of battle. In a paper aimed to find equations by which "a commander can calculate the maximum possible duration of effort at every horsepower level" for his soldiers, Wallace Fenn, a physiologist from the University of Rochester School of Medicine, ultimately saw his equations as unable to account for the other crucial side of maintenance of a soldier's energy output. Humans, quite simply, were not machines. "These equations describe the machinery or the means," Fenn stated in conclusion, "but the motivation and morale are equally or even more important—machinery and morale, and the greater of these is morale." As Whitehorn phrased it, "the psychiatrist must perforce acknowledge these physiological limitations and their variability in different individuals and under different conditions; just as the physiologist who would understand well the utilization or exhaustion of physiological resources needs some appreciation of the significance of motivation in determining the extent and pattern of effort and of stress."[67] In the effort to solve the very practical problem of keeping boots on the ground in combat situations, the full complexity of the stress response became apparent. Neither the mental nor physiological aspects could be left out of the equation.

The Psychoendocrine Approach: John W. Mason and Joseph V. Brady

The message from the 1953 Walter Reed Symposium on Stress regarding the need for an integrated psychophysiological understanding of the mechanisms underlying combat stress would have struck a chord with at least one attendee of the conference: David McKenzie Rioch, a psychiatrist and neuroscientist as well as the director of the Division of Neuropsychiatry at Walter Reed. The Division of Neuropsychiatry had itself been an outgrowth of lingering concerns over the problem of psychiatric casualties during World War II, a specter that appeared all the more ominous to the nation's security as hostilities in Korea broke out in 1950. Walter Reed recruited Rioch in 1951 to organize research that would help to understand how emotions such as fear and anxiety led to mental and physiological consequences, including the debilitating manifestations of combat failure.[68]

Within Rioch's division at Walter Reed, the research of John W. Mason and Joseph V. Brady, a neurophysiologist and a behavioral psychologist, respectively, exemplified the mixture of endocrine physiology, behavioral biology, and psychology that the Walter Reed symposium called for in 1953 and for which Walter Reed's neuropsychiatry division became renowned. Their work explored the relationship of psychological and emotional influences on the endocrine system through exhaustive primate studies in the 1950s.[69] Whereas Hans Selye's work focused on physical stimuli and hormonal responses, Mason's research emphasized psychological factors and behavioral stress responses. In lieu of older methods of histology and bioassays to detect the presence and metabolic action of certain hormones in the body, Mason and Brady's research also utilized the newest chromatographic techniques to directly measure the metabolic by-products of the stress hormones of the adrenal cortex.[70] Nevertheless, as Mason recalled in 1971, Selye's concept of stress held sway in the field of neuroendocrinology at the time Mason and Brady began their collaboration at Walter Reed in the early 1950s. In fact, Mason credited a comment by Selye that "mere emotional stimuli" could elicit the alarm reaction as the "point of departure in our own research."[71] The conclusions reached by Mason and Brady showed the hugely significant influence that emotional states could have on an animal's physiology. Further, the subtleties of endocrine responses to emotional stressors seen in Mason and Brady's experiments illustrated that, far from being the general and nonspecific phenomenon that Selye claimed, stress responses were quite specific to certain stressors, especially when those stressors were psychological.[72] Mason became involved in an increasingly broad swath of human psychoendocrine studies during his tenure as chief of the Department of Neurophysiology at Walter Reed from 1953 through 1974, which explored the psychosocial reason underlying individual variations in stress responses and ultimately accrued evidence that led him to call for the reevaluation of Selye's formulation of stress theory.[73]

On paper, Mason appeared a bit unsuited to take the reins of neuroendocrine research at the Walter Reed Army Institute of Research in 1953, since he came to the job without a doctorate in physiology or any extensive research training in the field.[74] Following the receipt of his medical degree from Indiana University in 1947, he completed rotations in pathology and surgery at the New York Hospital–Cornell Medical Center and worked as a pathologist at Fort Riley in Kansas and the Brooke Army Hospital in Texas.[75] Perhaps due to this lack of a specialized scientific background, Mason was open to the fruitful hybridization between endocrinological and psychological approaches that he pursued at Walter Reed.

Mason also began his career at Walter Reed at a moment when the institutional culture was particularly open to interdisciplinary collaboration, thanks to a large degree to the leadership of David McKenzie Rioch. Described by colleagues as a "brilliantly catalytic administrator" and a "research tycoon," Rioch capitalized on the generous funding and support for expanding research agendas that followed in the wake of World War II, as well as the opportunity to engage the brightest young doctors and scientists as they graduated from their degree programs and faced the prospect of conscription under the Selective Service Act of 1948.[76] The Division of Neuropsychiatry offered their recruits a safe place to discharge their service obligations and a well-equipped facility in which to pursue their scientific interests. In addition, Rioch actively encouraged dynamic, cross-disciplinary research topics and teams within his division, not only pairing psychologists and psychiatrists with anatomists and physiologists but also occasionally employing the expertise of social scientists.[77] All these factors contributed to the Division of Neuropsychiatry's reputation in the 1950s as a well-funded, well-staffed, and immensely creative research center on topics of neuroscience and psychiatry.

The importance of interdisciplinary collaboration was, in Mason's view, vital to progress in this field. When in 1959 he looked back on the interactions between psychological and physiological research that took place in the 1950s, Mason reflected on the accomplishments of the field but noted that in general this branch of scientific investigation had been hindered in two respects. First, he believed the wide acceptance of the homeostatic view that the body's visceral functions regulate themselves had resulted in resistance to the notion that metabolism might respond to both psychological and physical stimuli. More important, Mason argued, adequate methods and techniques with which to untangle the complex relationships between the mind and the body had been slow to develop, largely because they required interdisciplinary collaboration.[78] Mason may well have been in a privileged position to make such observations, given the fertile intellectual atmosphere he enjoyed at his home institution in the 1950s. In Mason's time at Walter Reed, the elements of collaboration and psychological experimental techniques would be supplied by his colleague Joseph V. Brady of Walter Reed's Department of Experimental Psychology and fellow member of an interdisciplinary neuroscience team set up by Rioch.[79] Together, they would produce a set of interdisciplinary studies that demonstrated that the endocrine stress response was much more sensitive and specific than previously thought. In addition, their experiments established the strong effect of the psychological on physiological processes, including an organism's endocrinological reaction to emotional stress.

Although Joseph V. Brady had just received his doctorate from the University of Chicago when he arrived at Walter Reed in 1951, he already held a strong record of experience in psychology, both in the laboratory and in the military. Prior to his graduate studies Brady had served a tour of duty in the army during World War II. From 1946 to 1948 he acted as the chief clinical psychologist at the Neuropsychiatric Center at the US Army's European Command in Germany. At Chicago Brady pursued research with Howard F. Hunt that developed and refined the work of William K. Estes and B. F. Skinner from the early 1940s, which elaborated a method for producing a conditioned emotional response, such as anxiety or fear, in rats.[80]

From the outset of their experimental work, Mason and Brady made several crucial choices in their experimental design. First, they decided to build on Brady's doctoral work with conditioned anxiety and fear responses in rats to produce a controllable psychological stress. Through experimental manipulation of an animal's behavior, the scientists could then measure changes in corticosteroid levels in the animal's blood and urine, thus correlating behavioral patterns to the activity of the pituitary-adrenal cortical system.[81] Second, Mason and Brady chose the rhesus monkey as an experimental animal. The choice of the monkey was due in part to animal's apparent amenability to the techniques of operant conditioning. The species had also proven useful in other studies on the physiology and anatomy of the brain, meaning that a great deal of reference information was already available for any potential experiments involving electrode stimulation or lesion production in the brain. Finally, due to their choice of animal subject and their wish to conduct the experiments on conscious monkeys, the Walter Reed scientists decided to design a special chair apparatus that would restrain the monkey for the duration of the experiment while keeping it relatively comfortable. While the chair enabled ease of handling during delicate tasks, such as drawing blood, its very use supplied several unforeseen observations that served as opportunities for important and novel conclusions to be drawn regarding the interrelationships of psychological and physiological responses to stress.[82]

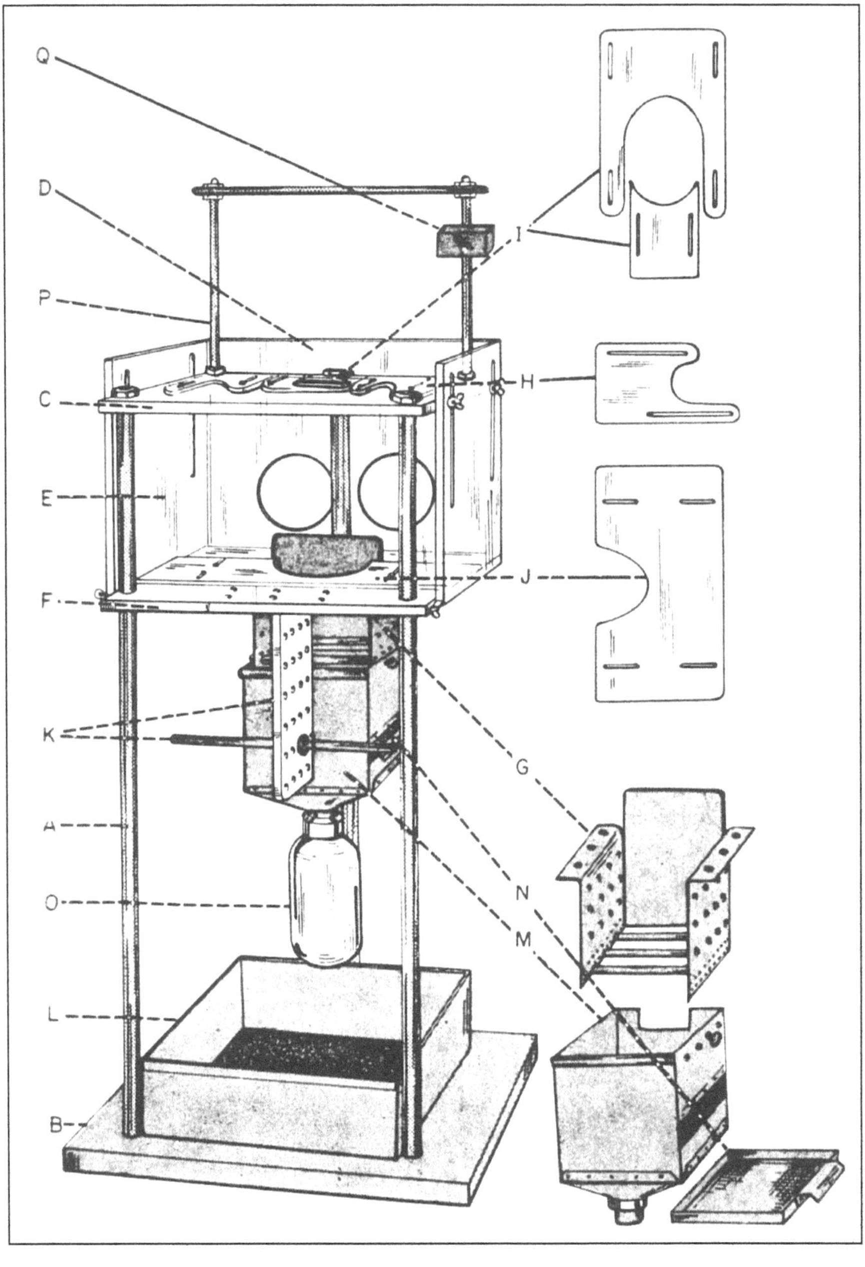

Figure 6.1. Schematic of John W. Mason's chair apparatus for psychoendocrine experiments on rhesus monkeys. Mason, "Restraining Chair for the Experimental Study of Primates," *Journal of Applied Physiology* 12, no. 1 (1958): 132. Reproduced with permission from the American Physiological Society.

Before any meaningful data could be obtained, however, there were many preliminary steps. Brady, along with another psychologist, Murray Sidman, began the intensive process of conditioning the monkeys. Once an animal had been trained to press a lever for a small reward of sugared orange juice, the psychologists imposed conditions to elicit two different behavioral patterns. An "anxiety" or "fear" response occurred when the monkey was conditioned to associate a clicking noise with an ensuing electric shock, causing a cessation of the normal lever-pressing activity, trembling, crouching, and other nervous behavior. The conditioning for "avoidance" behavior, on the other hand, taught the monkeys to press the lever to prevent a shock.[83] Meanwhile, Mason devised a chair apparatus that was fashioned out of a clear acrylic plastic box the height of the monkey's torso. The animal would be seated on a support just below the box with its waist extending through a loose hole at the bottom and its head through a hole in the top. The box was open in the front to give the investigator access to the monkey and hollow to provide the monkey's arms full range of motion within the box. Small apertures only large enough for the monkey's hands were placed in the top so that the animal could feed itself. Mason aimed to create an apparatus that would streamline the experiments and could allow an animal to remain relaxed while confined for days at a time.[84]

While standardizing the procedures with his new apparatus and allowing the animals to get accustomed to the chair, Mason observed that the very introduction of a monkey to the new environment of the chair caused a distinct and consistent rise in the animal's urinary corticosteroid levels. Indeed, he noted the same effect when a monkeys would be first handled, have blood drawn, or be moved from their home cage. Mason believed that this effect might be due to an emotional response elicited by the changes or stimuli from the animal's environment. Following this line of reasoning, Mason even kept several animals in the chair apparatus for several weeks and saw a marked decrease in their corticosteroid levels over the weekends, even when light, temperature, and feeding schedules were kept constant. What other factor could account for this observation besides the absence of the normal intensity of the laboratory activities that occurred on weekdays and the psychological response that accompanied such stimuli? These findings, though unanticipated in the original study plan, provided a valuable warning for Mason and Brady to be exact in their techniques and set careful baseline measurements in their studies to ensure they could obtain a true measure of psychologically induced stress in their conditioned animals despite any effect the environment might contribute. Moreover, the subtle influences of the environment pointed to the extreme sensitivity of the pituitary-adrenal cortical response to the myriad minute variations in an animal's milieu and, Mason believed, to the heightened emotional state that even those slight environmental factors could trigger.[85]

While Mason could only speculate about the psychological state that certain environmental factors might generate in the monkeys, Brady's conditioned animals allowed for the certain production of a specific mental state and the ability to quantify the stress that the emotion evoked in the animal. In both his anxiety-conditioned monkeys and those conditioned for the avoidance behavior, blood and urinary corticosteroid levels skyrocketed to levels as marked as those achieved after a large dose of ACTH. The close correlation between behavior and the hormone response was further confirmed when Mason and Brady tried altering the length and frequency of the conditioned emotion episodes, finding that the magnitude of the corticosteroid response also fluctuated in a similar fashion.[86]

On the basis of experiments such as these, Mason and Brady believed strongly that emotional and psychological factors played a role—and perhaps a major role—in the physiological stress response. But questions remained. Would all emotional situations spur the endocrine stress response into action and produce a rise in corticosteroid levels? If not, what features of a psychological situation prompted the physiological reaction? And, given the system's extreme sensitivity to environmental factors, did slightly different types of emotional stresses produce variations of the hormonal stress response? Or was the physiological reaction uniform and nonspecific, as Selye had been claiming for twenty years? Once again, Mason's chair apparatus permitted investigation of these kinds of questions. Due to the ease of obtaining samples from the monkeys while they were in the chair, Mason could take simultaneous measurements of a number of different hormones, such as the corticosteroids, epinephrine, and norepinephrine, and create a snapshot of an animal's endocrine profile in any given conditioned or unconditioned emotional response. The researchers found that their standard fear- and avoidance-conditioning situations produced elevated levels of all the hormones except epinephrine, while other situations "involving considerable uncertainty, ambiguity, or novelty" stimulated a flood of epinephrine in addition to the other hormones.[87] Rather than being consistent and universal, the stress response seemed to vary depending on the emotional stress the animal experienced.

Brady's operant conditioning of the rhesus monkeys had allowed the Walter Reed team to introduce a controllable psychological stress, which, using the tool of the pituitary-adrenocortical stress response, they had been able to quantify and tie directly to physiological function. But the conditioning experiments also produced a wholly serendipitous line of research, the so-called Executive Monkey studies that ultimately became much more widely known than the rest of the Walter Reed Neuropsychiatry Division's research. The Executive Monkey studies popularized the idea that ulcers were the result of certain forms of stressful experience. As the monkeys that had undergone intensive conditioning for the psychoendocrine stress studies died, autopsies of the animals revealed a high proportion of them had duodenal ulcers, a symptom that was nearly unheard of in most monkeys. Follow-up studies compared monkeys who had undergone the conditioning experiments in the chair apparatus and monkeys who spent the same amount of time in the chair apparatus but had not been subjected to conditioning. These studies showed a relationship between the behavioral conditioning and the appearance of ulcers and thus implicated psychological stress as a possible cause of ulcers.[88]

Extending this work, Mason and Brady designed a new variation of the chair apparatus that allowed monkeys to undergo a paired conditioning experiment. Each monkey pair would receive an electric shock every twenty seconds unless the lever was pressed to delay the shock. Only one monkey, called "the experimental 'avoidance' monkey" in the original publication, had access to the lever, making the other monkey in each pair a control for the avoidance behavior and the ulceration that Brady and Mason postulated such conditioning behavior caused. Six-hour "shock" sessions would be alternated with six-hour "off periods" around the clock for up to six or seven consecutive weeks. The researchers collected urine throughout the experiment, but corticosteroid analysis showed little marked elevation in hormone levels outside of the initial twenty-four-hour conditioning period. Autopsies of the animals, however, yielded the expected results in a dramatic and conclusive fashion. Four of the experimental animals, three of which died in the apparatus during the course of the experiment, had "extensive gastrointestinal lesions with ulceration," while "none of the control animals sacrificed for comparison with their experimental partners . . . showed any indications of such gastrointestinal complications."[89]

As early as the fall of 1957, the experimental "avoidance" monkey was masquerading under a new name, one that resonated with the American public in the 1950s and effectively carried Brady and Mason's message about the important link between mental and physical well-being. "You have heard about The Organization Man," a *New Scientist* article began, referencing William Whyte's 1951 bestseller about the rise of the corporation in the United States and its destruction of American individualism and character. "Has anyone told you about The Executive Monkey?" By October 1958 a more popular version of the research appeared in *Scientific American*, this time with the more striking title of "Ulcers in 'Executive' Monkeys" and with Joseph V. Brady as a solo author. "Of all the body's systems," Brady penned, "the gastrointestinal tract is perhaps the most vulnerable to emotional stress. The worries, fears, conflicts and anxieties of daily life can produce gastrointestinal disorders ranging from the 'nervous stomach,' which most of us know at first hand, to the painful and often disabling ulcers which are the traditional occupational disease of business executives."[90]

Though Brady stopped short in the article from speculating on the exact mechanism by which such stress-related ulcers formed, his account carried the same message that the Walter Reed Division of Neuropsychiatry had been hammering home all decade: physiological health was crucially linked to psychological health. This message resonated in the pressured work environment of America in the 1950s as much as it did for the military commanders concerned about combat failure. Even prior to the popularization of the Executive Monkey study, corporations and public health institutions were publicizing the dangerous consequences of unchecked psychological stress. The Oklahoma State Department of Health, for instance, produced the 1957 film, *Ulcer at Work*, which follows the story of an overworked corporate man whose single-minded ambitions at work and fractious home life have led him to develop an ulcer, a physical ailment that, the film suggests, has psychological causes and thus can be treated only through conscious changes in mental attitude and behavior (on the part of both the working man and his wife, who desires all the latest modern comforts).[91]

While Brady's work on the Executive Monkey struck a chord in the domestic sphere, the outgrowths of Mason's psychoendocrine work with Brady in their Walter Reed laboratory would ultimately bring stress research back to the front lines during the Vietnam War and lend endocrinological evidence to earlier assertions by military psychiatrists about the importance of individual variation and group dynamics in dealing with the problem of combat stress. In the late 1950s and early 1960s Mason collaborated with researchers at Walter Reed and elsewhere on a number of studies aimed at extending knowledge of the psychoendocrine response to stress to humans. Mason and his colleagues clearly could not subject people to the same conditioning experiments that he and Brady conducted with the rhesus monkeys. Instead, subjects were chosen who faced some kind of unusual or anxiety-inducing emotional state, including fear over upcoming surgeries, the experience of hospitalization, the anticipation by a parent of the death of a fatally ill child, mental illness, or even simply "novel or ambiguous situations." The findings of these studies closely mapped those that had emerged from the monkey studies at Walter Reed, concluding that adrenal-cortical secretion patterns responded to the intensity of an experience and emotional responses to changes in a given environment.[92] The central difference, however, was in the much higher degree of individual variation that human subjects in their endocrine response to a given stimulus compared to their primate counterparts. Although the researchers explored the possibility of standardizing the administration of an emotional stimulus using carefully selected motion pictures to aid in mitigating such wild variation, Mason's psychoendocrine experiments with humans soon began to focus on the variability of the stress response between individuals as the object of inquiry.[93]

Beyond a simple, linear influence of emotional states on endocrine function, these human psychoendocrine studies emphasized the many environmental, situational, psychological, and social factors that shaped an individual's particular emotional and hormonal response to a stimulus. Through psychological data obtained using interviews, diaries, observations, and standard checklist-style evaluations of mood, Mason and his colleagues attempted to evaluate all such individual factors and correlate them to patterns of hormone levels in blood, plasma, or urine. In studies examining parents dealing with the chronic threat of the death of a child from cancer, for instance, they used a combination of in-depth, qualitative psychological interviews and biochemical testing of urinary 17-hydroxycorticosteroid levels to examine the reasons that led some parents to be "high excretors" or "low excretors" of stress hormone by-products, indicating the activity of their adrenal cortical response to their child's illness. They found that many of the parents who mobilized some degree of denial or some other psychological coping mechanism tended to fall into the "low excretor" group. The physiological stress response was dependent not only on the emotions caused by stressful circumstances but on an individual's perception of those circumstances as well.[94] That perception, in turn, could be vastly influenced by an individual's particular situation or context.

In another study, college students volunteered to live in a hospital research unit for a period of several months to gauge their physiological and psychological reactions to the relatively mild stress of new surroundings and a different social environment. Most of the students quickly adapted to the hospital, experienced decreasing feelings of apprehension, and had consistently low corticosteroid levels. Others, who were struggling in school and short of money, displayed opposite psychological and physiological reactions. For these students, their hospital stay provided respite from the pressures of their daily life, and as their class schedules resumed and exams approached, they showed increasing anxiety and elevated stress hormone excretion. Mason and his collaborators concluded that both the physiological and emotional response to environmental stimuli must be filtered through an individual's prior experiences and situational peculiarities.[95]

Yet another group of human subjects that provided the scientists of Walter Reed with evidence for their psychoendocrine stress research would be members of the US Armed Forces fighting in Vietnam. As with the ORO's study during the Korean War, the conflict in Vietnam provided Mason and several colleagues in Walter Reed's Department of Psychiatry with an opportunity to apply and test their ideas about stress in the field in order to clarify the mechanisms underlying the ongoing problem of combat stress. In particular, Mason's focus on the relationship of psychological mechanisms to the functioning of the endocrine stress response allowed these studies to bring physiological tools to bear directly on long-standing ideas within military psychology, such as the importance of group coherence and individual personality and experience in determining a soldier's ability to withstand the pressures of combat. Two young army psychiatrists, Peter G. Bourne and

Robert M. Rose, also participated in the studies, with Bourne, the head of the army's psychiatric research team in Vietnam, taking the lead in the dangerous front-line fieldwork in 1965 and 1966.[96]

They followed two groups of army personnel serving in South Vietnam who were subject to the chronic threat of death or injury: a group of seven helicopter ambulance medics charged with evacuating combat casualties by air, often under heavy fire, and a team of twelve members of the Green Berets, the US Army's Special Forces, who had established a remote camp near the Cambodian border to intercept the traffic of weapons and men along the Ho Chi Minh Trail. In each case Bourne and an enlisted technician maintained close contact with their subjects for weeks at a time, even living in the Green Berets' isolated camp for the duration of May and June, to complete interviews, psychological tests, and urine sample collection. In comparison to the ambitious scale and scope of the ORO combat-stress study in Korea, these psychoendocrine studies in Vietnam were much simpler in design, involving only one test for urine 17-hydroxycorticosteroid levels and less formal psychological evaluation and interview strategies. Analyses for urinary corticoid levels were performed off-site, rather than in the field. In addition, Bourne, Mason, and Rose focused on much smaller groups of soldiers, making regular sample collections and thorough interviews much more feasible. Above all, the Walter Reed team's explicitly integrative psychoendocrine method approached the topic of combat stress as a problem of the whole organism and allowed an examination how the psychosocial factors of individual difference and group dynamics influenced the stress response of a soldier under combat conditions.

In the helicopter medic study, which took place over the course of three weeks in January 1966, Mason, Bourne, and Rose began by asking what happens to physiological and psychological stress reactions of an individual during acute stress situations when the subject is already enduring chronic stress. The seven medics had been stationed in Vietnam for several months at the time of the study, constituting the chronic stress situation, but some days saw them flying missions under heavy combat conditions while other days did not require them to fly at all. Analysis of the daily urinary samples taken under these conditions yielded a startling result. Whereas adrenal cortical secretion would be expected to increase on days the medics saw combat, there was very little fluctuation in 17-hydroxycorticosteroid levels, regardless of whether they were flying. In addition, the medics' levels of corticoid excretion remained at an unusually low level for the duration of the study.[97] The medics had not exhausted the capacity of their adrenal cortices to respond to stressful circumstances; indeed, the levels of one medic's corticoid excretion tripled when a wound on his head became seriously infected. Instead, the researchers concluded on the basis of their psychiatric observations that the medics had all devised highly effective psychological defensive mechanisms, ranging from religious faith to the act of retelling stories of "near-misses" and survival to reinforce a feeling of security and invulnerability. The notion that a soldier could create such psychological coping strategies was a concept promulgated as early as World War II, but substantiation from the endocrine evidence made visible the clear physiological benefits of such psychological defenses. Humans could adapt physiologically even to the most dire circumstances, the researchers argued, simply by modifying their perception of their situation. Stress, therefore, could not be seen as general, uniform, or universal; rather, the authors of the study viewed it as a conditional and relative response that could "only be defined in terms of the individual's interaction with the environment."[98]

The study of the Green Berets, conducted a few months later in May and June, built on the findings with the helicopter medics. Since the Special Forces team included ten enlisted men and two officers, the Walter Reed scientists were able to consider the influence of assigned roles and group dynamics in shaping the individual's response to stress. As with the medics, overall urinary 17-hydroxycorticosteroid levels were surprisingly low among the group. Even so, the excretion levels of the officers were significantly higher than the enlisted men, who, as a group, showed especially low and uniform response patterns. Evaluation of the men's various coping strategies once again showed a variety of defenses and suggested that the nature of the respective roles of officers and enlisted soldiers explained these differences in physiological responses. Among the enlisted men, whose normal daily tasks included highly specialized and routine activities, these defenses seemed to rest on confidence in their own abilities and the invincibility of the team based on past successes and survival, as well as diffusion of tension through outward behavior and occupation with their assigned tasks. The officers, with their duties encompassing higher-level, less standardized decision-making processes, not only felt responsibility to the demands of the group and pressure to prove themselves as leaders, but also had fewer options in the course of their work to diffuse tension. Although the officers encountered the same dangers that the enlisted men did, Bourne, Mason, and Rose believed that the additional pressure placed on them by their position made it more difficult to develop the same extensive psychological defenses as the enlisted men. In addition, the uniformly low levels of cortical excretion among the enlisted men suggested that that group cohesion and confidence in the team also helped to minimize the individual differences and render the team more adaptable to a chronically stressful situation. Due to group dynamics and the difference in the assigned roles of officers and enlisted men in the team, the authors concluded that the enlisted men altered their perception of the danger of an impending attack on the camp more than their superiors.[99]

Through use of biochemical techniques for measuring the physiological stress response to the psychological influences of war, these psychoendocrine studies in Vietnam represented a huge step toward the fulfillment of the type of interdisciplinary military stress research striven for in the ORO study and called for at the 1953 Walter Reed symposium. Mason's work finally brought the potential of physiological stress research into communication with the older psychiatric and psychological approaches to the problem of combat stress, contributing physiological evidence to the argument that psychological factors are crucial to helping the soldier remain effective on the battlefield. Experimental data from Mason's psychoendocrine research on the role of the mind in the physiological stress response also led him to actively question the stress theory espoused by Hans Selye. Although a number of the physiologists at the 1953 Walter Reed symposium had not hidden their skepticism of Selye's ideas, Mason complained in 1971 that most scientists had "simply tended to assume personal stands more or less intuitively concerning 'stress' theory" without making "sustained and systematic attempts to put specific points in 'stress' theory to rigorous experimental tests, particularly as new methods became available."[100] Mason's own research did make such an attempt, taking advantage of the new chromatographic techniques for corticoid quantification, as well as the uniquely collaborative environment at the Walter Reed Division of Neuropsychiatry. In the late 1960s and early 1970s he began to synthesize his experimental data from the past two decades to make an appeal for the critical reevaluation of stress theory and the revision of its claims that the stress response was predominantly a physiological and nonspecific phenomenon.

Mason's qualms with the stress theory that Selye had promulgated drew directly on the research discussed in this chapter and fell in two categories. First, Mason took issue with the importance Selye placed on physical and physiological stimuli without controlling for the psychological reactions that went along with them. Mason and Brady's work with the rhesus monkeys had clearly demonstrated the extreme sensitivity of the pituitary-adrenal cortical system to psychological stresses produced by even subtle changes in environment, such as the level of activity in the laboratory on weekdays versus weekends. But their own attempts to minimize psychological stress and isolate the response of an animal to a specific physical stimulus proved surprisingly difficult. For instance, the measurement of 17-hydroxycorticoid levels while depriving an animal of food was inadequate for studying the effects of fasting because the monkey might be responding to any number of other stimuli, from the discomfort of an empty stomach to frustration over neighboring monkeys receiving normal rations. To correct for this, Mason's group isolated the animal and gave it flavored cellulose pellets to mimic their normal feed and counteract hunger. Indeed, when steps were taken to control for such extraneous physical and psychological stimuli, the fasting monkey showed no increase in corticoid excretion in response to nutritional deprivation. "Fasting *per se*," Mason argued, "appears to elicit little, if any, adrenal cortical response, but the fasting *situation* as a whole may indeed evoke a marked 17-OHCS response if it includes factors which elicit psychological reaction."[101] While Mason acknowledged much more research needed to be completed along these lines, his experiments showed that psychological and emotional factors involved in the stress response could not be ignored. Stress was, in fact, a reaction of the whole organism.

Mason also expressed misgivings surrounding Selye's idea of stress as a nonspecific or generalized response of the animal to any number of threats or "nocuous stimuli." As discussed earlier, by tracking the subtle changes in the endocrine profiles of monkeys, Mason and Brady had shown that hormonal responses could differ depending on whether the animal had been conditioned for a fear response or was facing a novel situation. Even putting aside the involvement of psychological and emotional factors, Mason voiced concern over the assumption of the "non-specificity" of stress when the very physiological mechanisms by which environmental stimuli are translated into the cascading endocrine response of ACTH and cortisol were still unknown. What are the pathways by which all the various stimuli reach the anterior pituitary? Are there receptors in the body for these stimuli, and do they react nonspecifically?

Further, how can one account for the notion that so many diverse environmental factors, many of which, such as heat or cold, required very different metabolic reactions on the part of the organism, culminate in a single, generalized reaction? And what is the "first mediator" by which the environment interacts with the organism? In Selye's physiological schema, it had been assumed that this was a humoral or neural entity. But Mason, building on his experiments and following his convictions about the significance of the role played by the mind in an organism's response to stressful situations, suggested instead "that the 'primary mediator' underlying the pituitary-adrenal cortical response to the diverse 'stressors' of the earlier 'stress' research may simply be the psychological apparatus involved in emotional or arousal reactions to threatening or unpleasant factors in the life situation."[102] Not only was stress not predominantly a physiological response, Mason asserted, it might in fact be primarily a psychological one. As the physiologist Wallace Fenn had said of the two sides of the combat-stress problem nearly two decades earlier, successful adaptation to a stressful situation such as the battlefield required "machinery and morale, and the greater of these is morale."[103] Mason's research during the 1950s and 1960s, conducted within a military scientific community inspired by the potential of interdisciplinary pyschoendocrine research to help solve the operational problem of combat stress, would provide experimental evidence to support that view.

Getting Specific: Stress in the Military Context

In striving for practical solutions to the complicated issue of combat stress, the military research community of the early Cold War period sought to embrace both its established knowledge base regarding psychological manifestations of stress and the new ideas and methods of stress physiology. The orientation of military stress research toward the interrelationships between the physiological and psychological phenomena of the stress response seems to have continued through the 1950s and into the 1960s, through the collaborations of physiologists and psychologists, such as John W. Mason and Joseph V. Brady, at the Division of Neuropsychiatry at the Walter Reed Army Institute of Research. Just as many of the participants at the Walter Reed Symposium on Stress in 1953 had emphasized the importance of the individual experience, character, and behavior in shaping a soldier's reaction to the combat environment, Mason and Brady's psychoendocrine approach to the problem of stress highlighted the way in which many environmental, situational, psychological, and social factors shaped an individual's particular emotional and hormonal response to a stimulus. In so doing, this research moved the idea of stress further away from the overtly physiological, general, nonspecific concepts promoted by Hans Selye and readily adopted as an explanatory framework by earlier combat-stress studies, such as the ORO's 1952 study of combat stress in Korea. Instead, the work of Mason and Brady asserted the central role of psychological and emotional factors in an organism's physiological responses and to the overall adaptation of an organism to a stressful situation. In focusing on these psychological factors in their experiments with both monkeys and humans, the researchers also recognized such responses were highly individualized, given the nature of the stressful situation. By 1970 such research demanded a revision to stress theory that acknowledged this migration from "general" to "particular" and strove for a closer mind-body approach.

The military's goal of solving the problem of combat stress, I argue, was central in effecting this shift in thinking about stress theory in total. Both the ORO study and the discussions from the Walter Reed symposium in the early 1950s showed the desire on the part of military and operations research scientists to build on the psychological and psychiatric work on combat stress during World War II by integrating the new insights of physiology into the function of the pituitary-adrenal cortical system in the body's response to stress. The new Division of Neuropsychiatry at Walter Reed also shared this mandate and succeeded in constructing a highly collaborative research program using an integrative psychoendocrine approach. While operational concerns seem to have served as only an indirect motivation for much of Mason and Brady's research on psychological stresses of rhesus monkeys, the interdisciplinary institutional culture at

Walter Reed during their time there was most certainly fostered to understand how the workings of the mind led to physiological consequences and to forge a more holistic approach to dealing with the ongoing problem of psychiatric casualties. Such an environment made possible their collaboration and promoted serious consideration of the interactions between psychological and physiological factors during the stress response. Their data, bolstered by Mason's psychoendocrine studies on stress in Vietnam, suggested the inadequacies of Selye's generalized, nonspecific, and purely physiological notion of stress. In its place Mason and Brady constructed a picture of stress that incorporated the psychological as well as the physiological factors and transferred attention back to how specificity and individual variation affect the reaction of organisms—soldiers and monkeys alike—to the challenges of their environments.

In focusing on the individual, the work of Mason and Brady lent physiological evidence to the emphasis on personal character and situational context that military psychiatrists had long advocated as central to determining a soldier's reaction to the stresses of the battlefield. Mason and Brady's psychoendocrine stress studies in the 1950s and 1960s built on these older traditions in military psychiatry, but their research would also serve as important context for a future development in the field: the rise of post-traumatic stress disorder (PTSD) in the 1970s and 1980s. While the history of psychiatry's role in bringing about a formal category of combat-related neuroses during the 1970s has received scholarly attention, the differences and continuities between the psychoendocrine work described in this chapter and later studies of PTSD remain to be elaborated.[104]

One connection between the two bodies of research is John W. Mason himself. After serving as the head of psychoendocrinology at Walter Reed for twenty years, he was recruited by Yale University in 1974 to work with members of a neuropsychiatry group there that, in collaboration with psychiatric professionals working for the Veterans Administration, had become concerned that veterans returning from Vietnam were having their combat-induced symptoms misdiagnosed. The research by this Yale group helped to make PTSD an official diagnosis in the *Diagnostic and Statistical Manual of Mental Disorders* in 1980. Mason was critical to the first neuroendocrine studies in the 1980s that proved that the functions of the pituitary-adrenocortical axis are altered in cases of PTSD, once again contributing physiological data to enrich and quantify psychiatric observation.[105] Further study of the intellectual and methodological links between Mason's earlier psychoendocrine studies, particularly the Vietnam-field studies, and his later involvement in PTSD research at Yale would deepen the current psychiatry-focused literature on PTSD and shed additional light on how the interaction of physiological and psychiatric approaches to combat stress within the military context conspired to shape the evolving concept of stress in the twentieth century.

Notes

1. The contributions of psychology and psychiatry to the World War II effort have been well documented; see Ellen Herman, *The Romance of American Psychology: Political Culture in the Age of Experts* (Berkeley: University of California Press, 1995); Ben Shephard, *A War of Nerves: Soldiers and Psychiatrists in the Twentieth Century?* (Cambridge, MA: Harvard University Press, 2001); Edgar Jones and Simon Wessely, *Shell Shock to PTSD: Military Psychiatry from 1900 to the Gulf War* (New York: Psychology Press, 2005); Paul Wanke, "American Military Psychiatry and Its Role among Ground Forces in World War II," *Journal of Military History* 63, no. 1 (January 1999): 127–46; and Hans Pols, "War Neurosis, Adjustment Problems in Veterans, and an Ill Nation: The Disciplinary Project of American Psychiatry during and after World War II," *Osiris* 22 (2007): 73–82.

2. Russell Viner, "Putting Stress in Life: Hans Selye and the Making of Stress Theory," *Social Studies of Science* 29, no. 3 (1999): 391–410; Anne Harrington, *The Cure Within: A History of Mind-Body Medicine* (New York: Norton, 2008), 139–74.

3. Other forums such as the Macy Conferences on the Adrenal Cortex, held annually between 1949 and 1953, also display the disagreements and controversies surrounding the exact nature of the stress response. See Elaine P. Ralli, ed., *Adrenal Cortex* (New York: Macy Foundation, 1950–54).

4. Albert Glass, "Psychotherapy in the Combat Zone," in *Symposium on Stress* (Washington, DC: Army Medical Graduate School, Walter Reed Army Medical Center): 284–86.

5. Pols, "War Neurosis."

6. Roy R. Grinker and John P. Spiegel, *Men under Stress* (Philadelphia: Blakiston, 1945).

7. Thomas F. Gallagher, "The Synthesis of Adrenocortical Steroids," in *Advances in Military Medicine*, ed. Edwin C. Andrus, Detlev W. Bronk, G. A. Carden Jr., Chester S. Keefer, J. S. Lockwood, Joseph T. Wearn, and Milton C. Winternitz (Boston: Little, Brown, 1948), 659–63; Edward C. Kendall, *Cortisone* (New York: Scribner's Sons, 1971), 99–105; Dwight Ingle, "Edward C. Kendall, 1886–1972," *Biographical Memoirs of the National Academy of Sciences* (Washington, DC: National Academy of Sciences, 1975): 266–67; Nicolas Rasmussen, "Steroids in Arms: Science, Government, Industry, and the Hormones of the Adrenal Cortex in the United States, 1930–1950," *Medical History* 46, no. 3 (2002): 312–18.

8. Hans Selye, "The General Adaptation Syndrome and the Diseases of Adaptation," *Journal of Clinical Endocrinology* 6, no. 2 (1946): 117–230.

9. Stanley W. Davis, Fred Elmadjian, Lincoln F. Hanson, Howard S. Liddell, Algird A. Zilinsky, Muriel E. Johnston, John H. Kilbuck, et al., *A Study of Combat Stress in Korea, 1952–Preliminary Report* (Chevy Chase, MD: Operations Research Office, Johns Hopkins University, 1953), 144–46; Davis, "A Study of Combat Stress in Korea" (paper 10, Informal Seminar in Operations Research, 1953–54, Operations Research Office, Johns Hopkins University, December 15, 1953), 1.

10. Stanley W. Davis, "A Study of Combat Stress in Korea: Bio-Social Research in Operations Research," in *Case Histories, Methods, Information Handling*, vol. 2 of *Operations Research for Management*, ed. Joseph F. McCloskey and John M. Coppinger (Baltimore: Johns Hopkins University Press, 1956), 252–53.

11. On the history of operations research in the US Army and the founding of the Operations Research Office at Johns Hopkins, consult Charles R. Shrader, *1942–1962*, vol. 1 of *History of Operations Research in the United States Army* (Washington, DC: United States Army Center of Military History, 2006). For the British side of the development of the field, see Maurice W. Kirby, *Operational Research in War and Peace: The British Experience from the 1930s to 1970* (London: Imperial College Press, 2003).

12. Davis, "Study of Combat Stress: Bio-social Research," 250–51. For the proceedings that led to the organization of the 1952 ORO combat-stress study, consult "Fatigue and Stress and Their Roles in Military Operations" (ORO symposium, Johns Hopkins University Operations Research Office, Chevy Chase, MD, January 24–26, 1952).

13. Davis, "Study of Combat Stress: Bio-social Research," 251. This kind of short-term, operational attitude toward the impact of combat on military personnel seems especially striking in light of the fact that about three more decades would pass before the reality and severity of post-traumatic stress disorders were acknowledged by the medical community and by the military.

14. The uncertainty about precisely how many members of the team worked on each side of the problem stems from the fact that the exact specialties and biographical details of some members of the team have been lost to the historical record. Ernest R. Kolovos and George H. Longley are listed on the preliminary report as authors representing the Office of the Surgeon General of the US Army, though I have been unable to trace other aspects of their careers with certainty. In 1950 Kolovos had been a staff member of a team at the American Institute of Research in Pittsburgh that was under contract with the ONR to improve testing for the selection of their scientific research personnel. See Mary H. Weislogel, *The Development of a Test for Selecting Research Personnel* (Pittsburgh: American Institute of Research, January 1950). As for Longley, I must assume he was involved in the psychology investigation in Korea, since the 1956 published account of the study, which covered only the more successful physiology research, did not list him as an author. Conversely, Algird Zilinsky of the ORO was an author of this later study and, thus, likely a part of the physiology investigation. According to Stanley Davis, Zilinsky was a "medical technician"; see Stanley W. Davis, "Stress in Combat," *Scientific American* 194, no. 3 (March 1958): 35.

15. On the Worcester Foundation, see Leon Speroff, *A Good Man: Gregory Goodwin Pincus: The Man, His Story, the Birth Control Pill* (Portland, OR: Arnica, 2009); Dwight J. Ingle, "Gregory Goodwin Pincus," *Biographical Memoirs of the National Academy of Sciences* 42 (1971): 229–70; Hudson Hoagland, *The Road to Yesterday* (Worcester, MA: privately published, 1974).

16. For biographical information on Elmadjian, see "Elmadjian, Dr. Fred," in *American Men of Science*, ed. Jacques Cattell, 9th ed., vol. 2 (Lancaster, PA: Science Press, 1955), 318. For examples of his early work with Pincus and Hoagland, see Gregory Pincus and Fred Elmadjian, "A Study of the Diurnal Variations in Circulating Lymphocytes in Normal and Psychotic Subjects," *Journal of Clinical Endocrinology* 6 (1946): 287–94; Gregory Pincus and Fred Elmadjian, "The Lymphocyte Response to Heat Stress in Normal and Psychotic Subjects," *Journal of Clinical Endocrinology* 6 (1946): 295–300; Gregory Pincus, Fred Elmadjian, and Hudson Hoagland, "Stressful Psychomotor Performance and Adrenal Cortical Function as Indicated by the

Lymphocyte Response," *Journal of Clinical Endocrinology* 6 (1946): 301–11; Gregory Pincus, Hudson Hoagland, Harry Freeman, Fred Elmadjian, and Louise P. Romanoff, "A Study of Pituitary-Adrenocortical Function in Normal and Psychotic Men," *Psychosomatic Medicine* 11 (1949): 74–101; and Gregory Pincus, Hudson Hoagland, Harry Freeman, and Fred Elmadjian, "Adrenal Function in Mental Disease," *Recent Progress in Hormone Research* 4 (1949): 291–322.

17. "Minard, Dr. David," in Cattell, *American Men of Science*, 2:780.

18. On Nello Pace, see Ralph H. Kellogg, John W. Severinghaus, Arthur H. Smith, and Paola S. Timiras, "Nello Pace: Physiology and Anatomy: Berkeley," in *University of California: In Memoriam, 1995*, ed. David Krogh (Berkeley: University of California Academic Senate, 1995): 140–43. Pace's career in environmental physiology varied widely. During the 1950s and 1960s his interest in high-altitude physiology led him to help establish White Mountain Research Station in eastern California; participate in the California Himalayan Expedition to the world's fifth tallest mountain, Makalu; and extend his studies into gravitational physiology and the effects of weightlessness on monkeys during consulting work for the national space program in the 1960s.

19. The other ONR personnel included Lt. John H. Kilbuck, a chemist who specialized in analysis of food products, and Lt. Frederick L. Schaffer, a biochemistry researcher at Berkeley. For biographical information, see "Kilbuck, John H(enry)," in Cattell, *American Men of Science*, 2:610; and "Schaffer, Dr. Frederick L(eland)," in Cattell, *American Men of Science*, 2:1693. The ONR group also featured the unusual addition of two Navy WAVES, Lt. Muriel E. Johnston and Lt. Elaine Walker, marking the first time female naval officers were allowed into a combat zone. Both women were trained as physiologists, giving them "special technical qualifications" for the type of research undertaken in the combat-stress study. See Marjorie van de Water, "The Human Price of Combat," *Science New Letter* 64, no. 23 (December 5, 1953): 362.

20. "Davis, Stanley W(arburton)," *American Men of Science*, ed. Jacques Cattell, 9th ed., vol. 3 (New York: Bowker, 1956), 158.

21. For a published version of Davis's doctoral research findings, see Stanley W. Davis, "Auditory and Visual Flicker-Fusion as Measures of Fatigue," *American Journal of Psychology* 68, no. 4 (December 1955): 654–57.

22. "Hanson, Lincoln Flint," in Cattell, *American Men of Science*, 3:278.

23. On Liddell, see James D. Block, "In Memoriam: Howard S. Liddell, Ph.D., 1895–1962," *Psychosomatic Medicine* 25 (January 1, 1963): 1–2; and Frank S. Freeman, "A Reflection: Howard Scott Liddell, 1895–1962," *Journal of the History of the Behavioral Sciences* 21 (October 1985): 372–74.

24. Howard S. Liddell, William T. James, and Oscar D. Anderson, *The Comparative Physiology of the Conditioned Motor Reflex, Based on Experiments with the Pig, Dog, Sheep, Goat, and Rabbit* (Baltimore: Johns Hopkins University Press, 1934).

25. Howard S. Liddell, *Emotional Hazards in Animals and Man* (Springfield, IL: Charles C. Thomas, 1956).

26. Freeman, "Reflection," 372–73.

27. Davis et al., *Study of Combat Stress*, 9–10. Descriptions of the testing procedures are also detailed in the published version of the study. See Nello Pace, Frederick L. Schaffer, Fred Elmadjian, David Minard, Stanley W. Davis, John H. Kilbuck, Elaine L. Walker, et al., *Physiological Studies of Infantrymen in Combat*, vol. 10

of *University of California Publications in Physiology* (Berkeley: University of California Press, 1956): 2–6.

28. Davis et al., *Study of Combat Stress,* 107–8; Pace et al., "Infantrymen in Combat," 6.

29. Davis et al., *Study of Combat Stress,* 10.

30. Davis et al., *Study of Combat Stress,* 11–12; Pace et al., "Infantrymen in Combat," 2.

31. Davis, "Stress in Combat," 34.

32. Pace et al., "Infantrymen in Combat," 2.

33. From pictures and accounts in a popular article about the study, it is clear that lieutenants Schaffer and Kilbuck from the ONR certainly were among those who went to the front, accompanied by lieutenants Johnston and Walker, the WAVES. See Van de Water, "Human Price," 362. This is corroborated by Elmadjian, who mentioned that the group included "two Navy Ensigns (young ladies)," as well as others "capable of taking blood." Elmadjian admitted that he "was not actually at the front when the samples were taken. . . . The rest of us waited in the laboratory for the samples to come in." See "Adrenocortical Function of Combat Infantrymen in Korea," in *The Human Adrenal Cortex,* vol. 8 of *The Ciba Foundation Colloquia on Endocrinology* (Boston: Little, Brown, 1955): 645.

34. Davis et al., *Study of Combat Stress,* 10–12. Analysis of urine for 17-ketosteroid and corticoid was done by the Metabolic Institute of the University of California and the Worcester Foundation for Experimental Biology in Massachusetts. The Worcester Foundation, which was directed by the physiologists Gregory Pincus and Hudson Hoagland and served as Elmadjian's institutional home, was one of the preeminent sites for physiological research of the adrenal cortex in the United States, along with Cyril Norman Hugh Long's laboratory at Yale University, Edward Kendall's group at the Mayo Foundation, and the research group of Choh Hao Li and Herbert McLean Evans at the University of California at Berkeley.

35. Davis et al., *Study of Combat Stress,* 12–16; Pace et al., "Infantrymen in Combat," 6–9.

36. Davis et al., *Study of Combat Stress,* 151.

37. Davis, "Combat Stress in Korea" (paper 10), 7; Elmadjian, "Adrenocortical Function," 645–46.

38. Davis et al., *Study of Combat Stress,* 14–15.

39. Davis, "Combat Stress in Korea" (paper 10), 6.

40. Davis et al., *Study of Combat Stress,* 146.

41. Davis, "Stress in Combat," 34.

42. James Chimbidis, "Stress in Combat," *Johns Hopkins File 7* (television program), directed by Ed Fryers, aired April 10, 1960 (Baltimore: Johns Hopkins University, 2004), videocassette.

43. Davis et al., *Study of Combat Stress,* 154.

44. For the first two Walter Reed symposia, see *Symposium on Shock* (Washington, DC: Army Medical Graduate School, Walter Reed Army Medical Center, May 7–9, 1951); and *Symposium on Treatment of Trauma in the Armed Forces* (Washington, DC: Army Medical Graduate School, Walter Reed Army Medical Center, March 10–12, 1952).

45. John C. Whitehorn, "Introduction and Survey of the Problems of Stress," in *Symposium on Stress,* 7.

46. Pace et al., "Infantrymen in Combat," 1–48.

47. Notably absent are some of the major players in endocrinology and stress physiology. Selye did not attend the symposium, nor apparently did others cited repeatedly in the first day's presentations, particularly Cyril Norman Hugh Long, Dwight Ingle, and the scientists involved in stress research at Walter Reed in the 1950s (including John W. Mason and Joseph V. Brady). The participants listed in the beginning of the volume included only those who presented papers, however, so there may well have been attendees for whom there is no record. Selye is the one person whose absence was noted formally by Whitehorn in his opening remarks: "I wish particularly, however, to mention one person, Dr. Hans Selye, whose work has been of great historical importance in this field, who is not present in our symposium." See Whitehorn, "Introduction," 2.

48. Whitehorn, "Introduction," 2. I. Arthur Mirsky, "Metabolic Responses in Acute Stress Situations," in *Symposium on Stress*, 38–39. Mirsky devoted his career to bringing the methods of biochemistry and physiology to bear on problems in psychiatry and psychosomatic medicine. Perhaps his most important contribution was a biochemical study of pepsinogen (the precursor of the digestive enzyme pepsin), which resulted in new understandings of the psychological and physiological factors of peptic ulcers. See Herbert Weiner, Margaret Thaler, Morton F. Reiser, and I. Arthur Mirsky, "Etiology of Duodenal Ulcer: I. Relation of Specific Psychological Characteristics to Rate of Gastric Secretion (Serum Pepsinogen)," *Psychosomatic Medicine* 19 (1957): 1–10. On Mirsky, see Alvin P. Shapiro, "In Memoriam: I. Arthur Mirsky, MD, 1907–1974," *Psychosomatic Medicine* 37 (January–February 1975): 1–3.

49. Whitehorn, "Introduction," 3. For later dialogue regarding the importance of having a more rigorous definition of stress, see the open discussion following Daniel H. Funkenstein, Stanley H. King, and Margaret Drolette, "The Experimental Evocation of Stress," in *Symposium on Stress*, 317–18.

50. Mirsky, "Acute Stress," 37–44.

51. In the early 1940s two research groups, one led by Cyril Norman Hugh Long at Yale and the other led by Choh Hao Li at Berkeley, isolated and purified ACTH by several methods nearly simultaneously. This development and thus access to pure forms of the protein undoubtedly made possible much of the research described by Mirsky and others at the Walter Reed symposium. For a retrospective on the ACTH work in the 1930s and 1940s, see Nicole Kresge, Robert D. Simoni, and Robert L. Hill, "The Isolation of Adrenocorticotropic Hormone by Three Pioneers in Molecular Embryology: Choh Hao Li, Abraham White, and Cyril Norman Hugh Long," *Journal of Biological Chemistry* 280, no. 3 (January 21, 2005): 121–23. The original articles were published back-to-back: Choh Hao Li, Herbert M. Evans, and Miriam E. Simpson, "Adrenocorticotropic Hormone," *Journal of Biological Chemistry* 149, no. 2 (August 1943): 413–24; and George Sayers, Abraham White, and Cyril Norman Hugh Long, "Preparation and Properties of Pituitary Adrenotropic Hormone," *Journal of Biological Chemistry* 149, no. 2 (August 1943): 425–36.

52. Mirsky, "Acute Stress," 40–41. According to Mirsky, the researchers arguing against Selye were Long and his group at Yale and Marthe Vogt, a German chemist working in Britain.

53. Mirsky, "Acute Stress," 42.

54. Largely unknown now, Ingle had worked with Edward C. Kendall's group on the purification and activity of adrenal cortical extracts. Ingle went on work out

that adrenal activity was mediated by a negative feedback mechanism in which glucocorticoids secreted from the adrenal cortex restrict the output of ACTH from the pituitary. On Ingle, see Maurice B. Visscher, "Dwight Joyce Ingle, 1907–1978," *Biographical Memoirs of the National Academy of Sciences* 61 (1992): 247–68; and Mary F. Dallman, "Adrenocortical Function, Feedback, and Alphabet Soup," *American Journal of Physiology: Endocrinology and Metabolism* 289 (2005): E361–E362; as well as Ingle's own autobiography, *I Went to See the Elephant* (New York: Vantage, 1963). Although Ingle himself was apparently absent from the Walter Reed symposium, his idea of permissiveness was referred to numerous times throughout the first day. In addition to Mirsky, who in *Symposium on Stress* detailed Ingle's work on pages 39–40, Rachmiel Levine discussed Ingle on page 49, and John Symons Lyon Browne spoke to the concept on pages 60–61.

55. Mirsky, "Acute Stress," 40.

56. Whitehorn, "Introduction," 7.

57. Rachmiel Levine, "Metabolic Responses in Chronic Stress Situations," in *Symposium on Stress*, 51–52, quote on 51.

58. For more on George Thorn's life and career, see Jacques Lester Gabrilove and Bernard E. Simon, "Where You Go Depends on Where You Are: Early Investigations on the Use of Deoxycorticosterone in Addison's, a Historical Vignette," *Journal of Clinical Endocrinology and Metabolism* 83, no. 5 (1998): 1428–30; as well as "Dr. George W(idmer) Thorn," in *American Men of Science*, ed. Jacques Cattell, 7th ed. (Lancaster, PA: Science Press, 1944), 1783. Thorn's research focused on clinical applications of cortical steroids. In the late 1930s his work demonstrated the effectiveness of desoxycorticosterone as a treatment for Addison's disease and helped to unravel the pathology and physiology of the adrenal cortex. He collaborated with Dwight Ingle in the late 1930s and early 1940s, during which time they published a paper together that demonstrated the qualitative differences in adrenal cortical hormones. See Dwight J. Ingle and George W. Thorn, "A Comparison of the Effects of 11-Desoxycorticosterone Acetate and 17-Hydroxy-11-Dehydrocorticosterone in Partially Depancreatized Rats," *American Journal of Physiology* 132 (March 1941): 670–78.

59. George W. Thorn, Dalton Jenkins, and John Laidlaw, "The Response of Pituitary-Adrenal Systems to Acute Situations Evoking Stress," in *Symposium on Stress*, 53–61.

60. Hudson Hoagland, "Experimental Studies on the Pituitary Adrenocortical System in Situations Evoking Stress," in *Symposium on Stress*, 62–63. Under the workaday pressures of their duties, the pilots that performed most competently had much lower 17-ketosteroid outputs, while their colleagues who performed poorly registered "excessive" levels of the metabolic product, suggesting that "the efficient performers had to call upon their adrenals to a much lesser degree." As we saw in the ORO study, however, 17-ketosteroid analysis was in fact one of the complex and time-consuming tests that could not be done at the MASH laboratory in Korea; the analysis of those samples were in fact completed at the Worcester Foundation.

61. Levine, "Chronic Stress," 47–48.

62. Ibid., 48–52.

63. Curt S. Richter, "Behavioral Regulation of Homeostasis," in *Symposium on Stress*, 77–88.

64. Albert J. Glass, "The Problem of Stress in the Combat Zone," in *Symposium on Stress*, 91–94; Douglas D. Bond, "The Common Psychological Defense to Stressful

Situations and the Patterns of Breakdown When They Fail," in *Symposium on Stress*, 142–52.

65. Henry W. Brosin, "The Reciprocal Relations between Incentives, Motivation, and Strain in Acute and Chronic Stressful Situations," in *Symposium on Stress*, 210; Bond, "Psychological Defense," 142–52.

66. John P. Spiegel, "Psychological Transactions in Situations of Acute Stress," in *Symposium on Stress*, 110–12; Jurgen Ruesch, "The Interpersonal Communication of Anxiety," in *Symposium on Stress*, 161.

67. Wallace O. Fenn, "Acute and Sustained High Energy Output," in *Symposium on Stress*, 8–17, quote on 17; Whitehorn, "Introduction," 5.

68. Harry C. Holloway, "Commentary on 'Reflections on Sullivan and the Language of Psychiatry': Interpersonal Psychotherapy and Neuroscience," *Psychiatry* 66, no. 2 (Summer 2003): 100–101.

69. For an overview of Mason's work and the field in general, see John W. Mason, "Visceral Functions of the Nervous System," *Annual Review of Physiology* 21 (1959): 353–80.

70. The new analytical techniques were the 1952 Nelson-Samuels method of measuring blood plasma 17-hydroxycorticosteroid levels and the 1953 Glenn-Nelson technique for determining corticosteroids in urine. See: Don H. Nelson and Leo T. Samuels, "A Method for the Determination of 17-Hydroxycorticoids in Blood: 17-Hydroxycorticosterone in the Peripheral Circulation," *Journal of Clinical Endocrinology and Metabolism* 12 (1952): 519; and E. Myles Glenn and Don H. Nelson, "Chemical Method for the Determination of 17-Hydroxycorticosteroids and 17-Ketosteroids in Urine Following Hydrolysis with P-Glucuronidase," *Journal of Clinical Endocrinology and Metabolism* 13 (1953): 911. Mason would go on to modify and hone the Glenn-Nelson method for urine. See Nathan R. Rosenthal and John W. Mason, "Urinary 17-Hydroxycorticosteroid Excretion in the Normal Rhesus Monkey," *Journal of Laboratory and Clinical Medicine* 53 (May 1959): 720–28.

71. John W. Mason, "A Re-evaluation of the Concept of 'Non-specificity' in Stress Theory," *Journal of Psychiatric Research* 8 (1971): 325. While I was unable to find the exact passage to which Mason alludes, similar phrases can be found throughout Selye's writings. See, for instance, mention of "even more emotional stresses" in Hans Selye, *The Physiology and Pathology of Exposure to Stress: A Treatise Based on the Concepts of the General-Adaptation-Syndrome and the Diseases of Adaptation* (Montreal: Acta, 1950), 34.

72. For elaborations of these critiques of Selye, see Mason, "Re-evaluation," as well as John W. Mason, "A Review of Psychoendocrine Research on the Pituitary-Adrenal Cortical System," *Psychosomatic Medicine* 30 (September–October 1968): 576–607; Mason, "An Historical View of the Stress Field," pt. 1, *Journal of Human Stress* 1 no. 1 (March 1975): 6–12; and Mason, "An Historical View of the Stress Field," pt. 2, *Journal of Human Stress* 1 no. 2 (1975): 22–36.

73. William E. Bunney, Ernest L. Hartmann, and John W. Mason, "Study of a Patient with 48-Hour Manic-Depressive Cycles," *Archives of General Psychiatry* 12 (June 1965): 619–25; Peter G. Bourne, Robert M. Rose, and John W. Mason, "Urinary 17-OHCS Levels in Combat: Special Forces 'A' Team under Threat of Attack," *Archives of General Psychiatry* 19, no. 2 (1968): 135–40.

74. In 1953 the research components of the Walter Reed Army Medical Center were reorganized as the Walter Reed Army Institute of Research.

75. For what little biographical information there is on Mason, see "Mason, John Wayne," in *American Men and Women of Science*, ed. Andrea Kovacs Henderson, 28th ed., vol. 5 (Detroit: Gale, Cengage Learning, 2010), 283.

76. Mason likely entered into the service in this manner, since he did not appear to serve in World War II.

77. Kenneth Gaarder, "Commentary on 'Reflections on Sullivan and the Language of Psychiatry': The Times of David McK. Rioch," *Psychiatry* 66, no. 2 (Summer 2003): 104–6. See also the mention of Rioch's "attempt to transcend the conventional boundaries" of neurology and psychiatry with his interdisciplinary team, in W. Maxwell Cowan, Donald H. Harter, and Eric R. Kandel, "The Emergence of Modern Neuroscience: Some Implications for Neurology and Psychiatry," *Annual Review of Neuroscience* 23 (2000): 345–46.

78. Mason, "Visceral Functions," 353–54.

79. Rioch's neuroscience team was divided into a section devoted to the study of behavior (the experimental psychiatrists David Hamburg and Morton Reiser and the behavioral psychologist Murray Sidman, as well as Brady and Mason) and a section focused on the brain (the Dutch neuroanatomist Walle Nauta, the auditory physiologist Robert Galambos, and the Italian neurophysiologist Michael Fuortes). See Cowan, Harter, and Kandel, "Emergence," 345–46.

80. For biographical information on Brady, see William Hodos and Nancy A. Ator, "A Festschrift in Honor of Joseph V. Brady in his 70th Year," *Journal of the Experimental Analysis of Behavior* 61 (March 1994): 131–34. Brady's doctoral work appeared in a series of papers in the *Journal of Comparative and Physiological Psychology*. See, for instance, Joseph V. Brady "The Effect of Electro-convulsive Shock on a Conditioned Emotional Response: The Permanence of the Effect," *Journal of Comparative and Physiological Psychology* 44 (1951): 507–11; and Brady "The Effect of Electro-convulsive Shock on a Conditioned Emotional Response: The Significance of the Interval between the Emotional Conditioning and the Electroconvulsive Shock," *Journal of Comparative and Physiological Psychology* 45 (1952): 9–13.

81. John W. Mason, Joseph V. Brady, and Murray Sidman, "Plasma 17-Hydroxycorticosteroid Levels and Conditioned Behavior in the Rhesus Monkey," *Endocrinology* 60, no. 6 (June 1957): 741.

82. John W. Mason, C. Theresa Harwood, and Nathan R. Rosenthal, "Influence of Some Environmental Factors on Plasma and Urinary 17-Hydroxycorticosteroid Levels in the Rhesus Monkey," *American Journal of Physiology* 190 (September 1, 1957): 429.

83. Mason, Brady, and Sidman, "Plasma 17-Hydroxycorticosteroid Levels," 742–43.

84. John W. Mason, "Restraining Chair for the Experimental Study of Primates," *Journal of Applied Physiology* 12 (1958): 130–33.

85. Mason, Harwood, and Rosenthal, "Influence," 429–33; Mason, "Visceral Functions," 355.

86. Mason, Brady, and Sidman, "Plasma 17-Hydroxycorticosteroid Levels," 742–52.

87. Mason, "Visceral Functions," 356–57.

88. Robert W. Porter, Joseph V. Brady, Donald Conrad, John W. Mason, Robert Galambos, and David McKenzie Rioch, "Some Experimental Observations on Gastrointestinal Lesions in Behaviorally Conditioned Monkeys," *Psychosomatic Medicine* 20, no. 5 (1958): 379–94. Brady never directly claimed that emotional stress caused ulcers in his monkeys, but that implication would ultimately be subverted by

the finding in the 1980s that, in fact, most ulcers are not caused by emotional stress but by an acidophilic bacterium, *Helicobacter pylori.* See Barry J. Marshall and J. Robin Warren, "Unidentified Curved Bacillus on Gastric Epithelium in Active Chronic Gastritis," *Lancet* 321, no. 8336 (June 4, 1983): 1273–75; and Barry J. Marshall and J. Robin Warren, "Unidentified Curved Bacilli in the Stomach of Patients with Gastritis and Peptic Ulceration," *Lancet* 323, no. 8390 (June 16, 1984): 1311–15. Although *Helicobacter* might be the primary cause, recent research suggests that psychological stress might play a role in the pathology of the bacterium. The true etiology of peptic ulcers is likely multicausal.

89. Joseph V. Brady, Robert W. Porter, Donald G. Conrad, and John W. Mason, "Avoidance Behavior and the Development of Gastroduodenal Ulcers," *Journal of the Experimental Analysis of Behavior* 1, no. 1 (1958): 69–72, quote on 72.

90. John Lear, "Automation Aids the Post Office," *New Scientist* (December 19, 1957): 20; Joseph V. Brady, "Ulcers in 'Executive' Monkeys," *Scientific American* 199, no. 4 (October 1958): 95–100, 95.

91. *Ulcer at Work* (Oklahoma State Department of Health, 1957), archived in the Prelinger Archives, MPEG video, 28:38, http://www.archive.org/details/ulcer_at_work (accessed September 16, 2013).

92. Douglas B. Price, Margaret Thaler, and John W. Mason, "Preoperative Emotional States and Adrenal Cortical Activity: Studies on Cardiac and Pulmonary Surgery Patients," *Archives of Neurology and Psychiatry* 77 (June 1957): 646–56; Jacob R. Fishman, David A. Hamburg, Joseph H. Handlon, John W. Mason, and Edward Sachar, "Emotional and Adrenal Cortical Responses to a New Experience: Effect of Social Environment," *Archives of General Psychiatry* 6 (April 1962): 271–78; John W. Mason, Edward J. Sachar, Jacob R. Fishman, David A. Hamburg, and Joseph H. Handlon, "Corticosteroid Responses to Hospital Admission," *Archives of General Psychiatry* 13 (July 1965): 1–8. For the studies on parents of terminally ill children, see Stanford E. Friedman, John W. Mason, and David A. Hamburg, "Urinary 17-Hydroxycorticosteroid Levels in Parents of Children with Neoplastic Disease: A Study of Chronic Psychological Stress," *Psychosomatic Medicine* 25 (July–August 1963): 364–76; Stanford E. Friedman, John W. Mason, Paul Chodoff, and David A. Hamburg, "Behavioral Observations on Parents Anticipating the Death of a Child," *Pediatrics* 32 (1963): 610–25; Carl T. Wolff, Stanford E. Friedman, Myron A. Hofer, and John W. Mason, "Relationship between Psychological Defenses and Mean Urinary 17-Hydroxycorticosteroid Excretion Rates: I. A Predictive Study of Parents of Fatally Ill Children" *Psychosomatic Medicine* 26 (September–October 1964): 576–91. On studies of mentally-ill patients, see Bunney, Hartmann, and Mason, "Manic-Depressive Cycles"; and Edward J. Sachar, John W. Mason, Harold S. Kolmer, and Kenneth L. Artiss, "Psychoendocrine Aspects of Acute Schizophrenic Reactions," *Psychosomatic Medicine* 25 (November–December 1963): 510–37.

93. Ralph W. Wadeson, John W. Mason, David A. Hamburg, and Joseph H. Handlon, "Plasma and Urinary 17-OHCS Responses to Motion Pictures," *Archives of General Psychiatry* 9 (August 1963): 146–56.

94. See Wolff et al., "Relationship."

95. See Fishman et al., "Adrenal Cortical Responses."

96. Peter Bourne went on to have a varied career, which included studying anthropology at Stanford University, assuming the duties of adviser to President Jimmy

Carter on health issues and drug policy, becoming a consultant to various international nonprofit organizations, and serving as vice chancellor of Saint George's University in Grenada.

97. The researchers were drawing on their previous research conducted on basic-training inductees that developed a framework to predict the level of endocrine stress response based on factors such as body weight. See Robert M. Rose, Richard Poe, and John W. Mason, "Psychological State and Body Size as Determinants of 17-OHCS Excretion," *Archives of Internal Medicine* 121 (May 1968): 406–13. Based on the indices developed in that study, they expected their subjects in Vietnam to have higher levels of secretion.

98. Peter G. Bourne, Robert M. Rose, and John W. Mason, "Urinary 17-Hydroxycorticosteroid Levels: Data on Seven Helicopter Ambulance Medics in Combat," *Archives of General Psychiatry* 17 (July 1967): 110.

99. Bourne, Rose, and Mason, "17-OHCS Levels."

100. Mason, "Re-evaluation," 323.

101. Ibid., 326.

102. Ibid., 329.

103. Fenn, "High Energy Output," 17.

104. See Allan Young, *The Harmony of Illusions: Inventing Post-traumatic Stress Disorder* (Princeton, NJ: Princeton University Press, 1995); Shephard, *War of Nerves*; Edgar Jones and Simon Wessely, *Shell Shock to PTSD: Military Psychiatry from 1900 to the Gulf War* (New York: Psychology Press, 2005); and Wilbur J. Scott, "PTSD in DSM-III: A Case in the Politics of Diagnosis and Disease," *Social Problems* 37, no. 3 (August 1990): 294–310.

105. John W. Mason, Earl L. Giller, Thomas R. Kosten, Robert B. Ostroff, and Linda Podd, "Urinary Free-Cortisol Levels in Post-traumatic Stress Disorder Patients," *Journal of Nervous and Mental Disease* 174 (1986): 145–49.

Part Four

Work

Chapter Seven

Making Sense of Workplace Fear

The Role of Physicians, Psychiatrists, and Labor in Reframing Occupational Strain in Industrial Britain, ca. 1850–1970

JOSEPH MELLING

The Making of a Stressful World

At the beginning of the twenty-first century, Britain's Health and Safety Executive (HSE) estimated that five million UK employees experienced "stress" as a result of their work. Stress was defined as an individual's adverse reaction to external pressures, though such personal experiences varied in similar conditions. The impact of stress included high absenteeism, increased labor turnover, poor morale, difficult labor relations, and increased risks of accidents and illness. The cost of stress-related illness reported by half a million Britons was estimated at £3.7 billion per year.[1] Britain was only one among many developed countries swept by an epidemic of industrial stress that had become the single most important workplace illness.

The historical origins of this pandemic have recently attracted the attention of scholars, who have pointed to a growing interest in individual personality and the self during the twentieth century. This interest was encouraged in Britain by popularization of psychological ideas, the decline of older moral values, and the spread of holistic medicine during the later twentieth century.[2] This chapter shows that the advance of such ideas was, at best, partial and that notions of stress remained fluid, fragmentary and contested throughout the century. Nowhere is this more evident than in the development of knowledge about occupational stress, which was more usually (and arguably more accurately) understood as personal strain in the century before 1970. Not only were definitions and causal explanations ambiguous; they were also deeply contested, for the terms in which industrial disease was understood continued to be shaped and shadowed by the legal requirements of accident liability and the rigors of compensation law. The institutional framework by which occupational injury was recognized long resisted the idea of psychological injury at work, and occupational psychology established itself in the arena of compensation studies only late in the century.

The rise of occupational stress to primacy among workplace illnesses has been a recent historical development. Only in the 1970s did governments in Europe and the United States develop significant facilities for researching and addressing problems of psychological disorders at work. Britain's Health and Safety at Work Act (1974) established the HSE, which first employed psychologists in occupational research. This was a period when British trade unions pressed government to investigate mental health at the workplace, and the paucity of recent medical research became evident when the Department of Employment sought guidance from the Medical Research Council (MRC) on the nature and causes of industrial stress.[3] The United States had similarly developed job stress research, initially on a very modest scale, after the foundation of the National Institute for Occupational Safety and Health (NIOSH) following the Occupational Health and Safety Act of 1970.[4] When the World Health Organization (WHO) held a major international conference in the 1990s to survey the current knowledge of stress, they sought out historical antecedents by which to validate the concept of homeostasis. They found that physiologists since Claude Bernard had considered the *milieu interieur* in the 1870s, long before Walter Cannon developed the adrenomedullary model of "fight or flight," yet comparatively limited scientific notice was taken of Selye's popularization of these stress ideas before the 1960s.[5]

This chapter adapts Charles Rosenberg's proposal to understand the discovery of diseases as a "framing device," by which a domain of knowledge and expertise is assembled around perceived causal relationships in nature.[6] It views the eruption of interest in workplace stress and the identification of occupational stress as the expression of a specific historical ontology that provided a means by which experts and a lay audience came to comprehend specific kinds of biological, physiological, and psychological reactions to the work environment. Stress served thereby as an organizing principle for a fresh and expanding field of expertise, where different groups of experts measured conditions and objects to grant them significance.[7] The demarcation of such a realm of illness required a spatial as well as a temporal boundary, naming a disorder as belonging to a particular kind of place and to arise from relationships with people as well as with peculiar environmental conditions. The language of stress promised a scientific rationale for a range of perceived bodily changes in an environment that could be thereby designated as stressful, attributing sickness to a peculiar physical space.[8] The location of such bodily or mental disorders was not only a work of ideological or cultural construction: stress expanded in a world bounded by relationships of power and interest that ordered priorities of health and illness. As Gabrielle Hecht has noted, growing awareness of distinct workplace hazards has arisen not only in places bounded by physical terrain and the technological limits of resource exploitation but also in locations mapped by globalized trading relationships and political valuations of strategic materials, including the control of their extraction, handling, and processing.[9]

The present chapter suggests that workplace stress has come to denote a particular range of experiences in a peculiar period of history. The intellectual construction of workplace stress, and the ways it is understood, has been influenced by at least three distinct formations of knowledge in the twentieth century. There was the well-known introduction of models of physiology and biophysiology from the late nineteenth century but more particularly from the 1930s as Walter Cannon's ideas gained influence. Even in this period, the terms "fatigue" and "strain" continued to be used much more commonly than "stress" to depict the impact of work on the body and to denote a condition of anxiety related to the completion of tasks. A second intellectual current that contributed to the growth of post-1945 ideas about stress can be seen in changing assumptions in psychology and the practice of psychiatry concerning the liability of individual personalities to mental illness and to neurasthenia in particular. In the work of Frederic Bartlett and others we can see the beginnings of an effective challenge to biological and behaviorist, as well as older hereditarian, models of personal inadequacy. These changes had an uneven and inconsistent impact on the ways in which occupational fatigue and individual competence was understood more generally. Third, we can see post-1945 ideas of stress being linked to assessments of efficiency and performance within management and organizational theory that drew on ideas in physiology and psychology, but its practitioners were influenced by cybernetic theory and sought to develop behaviorist and sociological models of human relations.[10]

Each of these intellectual formations shared an interest in the stable, balanced personality as an expression of homeostasis in nature and in human organizations, though researchers in these fields rarely coalesced into networks around projects or personalities. These intellectual movements were also enclosed within social and political relationships that were themselves rarely the concern of researchers undertaking studies of workplace stress. Assumptions about class and gender, little noted in most studies before 1970, can be detected in many studies of workplace fatigue during the 1930s and 1940s, for example. The recognition of such differences contributed to the reappraisal of workplace relations in the 1960s and 1970s, when a vocabulary of stress extended across mature industrial societies as a viable way of framing mental, physical, and emotional experiences related to personal identity. The value of this extended word usage was enhanced by the ambiguities that continue to enfold the terminology of stress. For the term implied an etiological explanation for a bewildering array of conditions while reiterating the importance of the personal response to shared environments. The field or domain of stress gained utility as an imprecise, even opaque, vocabulary of existential concerns that owed little to the physiological or biological inquiries that devised the celebrated model of stress in the 1930s and 1940s. When industrial researchers in Britain and the United States came to test biological models of stress, they discovered remarkably little secondary discussion or primary evidence available. They turned to psychiatric records for ways of distinguishing sources of anxiety but found formidable legal and methodological obstacles to accessing such patient information. Even where medical research was forthcoming, there continued to be more emphasis on psychological theory than psychiatric practice and clinical evidence. We shall see that clinical psychiatrists made infrequent and inconsistent use of the medical terminology of "mental stress" (often eliding it with "mental strain"), from the early twentieth century.

Why then did occupational stress gain such currency in the late twentieth century? How did the workplace come to be seen as a space where specific forms of stress could be identified? It is clearly mistaken to view more recent outbreaks of workplace stress as a continuation of an older understanding of the nature and extent of workplace strain. For the field of workplace stress developed unevenly, and at different places and paces, during the later twentieth century. There was no underlying condition, primitively misunderstood as workplace strain, reassessed when medical discovery threw light on a new dark continent of stress. The political and popular appeal of stress arose, it is suggested here, from institutional and cultural needs that began in the postwar years, mostly beyond the scope or interest of scientific inquiry. Earlier occupational strain had served a different audience and was circumscribed by rather different institutional rationale than the more fluid language of individual stress. The transfer of attention from physical fatigue at work and mental strain in specific cases of mental illness to a less precise usage of personal stress cannot be explained simply, or mainly, in terms of scientific debate. The development of a globalized economy that required new forms of labor utilization and changes to arrangements for labor bargaining and the legal recompense of injured workers provided one important context for a reappraisal of the nature of personal anxiety. Regulatory bodies established by national states and transnational agencies did not trace a clear line of continuity between an older responsibility to protect workers against physical strain and fatigue and the fresh demands of investigating mental stress. The apparent surge of occupational stress is taken in this chapter to be a peculiar construction of a rationality grounded in specific forms of economic logic and commonsense understanding as well as scientific expertise.

Radical psychology challenged older explanations of mental illness and presented less stigmatized views of mental stress. But the consistency and impact of more liberal ideas of mental illness on society—or the workplace—before the 1970s should not be exaggerated. This chapter considers the growth of a distinct ontology of workplace stress by using evidence from institutional, organizational, and personal records to capture exchanges between doctors, researchers, and nonscientists in regard to the physical and mental health of the working population. Such materials provide historians with a rare opportunity to examine conversations and contests between professional and nonexperts. They show that ideas of occupational stress did not figure prominently in scientific debate, medical practice, or management discourse before the 1960s. Our analysis of the evidence begins with a brief review of recent scholarship that has considered industrial stress.

Narratives of Unease: Histories of Psychology and Stress

There has been limited specific research on the history of industrial stress. In his survey of mental illness, including depression and neuroses, Edward Shorter noted that "stress has become a kind of magic formula with which to explain psychic distress." Shorter's evidence indicates that the inability to work, rather than the strain of excessive or difficult employment, remained far more common in assessments of melancholy and depression.[11] Andreas Killen's study of neurosis among German telephone operators in the Wilhelmine and Weimar periods documents the initial willingness of psychiatrists to recognize mental anxiety arising from the physical trauma of electric shock. This orthodoxy was subsequently discredited by Fritz Giese, Ewald Stier, and others, who reiterated the importance of individual personality and self-control. More important, Killen shows the influence of legal procedure and compensation rules in medical assessments of the nature and severity of mental strain arising, not from an accumulation of fatiguing tasks, but from a specific and sudden shock.[12] Killen's "classic hysterical form" of madness exhibited by these operators affirmed a "rational, concrete myth," whose origins lay in the material "dislocations and stresses of technological modernity."[13] The advantage of this analysis is its displacement of assumptions about the chronological progression of scientific orthodoxy and specific forms of forensic proof, indicating that ideas about mental strain in particular occupations or tasks were themselves grounded in wider beliefs about gender and susceptibility to technological and organizational change.

Junko Kitanaka similarly argues that in Japan during the late twentieth century, earlier scientific assumptions, often drawn from Germany, regarding neurasthenia were replaced by biological models of depression and latterly to a recognition of the workplace environment as contributing to a renewed understanding of workloads and individual strain against the background of a long economic recession. Kitanaka suggests that the identification of workplace stress offered a means by which psychiatrists overcame the established dichotomies of biological and societal models of illness, providing biomedical categories that encompassed moral balance and personal responsibility. Nikolas Rose argued from a different perspective that the growth of industrial psychology and other "psy" sciences in the early twentieth century was related to management models of effort control, allocating responsibility for output to individual workers rather than groups or craft fraternities.[14] There is some parallel to Kitanaka's Japanese story and Rose's critique of early occupational psychology in the reassessment of occupational health models by European researchers in the 1990s, who argued that psychosocial and organizational factors in workers' health needed to be integrated in any assessment of stress.[15]

This scholarship provides clues as to the progress of psychological thinking in regard to occupational stress, though there remain few historical studies of treatment for those reported to be suffering employment-related strain or stress before the later decades of the twentieth century.[16] Nervous disorders and neurasthenia had long been associated in the nineteenth- and early twentieth-century medical literature with the excessive exertions of mental work, more particularly with female and male brain workers who were held to be susceptible to mental strain. There is some evidence from admissions to English mental institutions during the nineteenth century that groups such as governesses were notably overrepresented in the registers of fee-paying asylums, though the sources also suggest that descriptions of the social and emotional characteristics of such occupational groups were heavily influenced by contemporary cultural expectations and by institutional segregation of their treatment.[17] We know little about the perceived influence of those wider societal and organizational factors (including class, gender, ethnicity, and occupational community) in earlier incidents of work-related strain that later commentators considered so important.

Discussions about the psychology of workers and responses to industrial dangers can be found in Britain from the late nineteenth century. By the 1890s the psychiatric profession had elaborated its vocabulary of mental disorders beyond the staple diagnoses of mania, melancholia, and dementia, inspired in part by discussions about longevity and reflected in pamphlets such as James Collier's *Relation of Neurasthenia to the Duration of Life.*[18] In the early years of the twentieth century, asylums were provided with a basic guide to standard diagnoses and causes of insanity, which included mental stress. Diagnoses of "strain" related to conditions such as "hysteria" were not unknown in male as well as female admissions to asylums during the Victorian years, but such words appear far less frequently than "melancholia" or even "dementia" as descriptors of symptoms that came to be understood as "neurasthenia" or "neuroses" in many medical texts by the early twentieth century. By the 1920s the debates around Freudian therapy as well as detailed work, in Germany and elsewhere, on biological and physiological origins of mental disturbance were often noted, some medical commentators recognizing that "fear" and "nerves" could figure in the workplace and among manual as well as among brain workers in British industry.[19] Progress in recognizing the impact of physical and mental strain on the manual workforce remained extremely slow. Edgar Collis examined the relationship between industrial fatigue and the incidence of tuberculosis, though offering only the obvious conclusions that strenuous and dusty occupations left workers more susceptible.[20] Sir John Collie suggested in a 1933 *Lancet* article that industrial neurasthenia could be suffered by coal miners who went to assist injured other workers, though contemporary disasters make little mention of such shock.[21] The reasons for the limited attention devoted to occupational sources of mental strain are a major concern of the present chapter.

The following section adopts a chronological approach to the evolution of ideas about stress in psychiatry by considering how practicing psychiatrists and other medical authorities understood the relationship between occupation and mental strain from the late nineteenth century. Many diagnoses of patients were influenced by, if not negotiated with, a variety of other people involved in the identification of mental illness in these years, and "strain" figured in vernacular as well as scientific and professional discussions of mental unease.

The Complexions of Psy: Mental Disorder, Psychiatric Practice, and Work, 1855–1914

In the Victorian era British doctors recognized mental disturbance in the inability to work and a lack of diligence in regard to useful employment rather than in strain arising from work itself. Such assumptions were heavily gendered, though mental work undertaken by both males and females could give rise, it was recognized, to illness. William Young Sellar (1825–90), sometime professor of Latin at Edinburgh, became the subject of concerned correspondence between Florence Bairdsmith and Edmund Lushington in 1868. Florence observed Sellar suffering a "great deal of mental strain and gloominess about his own condition." He later recovered bodily health without corresponding relief from "the cruel depression" that flowed from "these dyspeptic derangements of the system." Florence did not attribute William's strain directly to his mental efforts but reflected sadly on the lack of the spirit of adversity that had enlivened their former exchanges.[22]

The rarity and opacity of such references to mental strain among even the intellectual middle classes during later Victorian decades is confirmed by an analysis of public (Poor Law–funded) and fee-paying mental asylums in England. Notes of "strain" and "overstrain" appear more often in explanations of the origins of insanity among middle class admissions to fee-paying asylums than Poor Law asylums before 1914. The use of such terms also became rather more common from the 1890s, though they were used in a relatively small number of cases and principally to describe female illness.

Among almost nine hundred female and eight hundred male admissions to one fee-paying institution in the later nineteenth and early twentieth centuries, there were only three or four female and one male case where a breakdown in health was directly attributed to "overstrain" arising from employment or mental exertion at work.[23] The term "fatigue" belonged to an earlier period than "overstrain" and was again used in very few cases, again primarily female.[24] More common were references to "overwork," and here the diagnosis of causes of mental illness was more commonly used for male admissions, with 7 percent of men having insanity partly attributed to overworking—predominantly in a mental rather than a physical capacity. Clergymen, educationalists, clerks, doctors, and lawyers were among those notably represented with "melancholy," the most common single diagnosis, closely followed by "mania."[25] The only references to physiology were among ten cases of "General Paralysis," subsequently attributed by medical experts to syphilitic infection. Among nineteen females said to have overworked, seven or eight were in education, though others were in occupations such as dressmaking or had no given occupation.

Even if we agree that "stress" and "strain" were uncommonly used to explain insanity before 1914, it could be argued that symptoms subsequently recognized as "stress" were characterized as "anxiety," overlapping with descriptions of overwork or fatigue. Such claims are difficult to sustain, for it is questionable to reallocate contemporary language to later diagnostic categories of mental illness. Even so, only small groups admitted to the fee-paying asylum in the five decades before 1914 were said to be ill because of "anxiety" (about 4 percent of female and 3 percent of male admissions). Female teachers again were noticeable, though with the portmanteau term "gentlewoman" assigned to more than half of these female sufferers and the care of others as a major source of anxiety. The small group of anxious males included lawyers, doctors, clerks, and teachers, with a station master said to be "anxious over work" and a butler displaying "anxiety on the death of his master." Nor did the association of insanity with "nerves" figure notably in the admissions to fee-paying asylums, with only 4 people of each sex suffering from conditions such as "nervous shock" (female) or "nervous debility" (male), and 1 clerk recorded as having a "nervous breakdown" and melancholia before admission in 1912.

Public asylums provide much less detail on the illness of the broader mass of the population admitted to tax-funded institutions before 1914. The case notes have fewer details, frequent repetition, and less consistency. Detailed examination of admissions for one asylum during 1880–82 shows about 60 percent of both female (168 of 276) and male (154 of 262) admissions recorded no known cause of insanity. Known causes included a few cases of "mental depression" (3 females) or anxiety (2 females). Males were noticeably more likely to have had accidents (12 cases) or sunstroke (4 instances). Work figured directly in 3 cases, though it was lack of work rather than excessive strain in 2 of them. "Over work" did feature in the case of a railway goods guard who complained of not being paid for overtime, though the medical diagnosis was "General Paralysis."[26] "Overstudy" was noted on 3 occasions, with 2 cases of anxiety at admission. William S. was anxious "as to Accounts," while Thomas G., a chimney sweep, suffered "mental anxiety" after being treated for genital disease (an occupational hazard for sweeps) and his wife's disappearance.

This limited comparison of fee-paying and public asylums before 1914 reveals that overwork and overstudy were more likely to figure among male admissions in fee-paying than in public asylums, though the latter catered for the broad mass of the laboring population. Work-related illness featured less prominently in female admissions to either kind of institution, and it was mental rather than physical exertion in the few cases of affliction noted for both sexes. Females in fee-paying institutions were more prone to "anxiety" than "overwork," and domestic and caring duties rather than employment figured in cameos of feminine distress. Bodily accidents and illness were more frequently connected to the onset of insanity in the public asylum, though even here work injuries were rarely noted.

The evidence of admission and diagnoses of insanity and mental illness gathered from institutions before 1914 suggests that "strain" and "stress" figured rarely in reported causes of insanity. Although the classification of such causes was codified and classified in 1907, as noted earlier, including the possible attribution of "mental stress," there is little evidence of its use for these hospitalized patients at this period. There were nonspecific references to "mental strain" in middle-class correspondence describing the "depression" and melancholy of intellectual acquaintances, with the first references to "mental breakdown" appearing before 1914. The onset of strain or overexertion at the industrial workplace was not recognized in psychiatric circles as a direct source of mental illness. The question of psychological factors in workplace injury arose from quite another quarter before 1914. This was in relation to the problem of determining legal liability for injury and illness at work and was linked by some writers to a much wider discourse about the disorders of industrial society. These discussions and the problems of output during World War I (1914–18) influenced the way in which psychological strain at work was understood before 1939.

Detecting and Deterring "Industrial Fear": Evidence of Strain at Work, 1910–40

Historians of occupational hazards have argued that we can understand the spread of modern technology and scientific expertise about disease within a transnational context, while also registering the distinct institutional practices and cultural values of different societies.[27] We can trace the medical and popular understanding of injury compensation along this perspective. Karl Figlio's assessment of occupational ailments, such as miners' nystagmus (caused by poor luminosity underground), suggests that the definition and understanding of injury remained a contested field of knowledge and that the testimony of workers was openly questioned.[28] The passage of workers' compensation legislation across Europe and in some US states in the three decades before 1914 gave rise to fresh areas of medical discourse and debate, more particularly after British law conceded the liability of employers for occupational illness as well as specific accidents. Thomas Oliver and other leading authorities on industrial disease helped to identify ailments that amounted to twenty-seven specific illnesses listed for compensation by Thomas Legge (the doyen of occupational disease experts) at Harvard in 1919.[29] Legge noted that disease descriptions were worded widely, to "sweep into the net all cases and not merely those with marked symptoms." There was no provision for traumatic shock of the kind covered in Germany, though there were provisions for repetitive strain suffered by telegraphists.[30] Deborah Palmer's research into British nursing before 1914 also suggests that it was not only female teachers who figured in reports of mental strain but also hospital nurses working long hours in London and elsewhere. The ethos of professionalism promoted by senior nurses and nurse leaders served to repress rather than express the hazards of overwork and strain in such nonmanual occupations.[31]

The threat of unionization of nurses before 1914 also complicated discussions of health at the workplace. The early years of the twentieth century saw the outbreak of unprecedented levels of industrial conflict in Europe and the United States, and it was with workplace strain and strife as much as the nature and implications of "trauma," or the relationship of physiology and psychology, that many commentators dwelled. The enlistment of the psychologists W. H. R. Rivers and Charles S. Myers for war and their subsequent departure from Cambridge left Frederic Bartlett with the burden of carrying laboratory psychology forward, though it was not until the 1930s that the Cambridge group (led by the brilliant Kenneth Craik) became directly involved in studies of fatigue and human decision making in conditions of psychological strain.[32] Although Henry Head and Rivers had engaged in pioneering research on sensory responses, collaboration of physiologists, psychologists, and medical experts on "strain" remained limited before Craik.

The distinctive impact of World War I on celebrated psychologists such as Rivers cannot explain these disciplinary distances, for physiologists as well as psychologists had often been personally affected by the experience of modern warfare. Scientists such as Walter Cannon of Harvard were clearly affected by the suffering, which contributed in part to his ideas in regard to the adrenal glands and the impact of emotions on the human body.[33]

It was the Industrial Health Research Board (IHRB), accountable to the MRC by the 1930s, which conducted the most detailed empirical investigations of workplace performance and mental attitudes, led notably by Stephen W. Wyatt. The impact of this work, and of debates about industrial injury and industrial conflict on the progress of medical discourse in regard to strain and stress, has been little noticed. These researchers approached the problem of strain in highly specific, nonmedical terms, where the problem was posed by others in terms of optimal output and physical efficiency of individual workers. The researchers involved in these studies made several assumptions about intelligence, class, and gender: they suggested more educated females were more likely to become bored with mundane and repetitive work, while less educated workers of both sexes were more liable to find the strain of intense machine pacing the greatest.[34] Vocational education and guidance became increasingly prominent during the 1930s, including Eric Farmer's research efforts encouraged by David Munro (secretary of the IHRB). Munro wished to monitor juvenile training in distressed areas of high unemployment and also persuaded Bartlett to take on Farmer, which led to important initiatives on the eve of World War II.[35]

Not only was research on industrial strain affected by various forms of social bias, but there were also fairly crude attempts during the early twentieth century to characterize industrial conflict as a pathological response of an unhealthy body of workers. The professor of neuropathology at Harvard, where Legge delivered his Cutter lectures, argued in the same year that they were published that "industrial medicine exists; industrial psychiatry ought to exist." He pointed to labor unrest as an expression of internal disorders within the production system, which the psychiatrists could address.[36] Writers discussing the relationship of traumatic injury to the onset of disease frequently slid into a discussion of mental illness after questioning the legal and moral implications of employees' conduct. Grahamsley Howitt's *Accident and Disease* (1914) suggested that venereal disease (particularly tabes) played a large part in claims for injury by affecting the nervous system of workers, including neuroses of which "Neurasthenia and Hysteria are the worst."[37] Notable experts in physiology, respiratory disease, and tuberculosis took part in discussions about traumatic injury, spurred by discussions about employers' liability under National Insurance and compensation laws. More sympathetic to the claims of workers, Dr. Frederick Parkes-Weber strongly advocated the German model of social insurance, arguing that compulsory insurance would ensure work was conducted "under the most hygienic conditions possible," as workers would be submitted to treatment by "the approved methods" rather than wandering between hospitals.[38]

In questions of injury, the rights, motives, and mental stability of workers in regard to compensation were widely discussed before 1914. During 1910 Sir Clifford Allbutt recalled his testimony of the 1870s in a successful claim for damages by a railway worker who had developed pneumonia after a chest injury.[39] The respiratory expert Arthur J. Hall of Sheffield described the case of an injured collier who developed acute phthisis (tuberculosis).[40] Hall had warned the employers that the Workmen's Compensation Act was "looming so large in the workmen's horizon" that they should settle the claim. Hall also confided to Parkes-Weber that he was satisfied that the "relationship between traumatism and Tuberculosis is considerably closer than the profession has hitherto recognized," despite the difficulty of providing conclusive proof of the onset of disease. Edgar Collis similarly took an active interest in respiratory diseases at work, including the relationship between industrial fatigue and the incidence of tuberculosis.[41]

The mental state of industrial workers and their vulnerability to "modern" neurasthenia interested several physicians critical of the impact of compensation legislation on malingering.[42] By 1914 a considerable literature on the problem of malingering and assurance had emerged, and insurance companies retained the services of doctors who provided an opinion on the likely illness of applicants for insurance. Not only insurance companies but friendly societies and trades unions examined the returns for sickness and superannuation, finding that sickness and pension rates declined in periods of high unemployment and that it required, in T. S. Ashton's words, a "high standard of character" among members if considerable malingering was to be avoided.[43] Parkes-Weber's 1911 article, "The Association of Hysteria with Malingering," drew on several cases at the German Hospital in London. Even the distinguished industrial health expert Thomas Oliver claimed in 1915 that "the rate at which traumatic neuroses are increasing among female workers in all trades is a noticeable feature of modern industrial life, and for this the Workmen's Compensation Act is no doubt partly responsible."[44]

Occupational injury specialists were willing to speculate about the nexus between physical trauma, psychological shock, and persistent illness, even when organic relationships remained obscure. It was the legal implication of accidents and ailments at work that raised acute problems of patient testimony for the physician faced with occupational sickness. Thomas Oliver told the Assurance Medical Society that there was "nothing in medicine more difficult to deal with than an illness in which the symptoms are purely subjective."[45] Testimony sharpened questions of self-certification and contested knowledge and alternative ways of knowing illness or dangers of injury, including the risks of phthisis. The evidence of workers became a basic component of compensation claims and contributed to debates on psychology and malingering. The relationship of physical illness such as pneumonia to the onset of psychosis provided another puzzle for clinicians, though the subject was surrounded by controversy as well as uncertainty.[46] Another tuberculosis expert, Hyslop Thomson, argued that the mentally ill sometimes imagined symptoms of consumption; in 1912 he suggested that "the modern neurasthenic" held pet delusions of tubercular illness.[47]

Medical discussions of the nature and severity of strain in the industrial workplace continued to be overshadowed during the interwar years by debates on incentives to malingering provided by national insurance and compensation laws and by assumptions about the demands of intellectual versus manual labor. The new physiology developed by Cannon and his predecessors in Britain left open the question of the relationship between physiological shocks and physical illness, though it was more in sympathy with behaviorist models of psychology than with the kind of pragmatic psychiatry practiced by those dealing with mental illness. Research into fear and mental strain made little obvious impact on discussions of workplace injury, even if physical fatigue had attracted considerable attention during the period immediately after World War I. Where employers could not demonstrate that workers were deliberately feigning illness to secure benefits, they were prepared to suggest that mental strain among nervous individuals led them to exhibit symptoms that simulated physical ailments. The tension regarding the denial of physiological and psychological illness became apparent in legal disputes over eyestrain among coal miners during the interwar years. Employers argued that many workers who appeared to suffer from nystagmus were in fact individuals predisposed to poor vision, possibly congenitally, and also nervous individuals unsuited to work underground. These symptoms were a form of nervous strain or neurosis. Dr. Llewellyn advised the north Wales coal masters that nystagmus originated in mental anxiety rather than the physical environment of the pit and that the best treatment was "to destroy the 'industrial fear' which the men had, and this was best done by work, light work on the surface at first then allowing the man to resume his former work."[48]

There were rare instances where eye disorders and mental illness appeared in the same patient. John Evans was suffering from nystagmus developed while employed at Westminster Colliery in north Wales when he was admitted to North Wales Lunatic Asylum at Denbigh in September 1914.[49] His claim was settled in early 1915, though the doctor retained by the employers argued that "the man's mental condition is still bad & the prospects of recovery is [*sic*] small" but "the Nystagmus has passed away." The employers' insurers added that this was also "the opinion of one of the Medical Attendants," whom their medical consultant spoke to during a visit to the asylum.[50] The reported testimony of the Denbigh attendant—attendants being usually untrained nurses—was flatly contradicted by the asylum's medical superintendent, who believed Evans still suffered from nystagmus and required examination by the certifying surgeon. The latter agreed the condition persisted, though the patient "could certainly do light employment" if his mental state improved.[51] Meanwhile, compensation continued and the employers required new employees to declare they had not suffered such industrial diseases, with the proviso that any "workman making a false declaration forfeits all claim to compensation."[52] Other miners in receipt of compensation were admitted to such institutions during the early twentieth century, though the cause of their illness was not always indicated.[53]

The coal-mining industry exemplified many of the issues that confronted any investigation of mental strain or stress at work, for communal and class values often reinforced an older view that it was lack of employment rather than the exertion of work that presented the greater threat to mental stability. Care is needed before reaching any general conclusions in this regard. George Orwell's account of a mining town in the 1930s noted working men's acceptance of "the strain of poverty" and their "psychological adjustment" to the risks of life on the dole.[54] Similarly, claims that neurasthenics were prone to faulty imagination and could not be relied on to provide authentic testimony of their illness, while more calculating individuals were suspected of malingering, should be placed in the context of contemporary political and moral disputes over the responsibility for absence from work. Diaries document feelings of individual isolation; one young unemployed person described being in "the midst of a sea of despondency," where thoughts of suicide alternated with feelings of angry desperation.[55] Communal and personal responses to injury, illness, and idleness in coal regions of south and north Wales during the interwar years reveal, however, a range of cultural values concerning family and social responsibility, personal privacy, and the stigma of illnesses among both young and old.[56]

It was not the fear of underground hazards that briefly concerned the South Wales Miners' Federation in 1938, but the impact of new technology on the workforce. Prominent communist official Arthur Horner replied to an inquiry from the Federation's compensation secretary in 1938, asking if members complained "about the nervous effects in consequence of working with pneumatic picks, or other coal-cutting machinery." Horner and other agents replied that pneumatic picks were not common and even cutting machinery was only recently introduced.[57] Given the long-standing battle of the mining unions to demonstrate the link between the physical environment of darkness, dust, gas, and water to the onset of disease, rather than individual neuroses, there may also have been reluctance to identify nervous strain as a widespread problem underground. The increased interest in workplace nerves could have originated with the Trades Union Congress

(TUC), for in 1938 its medical consultant reported Dr. Edward Snowden's experience with "cases of function disabilitics or neuroses," including "injury psychoneurosis" or "traumatic neurasthenia," which were generally ignored by doctors (though some progress was being made with the British Medical Association in 1939).[58]

By the late 1930s there was greater interest in mental capacity of the industrial workforce, including the value of vocational training on the productivity of labor, though no substantial medical or scientific research that considered the impact of workplace conditions or occupational environment on the mental or emotional health of employees. There remained an assumption that manual labor presented few intellectual or emotional strains. Discussions of injury rarely touched on mental well-being, with critics of insurance and compensation laws presenting two extreme examples of workers as unreliable witnesses of their own illness: at one extreme was the deliberate malingerer who exploited the opportunity to claim benefits and at the other was the neurotic individual whose inadequacies led them to imagine or invent symptoms that again qualified them for benefits.

This was the moment at which James Halliday began to publish his celebrated articles on psychoneuroses among benefit claimants that subsequently developed into a distinct psychosomatic model of illness. Scholars have located Halliday as a significant figure in holistic medicine and the restatement of the importance of emotional stress in personal health, as well as a contributor to the popularization of psychological ideas in British society during the twentieth century.[59] Halliday later drew on psychological ideas as well as American writings in psychosomatic medicine to emphasize the importance of internal struggles that were expressed in emotional stress and led sufferers to report physical ailments, though his earliest work was framed after critical observations of "mental and emotional maladjustment" among claimants of sickness benefits under the National Insurance scheme.[60] The Scots medical officer noted that the impact of "mental stress" on organic health had been known previously as neurasthenia but was properly understood as psychoneuroses, affecting a large section of the population.[61] It was the coal-mining population that again attracted the attention of this advocate of psychosomatic medicine, where he found "anxiety states" and "anxiety-hysteria" to be the most frequent specific expression in miners of the psychoneuroses he detected in much of the working population. The organic result was the recurrence of gastric as well as chronic respiratory ailments among miners. While Halliday identified fear of accidents and disease as a final factor in the illnesses induced or imagined by psychoneurotic anxiety, they figured alongside domestic troubles, economic problems, and fear of unemployment or difficulties in work relationships.[62]

Most writers have seen Halliday as a pioneer of psychosomatic thinking and a forerunner of changes in medical thinking from traditional to holistic approaches. From the perspective of occupational medicine, Halliday's concern was to demonstrate that changes in patterns of morbidity and physical ailments were the expression of broad shifts in societal expectations and neurotic anxiety states, which manifested themselves in apparent work-related diseases that could not be adequately explained in terms of specific environmental factors. In this respect, Halliday confirmed a conservative medical skepticism about the risks both of malingering and of neurotic anxiety that led to ill-founded claims of occupational injury and illness. It was the outbreak of another great military conflict and a brief resurgence of interest in workplace strain that encouraged more serious investigations of industrial environments and the impact of productivity drives on human relationships. These can be briefly considered along with the evidence of psychiatric treatment of strain and stress among the working population in the era of full employment and rising living standards.

Workplace Strain and Social Costs in the Transition from War to Peace, 1940–1960s

The director of the Cambridge Psychological Laboratory, Frederic Bartlett, had completed his major work, *Remembering* (1932), and published a popular book on noise by the time Kenneth Craik took over the leadership of cognitive laboratory research at the renamed Applied Psychology Research Unit.[63] The unit provided some of the most ambitious and influential studies of task performance and decision making under conditions of stress published in the postwar years, including Donald Broadbent's research on cognitive "filtering," which became the basis of his study *Decision and Stress.*[64] The Cambridge group had built on a series of workplace studies completed by the IHRB, continued during the war by Wyatt and Russell Davis, including Wyatt's study of variations in output and worker efficiency employed for different periods, funded by the MRC.[65] The outbreak of World War II and the drive for maximum productivity gave experts in occupational health and industrial psychologists a wider audience within government and in industry, including the British Employers' Confederation, which welcomed a survey into absenteeism at work, being convinced that as much as one-third of all illnesses in the United Kingdom was due to nonorganic causes.[66]

By the end of the war, industrial psychologists had become interested in the psychological well-being of manual workers, including Alastair Heron and Dorothy Braithwaite's study of "emotional stability in colliery workers," in which they used a model developed to assess levels of neuroses and emotional instability among soldiers.[67] These studies drew attention to the importance of military models informing such workplace investigations, as well as the tensions between technical and medical assessments of those monitoring and the progress of different production systems. The MRC funded Norah Davis in the early 1950s to examine "sources of strain" in the workplace, distinguishing physical fatigue and "mental strain" in machine workers employed on bonus wages. Davis followed Wyatt in using workers' own testimony to explore the language of strain. One employee told the researchers: "It's the ruin of men's health, physically and mentally. When the bonus system came on I worked so hard that I got pleurisy, with the sweating and then catching cold. Since then I've not bothered, for health is more important." Davis concluded that workers suffered not only from "nervous tension" but from a fear that they would be unable to continue working. Problems of workplace strain could be traced to poor work design but also arose from "often wholly unwarranted psychological assumptions about 'the worker.'"[68] The problem of gathering workers' opinions on their work may help to explain the restriction of so much psychological research into skill, work effort, and stress to highly technical laboratory studies of individual decision making and motor performance during the 1950s. When Hywel Murrell was commissioned by the MRC during the early 1970s to evaluate scientific and social research into stress and strain, he commented critically on the paucity and confusion of investigations since the war.[69] The consequence was that the most detailed scientific work remained disconnected from the contemporary study and practical conduct of management and labor relations in British industry.

Even if there was limited conversation between the scientific community and the parties employed in industrial production, it may be argued that ideas about workplace strain and stress were disseminated by medical services and publications that were undergoing significant change in the 1950s. Older models of custodial care for those with mental illnesses were changed by the introduction of new drugs and the adoption of more liberal regimes of hospital management. The records created by these agencies give us clues as to the opinions of relatives and friends concerning mental strain, as well as providing a professional narrative of medical treatment. The concluding section of this chapter draws on these sources and offers a point of comparison with the earlier survey of medical registers in regard to occupational illnesses.

Working Life and Mental Illness at the Dawn of the Age of Stress, 1945–70

Patient records were considered by Donald Broadbent as a key resource when he contemplated a new program of research on the mental health of industrial car workers in the mid-1970s, though problems of access and sampling presented insurmountable barriers to a contemporary study.[70]

Any retrospective analysis of the records of mental-hospital patients faces its own challenges, though these materials offer insights into contemporary attitudes to occupational distress not easily gleaned from other quarters. A study of mental hospitals in southwest England, based on many thousands of hospitals admissions from 1910–65, undertaken with my colleague Nicole Baur, indicates that "mental stress" was introduced as a contributory or main cause of mental illness from 1907 but not as a primary diagnosis.[71] This evidence suggests that stress was perceived as a primary or secondary cause of illness among a limited number of the thousands of admissions to one group of mental hospitals during the period under review. Not only did stress figure in a minority of admissions: its significance also rose and fell during the midcentury years, rising as a *primary* cause of 39 cases between 1931 and 1935 to 113 during 1945–50 and then falling consistently to 35 by 1955–60.[72]

During the early and middle decades of the twentieth century, it was much more common to attribute mental illness to heredity, biological imbalance, and the life cycle, accounting for a significant proportion of those for whom primary causes were assigned (and many admissions had no cause assigned). About 300 female admissions and just over 100 male admissions were recorded with "mental stress" as a primary cause of their illness. About half of each group were admitted compulsorily to the Devon asylums, though many were said to be suffering from such ailments as "senile psychosis" and "senile dementia" as well as "depression" and "schizophrenia," with schizophrenia and depression (as well as senile dementia) more prominent among males. Many patients were diagnosed as suffering from "mood disorders" (28.5 percent and 36.5 percent of single and multiple admissions, respectively), and about one-fifth of admissions were said to experience "anxiety disorders" of a neurotic kind.

In 298 female admissions "stress" figured as the primary cause of illness, with 273 being "prolonged mental stress." Prolonged mental stress was estimated by doctors and psychiatrists to be responsible for almost five times as many female hospital admissions in this period as the same condition among males, while the latter were twice as likely as females, thought the doctors, to suffer "sudden stress" prior to admission. Stress figured relatively rarely as a primary cause of illness for mental patients in the twentieth century, though it gained much more prominence as a "contributory" or secondary cause, particularly for males.[73] More than 1 in 5 females and almost twice this number of males were assigned "stress" as a contributory cause. The precision of the diagnoses and etiology remains questionable, because many of these "stressed" individuals were said to suffer from primary dementia as well as mania and "confusional" or "alternating [also "manic depressive" and later "bi-polar"] insanity," though these cases were mainly seen as melancholic or depressed.

The relationship between stress as a primary, or a contributory, cause of mental illnesses and the working lives of these patients is difficult to excavate from the medical case notes of patients. The evidence indicates that such links were tenuous and rarely recognized as a major factor in disease. A relatively small number of patients accounted for many admissions that were primarily attributed to "mental stress." Mary F. was admitted on twenty-two occasions between January 1930 and December 1955, suffering from "alternating insanity," "recurrent mania," and "manic-depression," caused in each case by "prolonged mental stress." On the first two occasions she was certified, but thereafter, probably reflecting the changes introduced by the 1930 Mental Treatment Act, she entered as a voluntary patient. Charles Z., a window cleaner, entered the hospital eleven times between October 1937 and July 1962, suffering "acute" depression, "manic-depression," and "recent mania," which resulted on each occasion from "sudden mental stress."[74]

Work was identified as a feature in the admission of fourteen males, half of whom were said to have suffered from "overwork" or "workload," three from unemployment, two from anxieties at work, and two from physical illness. Similarly, seven references to male employment related primarily to the loss of work, though David T., a civil servant, was said to be "unhappy in his job." Only one case directly linked "stress" and "overwork": William E., a hairdresser, entered the hospital with a "spasm of both eyes," though this singular case also involved the suspected infidelity of a wife. The few cases are difficult to place in a larger pattern of employment and illness. Our case study includes large numbers of male manual workers in regular, if moderately paid, employment during the period 1940–70. With the exception of "clerical work," no significant group of nonmanual employees entered the public asylum, most of the clerks having psychoses and less than one-third diagnosed as suffering neuroses. Among twenty-nine male admissions where "stress" figured as a primary cause of illness, most were laborers, though a quarter were skilled men and another quarter were in the armed services or nonmanual work. Slightly more male admissions with occupations were recorded as having stress as a contributory cause of illness, and there were fewer laborers and more skilled males and men in nonmanual occupations.

The picture for females admitted with illnesses due to stress differed from that of males. Work figured in the primary cause of illness for only 4 women and employment in 5 or 6 (including husband's unemployment, husband's low wages, and a refusal of reengagement for the patient). Betty B., a chambermaid, was unusually recorded as "unhappy in her job." Female patients in general were much less likely to be in waged employment, and the range of occupations in which they worked was more restricted. The majority of those admitted to the mental hospital were described as a "housewife" or given no occupational status, though a similar proportion of female as male admissions were nonmanual employees, representing a significantly greater proportion of the total employed. Teachers were a notable group among

Table 7.1. Selected occupations of single admitted and readmitted male patients, ca. 1948–65

	Male patients	
Occupations	Single admitted	Readmitted
Professional and clerical occupations	12.5%	15.9%
Agricultural work	10.9%	18.9%
Manual trades and related work	56.2%	48.3%
Not known	11.8%	6.7%
Unemployed	4.9%	5.4%
None	6.0%	5.4%

Source: Devon Record Office, Exeter: Mental Health Case Records, Unsorted Hospital Deposit, 2010–11.

admissions, with 170 admissions; more than half were diagnosed as psychotic, about a quarter were said to be suffering some form of depression, and very few exhibited neuroses. In addition to teachers, the other main group of skilled or professional females admitted to our mental hospitals in southern England was nurses: 171 nurse admissions appear in our study group, with more than half suffering from psychoses and few from neuroses, though 1 in 5 admissions were said to be in an "anxiety state." As in the late nineteenth century, nurses appear to be recorded as prone to mental and emotional strain, though even here it is rare to find a direct attribution of work as the primary or contributory cause of mental illness.

The information from mental hospitals places greater emphasis on domestic arrangements, marital relations, and family or kinship relations both in the identification of mental illness more generally and the incidence of stress among patients admitted. The number of housewives considered to have suffered prolonged or other mental stress is higher than their representation in hospital admissions, though all females were considered less prone than males to *sudden* stress attacks. One rare link made between a housewife's illness and her previous working life recorded an experience of "slave labor during the war" in occupied Europe.

The evidence gathered from hospital records indicates that doctors and psychiatrists dealing with the broad mass of mental patients in the postwar period rarely attributed serious mental illness to occupations or working life and more rarely still were inclined to characterize strain or mental stress to the workplace. The concern of this chapter has been with the nexus between scientific expertise and popular understanding of stress, and here again the records of mental hospitals provide a resource in the form of the recorded

Table 7.2. Selected occupations of single admitted and readmitted female patients, ca. 1948–655

	Female patients	
Occupations	Single admitted	Readmitted
Professional and clerical	14.4%	14.2%
Domestic occupations (including housekeeping)	13.3%	17.9%
Factory, manual, and shop work	9.8%	10.8%
Housewife	38.1%	42.2%
Unemployed	0.4%	0.6%
None	11.5%	8.0%
Not known	10.5%	5.9%

Source: Devon Record Office, Exeter: Mental Health Case Records, Unsorted Hospital Deposit, 2010–11.

testimony and opinions of the relatives, friends, neighbors, or community nurses who had cared for people admitted. The language of the recorded views of those related to the patients suggest that "stress" was used more rarely by lay individuals than medical personnel, with relatives attributing the illness of eight women and two men to "stress," all admitted after 1950 and often connected to the burden of bereavement or caring for others. Patients' relations and friends were rather more likely to refer to "strain," or even "mental strain," forty-two female admissions (involving twenty-four women) being attributed by relatives and others to "strain." The strain of caring for and nursing others appeared in eighteen female admission notes, difficult family relations being mentioned in five instances, including one who suffered "marital strain." In addition, the strains of war figured in eleven female admissions. For example, Eileen H. was admitted six times between 1945 and 1950, having fallen ill due to the "strain of war work," while Muriel W. had suffered "war strain" after her house was bombed, and Beatrice H. was admitted thrice between 1956 and 1961 with depression, having suffered war strain during World War I and also "overwork."

"Strain" was noted as a cause of illness by relatives in only twelve male admissions, again linked to military service in some instances. Richard C., admitted four times from 1950 to 1962, was said to suffer "strain" as a result of an "underwater collision" in 1929, as well as from convoy duties during World War II. Ernest H. was similarly admitted from 1945 to 1961 due to "strain under war conditions." The strain of work was commented on in the case of only two males, both in nonmanual employment. Nonmedical witnesses were more likely than doctors to link illness and overwork, though rarely phrased in terms of "stress" or even strain. In the cases of forty-two males (sixty-six admissions), relatives pointed to "overwork," though such references appeared among a variety of observations on domestic worries and disappointments. These males had a wide occupational profile, ranging from laborers to self-employed tradesmen and professional individuals. They included multiple-admission patients, such as a bus driver (a group whose gastric problems attracted research in the interwar years) and a cleaner whose conditions included, according to his wife, a gastric ulcer.

It is noticeable that the relatives of female patients were also more willing than medical staff to ascribe their worsening health to excessive work. Thirty-three female patients (sixty-five admissions) were said to have overworked, including women in higher-status occupations such as teaching and ladies whose life seemed to have led to genteel poverty and self-neglect, including the elderly Nellie K., a "Companion and Housekeeper," who arrived in 1953 suffering from overwork and undernourishment. A much younger woman who worked in a shop was said to have overworked and to have been affected by the death of Marilyn Monroe. Industrial workers rarely figured in notes of excessive working, in contrast to housewives, who accounted for one-third of those said to be overworked. Once again such commentaries were mixed with incidents such as the illness or abusive behavior of husbands or accounts of bereavement and wartime losses.

This brief survey of mental-hospital records in the middle decades of the twentieth century helps us to gain a firmer hold on the challenging question of how expert and nonexpert perceptions of strain and stress developed and interplayed in Britain during these years. Doctors referred to "prolonged" and "sudden" mental stress in assigning causes for mental illness, rarely referring to "strain" or attributing mental disorders to overwork. It is true that nonmanual groups, more particularly among female patients, were more likely to be associated with neuroses and with strain or stress than were manual workers, though this distinction should not be exaggerated, and the numbers of patients involved remained relatively small. The personal relatives and friends of patients were more likely than doctors to attribute illness to overwork and to strain, though they were not frequently connected in such commentaries, for domestic life, family connections, and personal disappointments continued to figure more strongly and consistently than working life in the biographical sketches of patients completed by their relatives and neighbors. It remained unusual for either medical staff or relatives and friends to identify work itself as an environment in which mental illness might develop. Accidents and physical injuries hardly figured in the same files, except for a handful of head injuries during car accidents and the only work-related injury being an accident with a farm bull. There are few signs in the mental-hospital records even of the 1960s of the eruption in the incidence and awareness of occupational stress during the last three decades of the century.

Reflections: Making Sense of Historical Strain and the Place of Work in Modern Stress

It is not easy to explain the arrival of a new age of stress at the end of the twentieth century. Within a relatively short period stress seemed to have become one of the most common expressions of unease and a shared experiential condition of modern society. This new age was not confined to Britain but appeared to be a malady found in every country in the developed world. The role of psychology and psychiatry in this process clearly deserves our attention. In early 1981 Dr. R. D. Laing was invited to become a member of the Scientific Advisory Council of the Stress Syndrome Foundation, a charitable trust established to research and educate on "all aspects of the human stress response in industrial societies," drawing in such bodies as the Institute of Directors as well as the BMA and Age Concern.[75] By this time Laing had become one of the best-known psychologists in Britain, figuring prominently in the challenge to clinical science during the 1970s by developing a critical existentialist psychiatry and suggesting the involvement of family and friends as well as medical professionals in the repression of those considered mentally ill. Medical historians of this period, notably Roy Porter, were influenced by, and participated in, this cultural and historical turn in the study of psychiatry that was associated with Laing but foreshadowed by Halliday's earlier call for a more holistic understanding of the body and the self as a social and cultural rather than merely a physical or scientific domain.[76]

These ideas have continued to resonate in the social history of medicine in the concern of historians to capture the contribution of the "popular" to the formation and growth of ideas about the medication of the body, including the dialectical progress of expertise and secular experience in relation to the mind and the history of emotional sensibility. This orientation to the cultural in historical writing provides a critical awareness of our own subjectivity in the explanation of popular sensibility. This chapter has argued that care is needed in examining the nexus between expertise, experience, and popular belief. In some settings popular or folk beliefs and medical practices sustained communal resistance to scientific practices (such as postmortem examinations in north and south Wales), which inhibited medical reform.[77] This chapter has also underlined the impact of social relations and practices within an unfolding discourse of personal strain and stress in British society. The ontology of stress has its peculiar technical as well as popular lineages, demarcated by the institutional fabric of scientific labor and the terms in which knowledge was attached to physical space, social authority, and different objects of attention. Laing shared with Halliday and Selye the distinction of being successful popularizers of unorthodox ideas while remaining clearly unpopular outsiders from the academy of science. They were excluded from the decision-making institutions of their profession, and their ideas were greeted with skepticism. The significant omission in the scientific investigation of strain was not the failure to grasp the opportunity presented by holistic medicine from the 1930s but the restricted engagement between leading physiologists, psychologists, and industrial fatigue researchers during the interwar years and after World War II. These experts rarely connected to exert a major influence on politics and industrial production, and often brilliant technical advances made limited contributions to popular opinion, social psychology, or clinical practice.

The understanding of strain and its relationship to different kinds of work registered not only the distinct institutional arrangements and practices of intellectual inquiry from the mid-nineteenth century but also the wider political economy in which labor was framed and performed. Manual work was culturally embedded in assumptions about health and purpose, impervious to mental strain of the kind associated with excessive intellectual labor and more particularly with females unsuited to the taxing effort of critical thought. MRC research studies in the 1950s revealed the presence of a customary language of "industrial fear" present in hazardous occupations such as mining. Such anxieties were rarely linked to mental strain, still less to the onset of mental illness, by the working population or medical advisers. The scope for such an understanding of workplace fear was constrained by legislative rules governing safe employment and injury compensation. Increased workers' rights under accident liability and compensation law introduced in Europe and beyond from the 1880s led physicians to reconsider the causal links between sudden injury and disease.

There was a reciprocal growth in professional skepticism in response to rising compensation claims that spawned the extensive literature on malingering, which persisted from the late nineteenth century into the interwar period. In resisting claims for physical injury, including damage to the nervous system, employers and their medical advisers composed a portrait of nervous and neurotic individuals who failed to cope with the acceptable demands of hazard and strain expected of employees, more particularly in male-centered occupations. Although James Halliday is often seen as an advocate of more inclusive, holistic approaches to the troubled body, the origins of his concern with psychosomatic disorders came directly from his skepticism about the organic diseases reported by National Insurance claimants. His research and his explanation of emotional stress among working people flowed with a strong current of medical and psychological thought that shifted the emphasis from industrial and social environment to frictions within the personality and emotional economy of the individual.

Similar assumptions appear to have informed scientific research and practical psychiatry in Britain during much of the twentieth century. Research on industrial fatigue, vocational training, and emotional strain among groups of workers conducted by distinguished field-workers such as Farmer and Wyatt betrayed clear bias when evaluating the significance of class, gender, and status in regard to personal capacity and the acquisition of essential skills. Wartime research expanded the horizons of such scientific evaluation at Cambridge and elsewhere, influencing the technical understanding of stress by psychologists such as Donald Broadbent, though studies such as those funded by the MRC did not generate a substantial reappraisal of the earlier quasi-military language of "morale," "fiber," and "leadership" that had figured in government and management publications of the 1940s. In the full employment and Fordist management models of the postwar years, more imaginative employers were receptive to the emerging literature on ergonomic design and peer leadership, often imported from US social science and management studies. There was little absorption of the language of social psychology, despite the efforts of such bodies as the Tavistock Institute, where Ronald Laing conducted some key research during this period.

Assumptions concerning class, status, and gender can be also detected in the records of mental hospitals in the mid-1800s and in similar admission papers more than a century later. Hospital psychiatrists infrequently used the lexicon of "mental stress" as a primary cause to explain mental illness even after 1907 and seldom attributed mental illness to workplace strain. Medical commentaries provided by hospital staff became more sophisticated after the 1930s, with "social histories" of patients (composed by social workers in the 1950s) providing a richer context of domestic background. Language moved from cruder diagnoses of "mania" and "dementia" to various forms of "depression," with "anxiety-state" becoming more common as a description. The psychotropic innovations of the 1950s also served to weaken and obscure the need for such sociological detail and renewed the reliance on a pharmaceutical fix for those suffering "mental stress." There are various descriptions to "overwork" and "overstrain" in patient notes, though references to difficulties at work remain remarkably sparse, and even those few said by doctors to be "unhappy at work" are often provided with concomitant sources of anxiety, such as infidelity or bereavement. The most likely association of stress and work was to be found in nonmanual female occupations, such as teaching and nursing, though here there were limited references to "mental stress," even when usage of such terms peaked in the mid-twentieth century. "Prolonged mental stress" was more characteristic of descriptions of ill housewives and used to describe the burdens of caring for others, personal disappointment, and difficult relationships.

The same institutional records offer rarely found insights into the language and testimony of large numbers of relatives and friends of hospital patients, where the references to "strain" and "worries" were more common than observations of "stress," though such witnesses were more willing than medical commentators to attribute personal distress to overwork, personal shocks, and the long-term impact of wartime and other historical incidents on the minds of their relatives. It may be objected that commonplace references to "stress" were more likely to be found in nonmedical social settings than in the clinical world of hospital psychiatry. It is argued here that the rarity of references to "stress" among relatives, friends, and neighbors of patients seeking to offer coherent explanations for poor mental health, suggests that such terms did not form part of the everyday speech of the shared culture of working-class communities in this period.

The conclusion of this chapter is that a series of social, institutional, and intellectual constraints served to restrict discussions of occupational stress before 1970, framing the incidence of workplace strain in various ways that served to limit professional and public attention. If this argument has some force, then the question remains: why should concerns about occupational stress have achieved a scale that led to commentaries on the "pandemic" of personal difficulties at work by the end of the century? This question clearly lies beyond the scope of this chapter, though a speculative suggestion can be offered. For the origins of recent workplace stress symptoms may be traced, in part, to the liberalization movements of the 1960s and 1970s, which viewed mental disorder as a response to a disruptive or authoritarian environment and where personal anxieties were recognized as a reasonable, and universal, existential condition by critical philosophers and psychologists. These ideas refreshed a language of personal stress that was extended and stretched to encompass feelings of strain, anxiety, and fear with the implication (hardly sustainable) of biological and psychological precision. In validating popular culture and experiences, the historical and cultural turn in psychology and social sciences helped to transform an older and customary acceptance of discomfort and hazard at work, permitting the expression of feelings of fear and loss even among working-class males who witnessed the passing of hazardous jobs with the manufacturing industries that had employed them.

These changes in the cultural landscape of industrial workers contributed to the new sensibility of stress at work, more particularly where male-centered manual work gave way to nonmanual employment in a host of service industries at the end of the long postwar boom in the oil crisis of 1971–73. There is little evidence here of a decisive change in social identity during or immediately after World War II or of a clear move to individualistic forms of sensibility and behavior. The intellectual and cultural shifts of liberalization in the 1960s were also grounded and registered in a larger political economy of labor and effort, whose rhythm was driven by a new international division of labor, moving goods and services within a reshaped global economy. The end of the long

Fordist boom was accompanied by movements among manual and nonmanual workers for greater control over their working environment, including a concern with health and safety that drew on, without depending on, the findings of expert investigators.[78] It seems appropriate that the first stirrings of demands for an investigation into "mental breakdowns" in industry should have come in the early 1970s from British assembly-line workers at the Ford motor plants.[79] Such movements alerted psychologists, psychiatrists, and others to the possibility of a new wave of popular discontent emanating from an arena of collective conflict.

Notes

1. Health and Safety Executive, "Making the Stress Management Standards Work: How to Apply the Standards in Your Workplace," http://www.hse.gov.uk/pubns/books/hsg218.htm (accessed September 16, 2013). See also "Stress," *TUC*, www.TUC.Org.uk/stress (accessed September 16, 2013).

2. Matthew Thomson, *Psychological Subjects: Identity, Culture and Health in Twentieth-Century Britain* (Oxford: Oxford University Press, 2006). Thomson critiques Rose's emphasis on management science; he argues for the influence of popular religious and traditional moral precepts on social identity and the self until a "crisis" in the 1940s gave way to postwar individualism. Rhodri Hayward, "Enduring Emotions: James L. Halliday and the Invention of the Psychosocial," *Isis: A Journal of the History of Science* 100, no. 4 (2009): 827–38; Andrew Hull, "Glasgow's 'Sick Society'? James Halliday, Psychosocial Medicine and Medical Holism in Britain, c. 1920–48," forthcoming. My thanks to Andrew Hull for allowing me to see his unpublished paper.

3. Colin Mackay, interview by Joseph Melling, HSE Head Office, Bootle, England, January 2008. Mackay worked for the Employment Medical Advice Service before HSE. He suggested Michael Foot decided that psychologists be employed under the 1974 legislation.

4. Lawrence R. Murphy, "Job Stress Research at NIOSH: 1972–2002," in *Historical and Current Perspectives on Stress and Health: Research in Occupational Stress and Well Being*, ed. Pamela L. Perrewe and Daniel C. Ganster (Bradford: Emerald, 2002), 2–6.

5. C. Liana Bolis, "Stress: Adaptation and Homeostasis," in *Stress and Adaptation: From Selye's Concept to Application of Modern Formulations*, ed. C. Liana Bolis and Julio Licinio (Geneva: World Health Organization, 1999), 1–2.

6. Charles E. Rosenberg, *Explaining Epidemics and Other Studies in the History of Medicine* (Cambridge: Cambridge University Press, 1992); Anne Hardy, "Reframing Disease: Changing Perceptions of Tuberculosis in England and Wales, 1938–70," *Historical Research* 76, 194 (2003): 536–56.

7. Ian Hacking, *Historical Ontology* (Cambridge: Harvard University Press, 2004); Lorraine Daston, *Biographies of Scientific Objects* (Chicago: University Of Chicago Press, 2000).

8. Michelle Murphy, *Sick Building Syndrome and the Problem of Uncertainty: Environmental Politics, Technoscience and Women Workers* (Durham, NC: Duke University Press).

9. Gabrielle Hecht, "Nuclear Ontologies," *Constellations* 13 (2006): 320–31; Gabrielle Hecht, *Being Nuclear: Africans and the Global Uranium Trade* (Cambridge, MA: MIT Press, 2012); Christopher Sellers and Joseph Melling, "Towards a Transnational Industrial Hazard History: Charting the Circulation of Workplace Dangers, Debates and Expertise," *British Journal of History of Science* 45, no. 3 (2012): 401–24.

10. Andrew Pickering, *The Cybernetic Brain: Sketches of Another Future* (Chicago: University of Chicago Press, 2010), 220–56.

11. Edward Shorter, *From the Mind into the Body: The Cultural Origins of Psychosomatic Symptoms* (New York: Free Press, 1994), 118, 132–33; cf. 22–23. Shorter also notes the reappearance of "fatigue" in diagnoses of "chronic fatigue syndrome."

12. Andreas Killen, "From Shock to Shreck: Psychiatrists, Telephone Operators and Traumatic Neurosis in Germany, 1900–26," *Journal of Contemporary History* 28, 2 (2003): 201–20. The move to personal responsibility also involved the promotion of "physical culture," which included exercise, control of diet, and healthy exposure to sunlight.

13. Ibid., 202, 207: "Traumatic neurosis emerged within a highly-charged social space constituted by the convergence of social insurance, clinical psychiatry and a new politics of the body as the site of labour power."

14. Kitanaka, "Work, Stress, and Depression," this volume; Nikolas Rose, *Governing the Soul: The Shaping of the Private Self* (London: Routledge, 1990); Nikolas Rose, *The Psychological Complex: Psychology, Politics and Society in England, 1869–1939.* (London: Routledge and Kegan Paul, 1985).

15. Tom Cox and Sue Cox, *Psychosocial and Organizational Hazards at Work*, World Health Organisation: European Occupational Health Series 5 (Copenhagen: WHO, 1993), 9–13.

16. Thomson, *Psychological Subjects*, summarizes and adds to this scholarship.

17. Helen Mabel W., case books Devon Record Office, Wonford House Asylum Archives, Devon County Record Office, Exeter. Helen Mabel W., an unmarried governess aged twenty-five, was admitted to the Wonford House asylum in 1895 with a predisposing cause of insanity as "Mental anxiety. Ill health" and an exciting cause of "Overwork." She had been in a "very hard situation as governess, was very hard worked & underfed, the poor financial conditions of her family preyed on her mind & she developed delusions." By the summer of 1909 she was described as "Demented & irrational. Excited & violent at times. Mostly dull." Joseph Melling, "Sex and Sensibility in Cultural History: The English Governess and the Lunatic Asylum, 1845–1914," in *Sex and Seclusion, Class and Custody*, ed. Jonathan Andrews and Anne Digby (Amsterdam: Rodopi, 2004).

18. James Collier, *Relation of Neurasthenia to the Duration of Life*, copy in FPW/B.226/2, Parkes-Weber Papers (hereafter cited as PWP), Wellcome Library, London.

19. Joseph Melling, "Labouring Stress: Trade Unions and Attitudes to the Incidence of 'Stress' at the Workplace, 1939–1980," in *The Stress of Life* (Chatto and Pickering), ed. Mark Jackson forthcoming, 2014.

20. Edgar L. Collis, "Industrial Fatigue in Connection with Tuberculosis," *Tubercle* 8 (1926–27): 49–58, 52–54. Although little attention has been given to the impact of the new physiological studies of John Scott Haldane and others on the understanding of bodily strain during the early twentieth century, such work contributed to detailed

studies of physical and mental endurance before and during World War I. Martin Goodman, *Suffer and Survive: Gas Attacks, Miners' Canaries, Spacesuits and the Bends: The Extreme Life of Dr. J. S. Haldane* (London: Simon and Shuster, 2007). The work of the Health of Munitions Welfare Board and the Industrial Fatigue Research Board was absorbed in studies of shell poisoning but also undertook postwar research into "industrial" disease such as tuberculosis in the boot and shoe industry.

21. Sir John Collie, "Workmen's Compensation: Its Medical Aspects," *Lancet*, December 30, 1933, 1463, copy in B.360/2/1–3, PWP. When 256 miners died in a single, devastating explosion at Gresford Colliery in 1935, there was little discussion of psychological damage to the survivors or those who retrieved the burned and asphyxiated bodies, though Stafford Cripps secured £85,000 for the miners in compensation for physical injuries. There were 256 cases and £82,972 compensation; after indemnity was deducted and court fees paid then the total was £85,469. Minutes, October 21, 1935, North Wales Mutual Indemnity, vol. 7, Haswell Collection, National Library of Wales, Aberystwyth.

22. Florence Bairdsmith to Edmund L. Lushington, September 26, 1868, MS GEN 557/2/1/2, University of Glasgow Library, Special Collections. Florence was the daughter of Thomas de Quincey.

23. Admission registers, 1855–1914, Devon Record Office, Wonford House Asylum Archives, reveal "mental strain" and "overstrain" entered for "origins of insanity" in fourteen female admissions (thirteen patients) and four male admissions, almost all between 1893 and 1902. Three female cases referred to "strain of nursing." One female and one male case referred to overstrain related to examinations.

24. Ibid. There were five instances (1861–80) for four female and one male admission where "fatigue" figured in "cause of insanity," with one governess (Susanna R.) said to be overfatigued from teaching.

25. Melancholy was found in fifteen male cases of overwork, with mania accounting for thirteen and acute mania ten, among a group of fifty-nine admissions.

26. All public asylum evidence is from detailed analysis of the admissions of the Devon County Lunatic Asylum, held at the Devon Record Office. The 1880–82 study was completed with the assistance of Robert Turner.

27. Christopher Sellers and Joseph Melling, "From Dangerous Trades to Trade in Dangers: Towards an Industrial Hazard History of the Present," in Sellers and Melling, *Dangerous Trade*, (Templeton University Press, Philadelphia, 2012) 1–13.

28. Karl Figlio, "What Is an Accident?," in *The Social History of Occupational Health*, ed. Paul Weindling (London: Croom Helm, 1979), 180–206, remains an excellent introduction.

29. Sir Thomas Oliver, *Some Medical and Insurance Problem Arising Out of Recent Industrial Legislation* (London: Life Assurance Medical Officers Association, 1909); Robert J. Collie, *The First Line of Defence in Workmen's Compensation Act, 1906* (London: Gray, 1910), 270. Collie claimed that the 1906 Act discouraged employment of older workers (aged fifty to seventy), noting Dr. Percy Dove's views, "I certainly think that you are very much more likely to meet with a malingerer over 40 or 45 than you are between 20 and 40." Byrom Bramwell, "Malingering, Valetudinarianism," *British Medical Journal*, April 19, 1913, 805–9, copies in B.360/2/1–3, PWP. Thomas M. Legge, "Industrial Diseases under the Workmen's Compensation Act," *Journal of Industrial Hygiene* 1, no. 11 (May 1920): 25–32.

30. Legge, "Industrial Diseases," 25–26. Legge later became a victim of overwork and strain, resigning as a medical inspector after having failed to persuade the government to approve a League of Nations ban on white lead use in industry.

31. Deborah Palmer, "Nursing and Occupational Health" (PhD diss., University of Exeter, 2008).

32. "A Note on the Early Signs of Skill Fatigue," n.d.; "Psychological Aspects of Industrial Productivity," n.d., B.72; Hull, "Men, Machines and Industrial Productivity," April 28, 1948, all in GBR/0012/MS Add.8076, B.46, Frederick C. Bartlett Papers, Department of Manuscripts, Cambridge University; L. A. Reynolds and E. M. Tansey, eds., *The MRC Applied Psychology Unit: The Transcript of a Witness Seminar Held at the Wellcome Trust Centre for the History of Medicine at UCL, London, on 12 June 2001* (London: Wellcome Centre for the History of Medicine, 2002).

33. See Walter B. Cannon to Sir Charles Sherrington, February 14, 1916, folder 836, box 63, H MS c 40, Walter B. Cannon Archive, Countway Library, Harvard University, regarding the "Freudian symbolism" of Cannon's dreams of war after hearing of Dardanelles campaigns. Thanks to the staff of the Harvard University libraries.

34. See Stephen Wyatt and John N. Langdon, *MRC, IHRB, Report 77: Fatigue and Boredom in Repetitive Work* 28, NA Medical Research Council Publications, FD 3/77, pp. 49–56, for the report stating that the fear of unemployment was the greatest single factor influencing workers, though work fatigue was a more important cause of dissatisfaction.

35. David Munro (unsigned), "Joint Experiment in the Application of Psychological Method to Vocational Guidance by the Industrial Health Research Board and the Ministry of Labour" and "Industrial Psychology: Memorandum by the Secretary on Scheme of Research . . . for the Industrial Health Research Board," December 1934, LAB 19/10, Ministry of Labour and National Service, National Archives, Kew, London (hereafter cited as NA), 5; Frederick Bartlett, "Selection of Industrial Workers in War Time" [File inscribed, "Psychological Work—Cambridge: General"], "Progress Report, 1940–41," NA FD 1/4006, MRCP; Eric Farmer to Landsborough Thomson, March 2, 1942, Medical Research Council.

36. Edward Southard, "The Modern Specialist in Unrest: A Place for the Psychiatrist in Industry," *Journal of Industrial Hygiene* 11, no. 1 (1920): 11.

37. Grahamsley Howitt, *Accident and Disease* (London, 1914), 60–62, copy in B.360/2/1–3, PWP.

38. Frederick Parkes-Weber, "Medical Aspects of Compulsory Insurance of Working Classes," *British Medical Journal*, February 13, 1897, copy in B360/1 (box 166), PWP.

39. Clifford Allbutt to Frederick Parkes-Weber, August 1, 1910, B.345/2, PWP. This followed publication of an article in the *British Medical Journal*.

40. Frederick Parkes-Weber, "Traumatic Tuberculosis," *Clinical Journal*, July 1916, B.345/2, PWP, in which author uses the Allbutt case, 19, 22–23; letter of local physician to *British Medical Journal*, August 26, 1911, 444, concerning tuberculosis and accidents; Thomas D. Lister, "Industrial Tuberculosis" *Lancet*, October 15, 1910, 1122–26; cuttings from *Lancet*, October 23, 1926, 848, for Workmen's Compensation for tuberculosis injury.

41. Arthur J. Hall to Frederick Parkes-Weber, May 20, 1910, B.345/2, PWP, concerning the latter's *British Medical Journal* article; Collis, "Industrial Fatigue," 49–58, 52–54.

42. Leonard Williams, "The Real Neurasthenia," *Practitioner*, July 1917. Williams declared, "The real neurasthenia has deserted Harley Street, and now resides almost exclusively in that abominable architectural monstrosity known as the Royal Courts of Justice" (3). Douglas Knocker, *Disease in Relationship to Accident* (London: Life Assurance Medical Officers Association, 1912), 184: "Until the medical referee sat as assessor with the judge, there was an enormous amount of malingering and exaggeration in connection with this disease [neurasthenia]. . . . Nervousness and nerve shock have replaced her in the affections of workmen."

43. Thomas S. Ashton, "The Relation between Unemployment and Sickness," *Economic Journal* 26, no. 10 (1916): 398, for the "psychological cause" of sickness during unemployment.

44. Frederick Parkes-Weber, "Two Strange Cases of Functional Disorder with Remarks on the Association of Hysteria and Malingering," *International Clinics* 1 (1912): 125–38; Parkes-Weber, "The Association of Hysteria with Malingering," *Lancet*, December 2, 1911, 1542–43, copies in B.207, PWP; Sir Thomas Oliver, "The Role of Traumatism in Disease Calling for Compensation," *Transactions of the Assurance Medical Society*, May 5, 1915, 172.

45. Oliver, "Role of Traumatism," 172.

46. Donald Bellamy, case notes, April 8, 1931, March 25, 1931, 251/2, PWP. Bellamy, aged twenty-five, was admitted March 22, 1931, and developed "Psychosis after pneumonia?" and melancholia.

47. Thomson, quoted in Linda Bryder, "'Not Always One and the Same Thing': The Registration of Tuberculosis Deaths in Britain, 1900–1950," *Social History of Medicine* 2 (1996): 259.

48. Dr. Llewellyn, Minute book, September 23, 1935, BA1/2/1, North Wales Mutual Insurance (NWMI), National Library of Wales. Aberystwyth, Haswell Collection, North Wales Mutual Indemnity: Volume 7.

49. Letter Book 2 (LB2), February 17, 1915, case of John Evans, certified as of unsound mind, September 14 and November 10, 1914, NWMI.

50. LB2, April 19, 1915, NWMI.

51. LB2, April 23–28, 1915, NWMI.

52. LB2, April 28, 1915, June 18, 1915, June 29, 1915, NWMI.

53. LB2, February 3, 1915, NWMI. See also the case of John Roberts, February 3, 1915, April 7, 1915, NWMI.

54. George Orwell, *The Road to Wigan Pier* (London: Victor Gollancz, 1937): "A working man does not disintegrate under the strain of poverty as a middle-class person does. . . . It may be that the psychological adjustment which the working class are visibly making is the best they could make in the circumstances, 93.

55. Frank Forster diary, Ms. 364.4, July 13–August 12, 1936, Modern Record Centre, University of Warwick, Coventry, England (hereafter cited as MRCW).

56. Enid M. Williams, *The Health of Old and Retired Coalminers in South Wales* (Cardiff: University of Wales Press, 1933), 1–4.

57. Arthur Horner to Evan Williams, February 5, 1938, SWCC/MNA/NUM/5/14: Correspondence, South Wales Miners' Federation Papers, Swansea University Archives, Swansea (hereafter SWMFP).

58. Dr. Hyacinth B. Morgan to James L. Smyth, March 1, 1938, April 28, 1938, "Rehabilitation" Memorandum, 292/142.1/2, Trades Union Congress Papers

(hereafter cited as TUC), MRCW; Snowden to James Smyth, February 18, 1939, 292/143.6.6, MRCW. Morgan succeeded Legge as medical consultant to TUC in 1931. Snowden, formerly of Bart's Hospital, unsuccessfully offered his services to the Interdepartmental Committee on Rehabilitation. Morgan proposed the TUC's Workmen's Compensation and Factories Committee take up the matter of "nervous system" injuries, since "functional nervous restoration" was the necessary counterpart to physical rehabilitation.

59. See Hayward, "Enduring Emotions."

60. James L. Halliday, "Psychoneurosis as a Cause of Incapacity among Insured Persons," *British Medical Journal*, March 9, 1935, 85–88; Halliday, "Psychoneurosis as a Cause of Incapacity among Insured Persons: A Preliminary Enquiry," *British Medical Journal*, March 16, 1935, 99–102.

61. James L. Halliday, "Some Reflections of a Regional Medical Officer on Medical Certification," *British Medical Journal*, November 24, 1934, 261–64.

62. James L. Halliday, "Dangerous Occupation, Psychosomatic Illness, and Morale: A Study Based on the Investigation of Incapacitation Disorders in Underground Miners," *Psychosomatic Medicine* 1 (1943): 72–75.

63. Frederick Bartlett, *Remembering: A Study in Experimental and Social Psychology* (Cambridge: Cambridge University Press, 1932; repr. 1977); "Notes on the Work of the Medical Research Council Applied Psychology Unit, 1944–1997," Papers for Wellcome Witness History, series 2003, GC/253/A/16, MRC Applied Psychology Unit, Wellcome Library; Alan Costall, "Frederic Bartlett and the Idea of an Historical Psychology," *Ethnographic Studies* 11 (2009): 24–32.

64. Donald Broadbent, *Decision and Stress* (London: Academic Press, 1971).

65. Copy of Stephen Wyatt, *A Study of Variations in Output* (London: Industrial Health Research Board, Medical Research Council, 1944), 200/B/3/2/C693, British Employers' Confederation (hereafter cited as BEC), MRCW.

66. Letter to Forbes Watson (sender illegible), May 10, 1943, BEC 200/B/3/2/C693, MRCW.

67. Alastair Heron and Dorothy Braithwaite, "Emotional Stability in Colliery Workers," *British Journal of Industrial Medicine* 10 (1953): 27.

68. Norah M. Davis, "Some Psychological Conflicts Caused by Group Bonus Methods of Payment," *British Journal of Industrial Medicine* 10 (1953): 18–26, 25, 26.

69. "Literature Survey of Mental Stress in Industry," minutes of an informal meeting at MRC to discuss the survey of the literature on mental stress in industry, January 27, 1976 (minutes dated February 18, 1976), FD 9/4367, MRCP, NA.

70. Donald Broadbent, "Proposed Study of Assembly-Line Workers," report of a meeting, December 14, 1976, Mental Stress in Industry: Potential Commissions from Department of Employment, MRC, FD 9/4159, MRCP, NA; copy of minutes of a meeting on Mental Stress in Industry at MRC, April 18, 1975, attended by Broadbent, 292 D/847.38/2, TUCP, MRCW.

71. This research was funded by the Wellcome Trust and undertaken with Dr. Nicole Baur, whose major research efforts are warmly acknowledged. The data included 16,317 female case notes, of whom 4,968 entered the hospital as "voluntary" patients and 3,948 were admitted as "informal" patients. Slightly less were formally certified (3,832) and 1,919 were brought under section 20 of the 1959 act. Among the 10,677 male admissions, 4027 (or 38 percent) were admitted on a "voluntary"

basis, with almost equal numbers of certified and informal admissions (2,194 and 2,182).

72. The main group of admissions took place in 1948–65.

73. Among 456 females for whom contributory causes were assigned, "prolonged mental stress" was given in 101 cases. More remarkably, among 435 male admissions, "prolonged" stress figured as a "contributory cause" in 163 cases and "sudden" stress in 13 more.

74. Devon County Record Office, unlisted deposits for patients analyzed by Nicole Baur and Joseph Melling.

75. Dr. Audrey Livingston Booth to Ronald Laing, January 19, 1981, L330/5; and Mary Kendon for Laing to Audrey Booth, May 11, 1981, L330/6, both in Ronald D. Laing Papers, Glasgow University Library.

76. Massimo Piattelli-Palmarini to Ronald D. Laing, December 11, 1979, December 22, 1980, GP 9–20, Ronald D. Laing Papers, enclosing Porter's essay on quacks, and October 28, 1981, urging Laing's contribution to a social history of biomedical sciences, because he had "historically and factually, a leading role in advocating a social outlook on the problem of mental disease."

77. Linda Bryder, "Tuberculosis, Silicosis, and the Slate Industry in North Wales, 1927–1939," in Weindling, *Social History*, 108–9.

78. Sellers and Melling, "Transnational Industrial Hazard History."

79. David Basnett to Victor Feather, September 5, 1973, and Larry Whitty to Trevor Mawer, September 22, 1975, both in 292 D/847.38.7, TUCP, MRC. The GMWU (General and Municipal Workers' Union) recruited only a limited section of the Ford workforce, which was largely represented by the Transport and General Workers' Union, the Amalgamated Engineering Union, and other manual employees' organizations.

Chapter Eight

Work, Stress, and Depression

The Emerging Psychiatric Science of Work in Contemporary Japan

JUNKO KITANAKA

Work, Stress, and Depression

In Japan, amid a prolonged economic recession since the 1990s, psychiatry has suddenly gained popular appeal by depicting depression as a quintessential illness of stress. Concerns about stress-induced depression have heightened after an epoch-making lawsuit in 2000, in which the Supreme Court ordered Dentsū, Japan's biggest advertising agency, to pay to the family of a deceased employee the highest amount ever to be paid for a worker's death in this country.[1] The court determined that the employee was driven to suicide because of depression, which had been caused by chronic work stress.[2] As the rising discourse about overwork depression coincided with an aggressive campaign for new antidepressants beginning in the late 1990s, a stress-based notion of depression quickly permeated Japanese society, turning it into one of the most talked-about illnesses in its recent history. In response to legal disputes and the rising number of the depressed particularly in the workplace, the government has made changes in labor policy to address the psychopathology of work. Most notable in this regard is the creation of Stress Evaluation Tables, which has done much to firmly establish psychological stress in the workplace as a legitimate reason for economic compensation.[3]

The Japanese situation seems to provide an intriguing contrast to that of the United States, where the rise in diagnoses of depression, probably linked to the advent of antidepressants, has raised concerns about the promotion of another form of medicalization, whereby a problem of living—indicating social origins and social contradictions—comes to be redefined as a problem of individual biology.[4] Critics have argued that, through this process, psychiatry is instilling in people a false sense of control by encouraging them to take pills to fix their personal "defects." By implicitly promoting the idea that workers should actualize a desirable selfhood through biological means, psychiatry, some contend, is complicit in the current neoliberal order that is imposing increasing demands on individuals in the workplace.[5] Given that Japanese psychiatry has certainly been criticized for biological individual reductionism in the past and given that its attempts at expanding into the realm of everyday distress have been strongly resisted by lay Japanese, it seems significant that psychiatry has been able to persuade Japanese to accept the diagnosis of depression. This, I argue, is partly due to the way it has successfully located depression not only in the individual brains but also in the stress-inducing workplace, thereby calling attention to how psychopathology can be socially produced.

This chapter examines how this conceptualization of depression as a product of stress has come about in Japan and what kind of political implications this may have. Anthropologists have of late called attention to emergent forms of biomedical legitimization, whereby a medical diagnosis or a patient identity becomes a means for the socially weak to collectively claim their victimhood and gain legitimacy for their suffering.[6] Here, I examine the brief history of overwork depression and suicide in Japan to discuss how this new form of legitimation has been made possible.[7] By illuminating the link between depression and work stress, psychiatrists have become engaged in a social movement against overwork that has brought doctors, lawyers, depressed workers, and their families together. Psychiatry is thus at the heart of important social changes, at times used to urge Japanese to question the status quo, particularly where model workers who have internalized a strong work ethic are driven to suicide. I also show, however, how psychiatrists' attempts to address social causality through the notion of stress are creating epistemological tensions within the medical community, where psychiatrists—faced with moral, rather than scientific, arguments about the nature of workers' psychiatric suffering—ultimately remain unsure of how to conceptualize the "social."

Socializing the Biological

Biomedical attempts to address social ills—particularly of the workplaces—have been fraught with moral ambiguities, as they repeatedly evoke questions about whether or not an illness is rooted in individual biology or in a pathogenic environment. In late nineteenth-century Europe, left-leaning doctors' attempts to address social ills through the biomedical language of "nerve diseases" gained political force, particularly as these doctors began to link up with workers' movements. In helping establish workers' compensation and welfare laws, these doctors made significant contributions in calling attention to the social etiology of psychopathology.[8] But an increase in the number of people with work-related neurosis eventually led to individual reductionism, as seen in the new label of "compensation neurosis," suggesting the idea that it was not the burden of work but the Welfare State itself that was creating mass addiction to neurosis among "weak" individuals.[9]

The question about the social etiology of mental illness—this time depression—surfaced again in Germany in the 1950s. Psychiatrists were then faced with the question of how to assess the nature of "depression" prevalent not only in returning soldiers but also in Holocaust survivors, many of whom had led "normal" lives before the war. These psychiatrists were being asked to determine the precise etiology of these people's depression, particularly in legal cases where survivors demanded economic compensation for their suffering. This led to a number of heated debates within German psychiatry about whether or not genetic factors are always at work in psychopathology (as their prewar biological determinism would have presupposed) or if a stressful situation alone can serve as a cause for psychopathology. This medical debate remained ultimately unresolved, while the immediacy of the problem gradually faded, as it was resolved through not scientific but rather political means.[10]

Also disturbing is the way that "social" discourse can be used—as elucidated by Arthur Kleinman in his ethnography of medicalization in post–Cultural Revolution China—by the state as a means for collectively managing people's dissent. The use of "neurasthenia" both as a medical and political category allowed people to express their *anger* against political injustice while serving to funnel their potentially disruptive emotional force into an officially sanctioned discourse that would keep the political machinery intact.[11] This sort of employment of the "socializing" discourse serves to assemble an inchoate mass of realities as an "illness" and place dissenting individuals under the supervision of medical experts, who then provide (and at times overdetermine) the meaning of patients' suffering while keeping them from fundamentally challenging the status quo. Given the tension that reoccurs in the history of psychiatry, one has to ask in what ways the use of stress in the Japanese discourse about depression departs from these historical precedents.

The Rise of Overwork Depression

The discourse about overwork depression in Japan is significant in the sense that it has established the seemingly mundane, daily *psychological stress of work* as a valid cause for psychiatric breakdown. The landmark lawsuit that first established this is the aforementioned Dentsū case, in which an employee's suicide was determined to have been caused by excessive work stress.[12] Psychiatrists aiding the plaintiff in this case departed from their traditional arguments by helping demonstrate that the worker's depression had been a result not merely of his biological vulnerability but also of the stress-laden work environment. In so doing, they seem to have succeeded in reshaping psychiatry as providing a voice for the weak and helping workers question the pathogenic nature of their workplace. Yet, as one of the plaintiff's attorney attested, the seemingly "commonsensical idea"—that too much stress may cause mental illness—turned out to be rather difficult to prove when they initially resorted to psychiatric theories for explaining such a mechanism.[13] In fact, the legal proceedings in the Dentsū case became a battle ground for competing psychiatric theories of depression and its precise etiology.

When the psychiatric concept of depression was first imported to Japan from German neuropsychiatry in the late nineteenth century, depression was conceptualized primarily as a genetically based disease. What modified this notion was a distinctive theory of "premorbid melancholic personality" proposed by Shimoda Mitsuzō, a renowned psychiatrist at Kyūshū Imperial University. In the 1930s Shimoda's group observed that there were a significant number of patients who exhibited neurasthenic symptoms but who differed from the neurasthenics in the sense that these patients exhibited a set of distinctive personality traits: hardworking, diligent, thorough, and responsible. Often praised as "model employees," these people tended to push themselves to overwork beyond their limits and fall into depression at the height of their exhaustion.[14] In contrast to the neurasthenics, who had by then become stigmatized as embodying a weak personality, Shimoda reconceptualized the depressed as overly adaptive, normative Japanese, whose particular personality, when faced with an overwork situation, would drive them to excessive fatigue and eventually to depression. Though he regarded such a personality as genetically determined (an assumption adopted by subsequent traditional psychiatrists), Shimoda's theory of the premorbid melancholic personality opened a path for the later reconceptualization of depression as a product of both individual genetics and society.[15]

What came to reshape this personality theory of depression in Japan was the adoption of a German psychopathologic concept of Typus Melancholicus, which closely paralleled Shimoda's notion and became further developed by Japanese psychiatrists during the vehement antipsychiatry movement of the 1960s and 1970s.[16] During this time prominent psychiatrists began to argue that such personality traits are not merely a matter of genetics but rather socially constituted, even a specific historical product of the Japanese workplace. Noting that it is often the normative, even ideal, workers who are susceptible to depression, some psychiatrists began to discuss how Japanese society came to reproduce and reward the depressive types and their self-sacrificing devotion to the collective to such an extent that they begin to take their responsibility too much to heart. Japanese psychiatrists at the time also came to problematize various kinds of social stress and pathogenic situations that they saw as triggering depression—such as workers' forced relocation and the alienation of homemakers in the nuclear family.[17] Their discussions about various forms of stress resonated with general attempts among psychiatrists at the time to engage with social causes of mental illness, some of whom began to engage in a workers' movement that was, from the 1980s, beginning to address work stress as an important cause for psychopathology.

These competing interpretations of depression—genetically based or stress-induced—came to be played out against each other in the proceedings of the Dentsū case. At the Tokyo District Court, the dispute initially centered around how high the employee's stress level had been and whether or not he was really depressed. Thus, once the presence of excessive stress (as shown in the excessive hours of overwork) was established, the court granted without too much conceptual debate the diagnosis of "fatigue depression." In the subsequent proceeding at the Tokyo High Court, however, the defendant aggressively rebutted the plaintiff's argument by questioning the exact nature of the employee's "depression," arguing that his genetic vulnerability, and not work stress, was the cause of depression. The Tokyo High Court partially accepted this argument and introduced comparative negligence by reducing the amount of compensation by 30 percent.[18] In the final round of disputes at the Supreme Court, what helped bring the all-out victory for the plaintiff was the social interpretation of depression. Echoing social psychiatrists' existential framing of depression, the verdict even ventures into the psychological state of the employee right before his death, stating that the completion of a project at work suddenly relieved him of one psychological burden, while, at the same time creating in him dreadful anticipation (and despair) for the kind of life that awaited him from that day on. The judges concluded that the employee thus committed suicide impulsively and accidentally, under the influence of depression that had affected his way of thinking.[19] The Supreme Court's verdict was intended as a public warning for employers to be responsible for protecting their employees' mental health at the workplace and for not letting their stress accumulate beyond a reasonable limit. Depression thus came to be legally established as an illness of stress, even an evocative sign of existential crisis.[20]

Defining Pathogenic Stress

The effect of the legal concept of stress-based depression has been profound, particularly in the realm of mental health and labor policies.[21] First of all, the Ministry of Labor has officially abolished the traditional psychiatric classification for diagnosing mental illness in workplaces and replaced it with the "stress-diathesis model," which clearly conceptualizes mental illness as a product of interaction between individual and society. Second, to formally recognize (and measure) the serious toll work stress has on workers' mental health, the ministry created the Stress Evaluation Tables.[22] These tables consist of thirty-one items for both work- and nonwork-related stressful events. These potentially stressful events such as a trouble with a client, a change of boss, promotion, as well as a death in the family, divorce, even a child's school entrance examination are each given a predetermined number of points. Experts can simply extract stressful events from a worker's record, add up the points, and see which stress—either at work or at home—was the greater contributing factor for the worker's mental breakdown or suicide. If it is then determined that the work stress outweighed that of home and that the worker suffered a mental illness or suicide as a consequence, then the case is approved for workers' compensation. By predetermining these points, the ministry initially emphasized that the stress evaluation has to be *objective*, that is to say, examiners should base their judgment on not how the particular worker *subjectively* responded to the event but determine *objectively* how the same event would be experienced by any average worker. This was meant to avoid the multiple and often competing interpretations that psychiatrists tend to make and to speed up the diagnostic process by quantifying and *standardizing* how to measure stress.[23]

But in the following legal debates, the government's assumptions embedded in the Stress Evaluation Tables came under harsh criticism for their claim to objectivity, their quasi-scientific nature, and their attempts to standardize human suffering. Most important, in a lawsuit regarding the suicide of a Toyota employee, the corporate—and the governmental—assertion of "objective stress" came to be challenged.[24] In this case a thirty-five-year-old employee, who was by all account an ideal "Toyota Man," committed suicide while under a heavy workload. What complicated this case, however, was that under Toyota's policy to reduce overwork hours, the actual hours he spent in the office did not seem much longer than that of his peers. Thus, while the defense argued that his suicide was an act of free will, the plaintiff instead emphasized how work intensified under the company's new policy and that it is not the quantity but rather the *quality* of work that should be considered. The judges accepted that what matters is not how each stress is "objectively" scored—as in the Stress Evaluation Tables—but how the worker subjectively experienced the stress. Furthermore, in response to the defense's argument that the worker's alleged depression was caused by his own biological vulnerability (i.e., "melancholic premorbid personality"), the verdict at the Nagoya District Court stated that the work conditions should be set to accommodate not the "average" worker—as the ministry's guidelines state—but rather those who are "most vulnerable to stress," as long as their personalities remain within an acceptable range found among the workers doing the same kind of jobs.[25] In arguing for this radically "subjective" approach, the judges stated that the causal mechanism of depression is yet to be scientifically proven and that the government's guidelines, and by implication psychiatrists', fall short of providing a clear and sufficient standard for objectively diagnosing mental illness at work.[26]

Though the government initially reacted strongly against this juridical decision, it has since succumbed after facing repeated losses in similar lawsuits. In fact, over the last fifteen years, the workers' side has continued to accumulate legal victories by arguing for corporate responsibility over individual vulnerability. For instance, a worker with a history of recurrent depression, which before would have surely been taken as a sign of innate biological vulnerability, was judged to have been driven to depression from overwork. The family of an anesthesiologist who had a history of epilepsy was likewise awarded compensation for her overwork depression and suicide.[27] As the notion of individual biological vulnerability has become reconceptualized in terms of social causality, the range of definitions of "pathogenic stress" has also expanded. In 2003 a worker who had become depressed not because of excessive work but lack of work (as his company had deprived him of any meaningful work as a way of pressuring him to resign) successfully held his company liable by arguing that this was a form of *psychological bullying*.[28] Other similar cases involving sexual harassment and what Japanese call "power harassment" (a term that signifies a wide range of harassments that occur particularly in workplaces and often take the form of verbal abuse) have also brought victories to workers.[29]

In response, the government commissioned its own empirical survey on pathogenic stress, interviewing six thousand employees about what kind of events are subjectively experienced as most stressful.[30] Based on these findings, the government revised the Stress Evaluation Tables in 2009, upgrading certain events to the category of "the most stressful events" and adding new criteria for sexual harassment and power harassment, thereby significantly expanding the notion of what counts as pathogenic stress.[31] By incorporating workers' own voices in its policies, the government seems to be accepting that stress is something relative and subjective and that the Stress Evaluation Tables are an evolving document that reflects the changing notions of stress over time.

Contradictory Effects of Medicalization

The radical normalization of depression through these legal and policy debates since the late 1990s has brought depression to the center stage of public discourse, turning it into what the Japanese media has come to call a "national disease" of the recession era. Psychiatrists have successfully destigmatized depression by emphasizing that depression is not a sign of genetic weakness or a mere psychological problem but a *physiological illness* (often described as a "cold of the heart") that one becomes susceptible to when placed under excessive stress. Redefining depression as a problem of somatic and social origins, they have offered both antidepressants and ample rest as the cure—a persuasive prescription for people who feel thoroughly overworked and wish to have it recognized. In the meantime sales of antidepressants have continued to rise, from approximately 17 billion yen in the 1990s to exceed 100 billion yen by 2007. The number of depressed patients as of 2010 was over a million, an increase of 2.4 times in the past ten years.[32] The impact of the labor-policy changes has also been profound. Prior to 1999 cases of workers' mental illness were rarely approved for workers' compensation, and few workers would even imagine holding their company legally liable for their psychiatric breakdown. After the Stress Evaluation Tables were established in 1999, the number of approved cases (a significant portion of which involves depressed workers) suddenly went up to 26 (19 suicides) in 2000, 100 (43 suicides) in 2002, and as many as 475 (93 suicides) in 2012.[33] Depression is now one of the most frequently cited reasons for taking long-term sick leave. This is remarkable, especially for a society whose own psychiatrists had assumed until the mid-1990s that depression was a rare occurrence.

Yet as workers' compensation has begun to be distributed more widely than before to cover the mentally ill at work, psychiatrists have been confronting the century-old question of how to tell a "malingerer" from the "truly depressed." Some psychiatrists, faced with a sudden overflow of patients in their clinics, have begun to relegate some of these patients to diagnoses with derogatory implications (such as "immature type depression," "escaping depression," and "new-type depression"). Echoing the earlier psychiatric discourse about neurasthenia, they seem to be trying to impose an intellectual boundary control, preaching to the public to strictly distinguish the *real* (biological) depression from other (merely psychological) depressed states. Given that these boundaries had long dissolved when psychiatrists adopted the *DSM*s, however, such attempts seem belated, even futile.

Other psychiatrists, however, are increasingly expressing concern that by fueling therapeutic optimism, they may have given rise to a massive number of what Ivan Illich called "iatrogenesis"—a false illness of doctors' own making. These patients are not only being (falsely) labeled "depressed" but also experiencing what Ian Hacking calls "biolooping effect," whereby the act of taking antidepressants is literally altering the chemical condition of patients' brains and changing the nature of their "depression" itself.[34] Since the mid-2000s Japanese psychiatrists have been seriously debating whether antidepressants are curing people or if they may well be producing chronically depressed "intractable" patients. As these patients' painful struggles with "depression" are being increasingly problematized in the media, the biomedical cure that involves mind-altering drugs has become morally suspect, leaving psychiatry's therapeutic power and its promise of rational control increasingly in doubt.

The Emergent Psychiatric Science of Work

As if to provide a remedy where traditional clinical psychiatry has failed, there is now a developing field of science—or, following Anson Rabinbach, what I would like to call the *psychiatric science of work*.[35] While occupational medicine as a whole has been mainly concerned with physical illnesses, the psychiatric science of work as its branch is trying to assess the nature of stress and psychopathology in the workplace. At the same time, while medical and forensic experts have done much to shift responsibility from the depressed, instilling a "blame-free self of the therapeutic model," the experts involved in this field seem to be readdressing it by reconceptualizing depression as a product of stress and a form of *risk* that threatens every worker.[36] Depression defined in this way becomes something preventable by rational management at both collective and individual levels—an idea increasingly adopted by the government and corporations as they search for effective means of dealing with the rapid increase in the number of depressed workers. In so doing, they are beginning to address what has been left unresolved in medical and legal debates, that is, the question of individual *agency* in the making—and managing—of depression.

While it is still premature to say how this field of science is going to develop, its effect may be a double-edged sword for workers. Recent legislative changes have generated a more restrictive, bureaucratic system of evaluation, bringing to the care of the depressed new expectations and demands, suggested in the way depressed workers' recovery is now assessed in terms of *industrial time* rather than *clinical time*. Before mental health became strictly mandated in workplaces, Japanese corporations used to offer a highly generous and flexible system of sick leave. This system operated with the Parsoninan idea of a sick role, where stressed workers were expected to recover under the jurisdiction of medical experts who determined what the "natural" recovery process should be. Today, as mental health comes to be seen as not only a matter of medical jurisdiction but also an object of corporate risk management, some companies are introducing much more rigorous systems for evaluating workers' stress levels and mental health to promptly restore their health and productivity. Given the prolonged recession, where both personnel staff and workers are coming under increasing pressure to return the afflicted to a healthy state, they have to negotiate between the ideals of clinical time that prioritizes a natural recovery and the demands of industrial time that constantly seeks, even for a therapeutic process, the principle of efficiency.

The ideal of efficient recovery may also be relegating those who remain out of line with industrial time into new categories of Otherness. The industry is now taking steps to deal with depressed workers using means that introduce various degrees of estrangement. First of all, instead of trying to take care of the depressed inside the company, more and more companies are now choosing to outsource the care of the depressed to specialized clinics that also provide occupational training, thereby dealing with depression as an individual problem rather than confronting stress-laden work conditions. Second, some companies are also exploring ways to let go of workers who do not easily recover—yet this can be a risky and costly measure for companies when they are legally challenged. Tension of this kind surfaced in 2009, when a female worker took Toshiba (a megaelectronic company) to court and successfully challenged its decision to fire her after she had been on sick leave for three years.[37] Thus, a third tactic that has recently emerged is to rehire depressed workers through the category of *disability employment*. This is now much talked about because of recent legislative changes that the government has made to pressure companies to fulfill the 1.8 percent disability employment quota. Some company personnel staff are now discussing how to fulfill the required quota with depressed workers, preferably those who are already employed through a "normal" route and who have since become ill and obtained a disability certificate from the government. While they think it would be easy to fill up the quota this way (as there are already so many depressed workers), they cannot urge employees to obtain a disability status (or to "come out" and declare that they actually applied for the certificate), as this might be considered a violation of their human rights. Given the scientific uncertainty of its definition, depression as a form of disability is still in the making, leaving the afflicted vulnerable to competing interpretations about their social, economic, and political status beyond their control.

On Individual Agency, Vulnerability, and Stress

Part of the current confusion both in the clinics and in the industry stems, it seems, from the oversimplified, optimistic assumptions about depression and its stress-based definition, which has come to largely eclipse previous psychiatric discussions about vulnerability. Traditionally, Japanese psychiatrists have rejected the idea that there is a simple model of direct cause and effect between work stress and psychopathology. Instead, they have been trained to pay close attention to individual differences and individuals' specific vulnerabilities. In this regard, their theories of premorbid melancholic personality have provided a framework for concretely analyzing how genetics shapes a particular personality, which then interacts with the environment in a certain way, at times giving rise to the pathogenic situation. Yet when it comes to analyzing—and therapeutically engaging with—individual vulnerability, psychiatrists are far from having an adequate model for conceptualizing individual specificity.

This lack was already evident in 1999, when psychiatric experts were asked to establish the Stress Evaluation Tables. While creating precise scales for social stress, they did not produce a similar one for assessing individual vulnerability. These experts, as I was told by one of the psychiatrists involved, decided that it would be nonsensical to call those who are prone to depression "vulnerable" (with its negative connotation of weakness), as the depressed often embody what is normal, even ideal, in Japanese society. Such vulnerability is seen to be rooted as much in socialization as it is in genetics and might manifest itself as pathology only when the individuals are placed in an unaccommodating environment or at a time of social change. While this certainly has liberating implications for the depressed, it also homogenizes them and reduces the complexity of clinical realities, while shifting the focus from individuals' actual ailments to abstracted notions about a collective predicament. Indeed, despite their high-minded, left-wing ideas about how individuals are victims of social forces (from which they can supposedly be emancipated to become agents of their own), these psychiatrists have largely fallen short of developing a therapeutic approach that helps people to cultivate their own power of self-transformation. By defining the depressed as a product of both innate personality and social environment, Japanese psychiatrists seem to have created a curious blend of biological and social determinism.

Furthermore, in attempts to normalize depression and dispel its residual image as a genetic disease marked by irrationality, psychiatrists may have gone to the other extreme by portraying depression as a straightforward, all-too-rational illness that can be easily induced by social stress. Contrary to the popularized image, however, depression is far more complicated in its etiology and often leaves a mark on the afflicted, at times fundamentally altering their bodies and their sense of identity. Because of the optimistic understanding about the prognosis of depression, workers who long remain depressed appear to patients' family and personnel staff as puzzling and unpredictable. This is particularly problematic for chronic patients, for whom "depression" remains irregular, irrational, and unpredictable and for whom a certain period of social disengagement may even be crucial for recovery. Thus, an overly normalized understanding of depression seems to be generating new forms of disability and stigmatization against those who fail to live up to the idealized view of the depressed. Psychiatrists themselves have become keenly aware of the limit of biomedical intervention into what they regard as social and political problems. Yet they seem increasingly helpless as they watch the machinery of medicalization at work, trapped in the contradiction they themselves have been complicit in creating.

Beyond Local Knowledge

Beneath the surface of the global "biologization" of depression thus lie rich undercurrents of local discourses about depression and stress. But can such discourses go beyond being local knowledge, while giving rise to a new theoretical foundation of psychiatry with a social perspective? In 1980 Allan Young showed that the discourse of stress in the United States, which can serve to signal the social implications of one's suffering, instead ends up reproducing abstract individualism and biological and psychological reductionism, because the scientists themselves rely on and reproduce tacit knowledge about the society in which they live. Furthermore, when the knowledge they produce becomes invested with the scientific aura of neutrality and gains popular currency, stress helps conceal social contradictions and takes on the status of universal knowledge seemingly devoid of the particularities of its local production.[38]

At the same time uses of biomedical categories such as "stress" depend on a delicate moral balance, as those who claim legitimacy for their social suffering through a biomedical category are also subject to biomedical experts' interpretations about the nature of their ailment that can at any time redefine what *really* lies behind their pathology. In tracing the history of post-traumatic stress disorder (PTSD), Young has further shown how this diagnosis was adopted by Vietnam veterans and resulted in their asserting their victimhood, obtaining public recognition of their plight as a group, and gaining governmental compensation. Despite its political effectiveness, however, Young has also shown the emotional and moral price that the veterans have had to pay in adopting the PTSD discourse for expressing their pain, because it ultimately deprives them of the historical, political implications of their experience and trivializes the moral meanings of their *anger.* With the recent rebiologization of psychiatry, patients with PTSD also face the possibility of having their ailment reinterpreted as a sign of biological vulnerability. The lack of dialogue between the local, clinical realities and laboratory science thus becomes a serious problem when the latter further moves the data away from the realm of local, clinical practices, replacing patients' narratives (which leave the possibility for raising contradictions) with fragments of voiceless material bodies in the laboratory. In this last phase of biopsychiatrization, when the dislocation of the ownership of self-knowledge becomes complete, local subjectivity may no longer matter.[39]

But Young has also demonstrated the way in which the conceptual control of such biomedical concepts may be breaking down, losing the aura of scientific neutrality. Instead, it is becoming increasingly recognized that biomedical concepts such as PTSD and depression are bundles of localized concepts whose meanings are constantly negotiated and redrawn by various actors—including pharmaceutical companies, physicians, and public administrators, as well as lawyers and judges who are playing a part in medicalization.[40] Such local heterogeneity has largely remained undiscussed in biomedicine partly because of the divide between global scientific psychiatry and local clinical practice.[41] This dual structure has made it easy for both global psychiatry and local psychiatries to proceed with business as usual in the face of growing gaps and contradictions.[42] In this regard, the new forms of "scientific" knowledge articulated through the depression discourse in Japan—as represented by the Stress Evaluation Tables—remain (consciously) malleable, negotiable, and highly localized. The emergent local discourses about stress and psychopathology may thus provide a unique blending of the subjective and the objective, the biological and the social, in the sense that it provides a pathway for local subjectivity to become part of universal scientific knowledge.

Notes

This chapter is adapted from my *Depression in Japan: Psychiatric Cures for a Society in Distress.*

1. "Karō jisatsu soshō de wakai: Dentsū shain izokugawa 'zenmenshōri no naiyō'" [Resolution for overwork suicide lawsuit: Dentsū employee's family "all-out victory], *Asahi Shimubun*, June 23, 2000.

2. Shigeru Fujimoto, "Karō jisatsu to shiyōsha no songai baishō sekinin" [Overwork suicide and the liability of employers], *Bessatsu Jurist* [Jurist supplement], 165 (2002): 142–43.

3. "Karo de jisatsu rosai nintei kijun wa: Sutoresu dō 31komoku de sokutei" [What are the standards for determining overwork suicide? The level of stress measured by 31 items], *Monday Nikkei*, December 27, 1999.

4. Carl Elliott and Tod Chambers, *Prozac as a Way of Life* (Chapel Hill: University of North Carolina Press, 2004); cf. Peter Conrad and Joseph W. Schneider, *Deviance and Medicalization: From Badness to Sickness* (Saint Louis: Mosby, 1980).

5. See Nikolas Rose, *The Politics of Life Itself: Biomedicine, Power, and Subjectivity in the Twenty-First Century* (Princeton, NJ: Princeton University Press, 2007).

6. Allan Young, *The Harmony of Illusions: Inventing Post-traumatic Stress Disorder* (Princeton, NJ: Princeton University Press, 1995); Adriana Petryna, *Life Exposed: Biological Citizens after Chernobyl* (Princeton, NJ: Princeton University Press, 2002).

7. My analysis of the rise of overwork depression in Japan is based on anthropological research that stretches from 1998 to early 2010, a decade that covers before and after the onset of the medicalization. This included observing the proceedings of several overwork death and overwork suicide court cases at the Tokyo District

Court and attending conferences and a series of study groups held by the lawyers and psychiatrists involved in such cases. For archival research I examined the *Japanese Journal of Psychiatry and Neurology* from its first issue in 1902 to the present, as well as a number of popular journals and a few of newspapers from the 1870s to the 2000s. I also used Japanese legal journals such as *Jurist* and *Hanrei Times* to investigate the legal discourses regarding overwork depression and overwork suicide.

8. Anson Rabinbach, *The Human Motor: Energy, Fatigue, and the Origins of Modernity* (New York: Basic Books, 1990).

9. Heinz-Peter Schmiedebach, "Post-traumatic Neurosis in Nineteenth-Century Germany: A Disease in Political, Juridical and Professional Context," *History of Psychiatry* 10 (1999): 27–57. The situation differed little in Japan, where the imported notion of neurasthenia became widely known by the 1900s as a quintessential illness of overwork. Yet it acquired derogatory implications by the 1920s, as it came to signal individual biological vulnerability, while gradually losing its legitimacy as an illness of social origin; see Junko Kitanaka, "Questioning the Suicide of Resolve: Medico-Legal Disputes Regarding 'Overwork Suicide' in Twentieth-Century Japan," in *Histories of Suicide: International Perspectives on Self-Destruction in the Modern World*, ed. John Weaver and David Wright (Toronto: University of Toronto Press, 2009), 257–80.

10. As they investigated the impact of the war on these patients, German psychiatrists turned to concepts such as "uprooted depression" and "existential depression" in an attempt to do justice to the magnitude of social suffering people had experienced. Waichirō Omata, *Doitsu seishin byōrigaku no sengoshi* [The history of the postwar German psychopathology] (Tokyo: Gendai Shokan, 2002).

11. Arthur Kleinman, *Social Origins of Distress and Disease: Depression, Neurasthenia, and Pain in Modern China* (New Haven: Yale University Press, 1986).

12. Hiroshi Kawahito, *Karō jisatsu* [Overwork suicide] (Tokyo: Iwanami Shoten, 1998).

13. Tadashi Fujimoto, *"Jisatsu karōshi" saiban 24 sai natsu adoman no ketsubetsu* ["Overwork suicide" lawsuit: 24-year-old advertisement man's departure] (Tokyo: Daiamond Sha, 1996), 162.

14. Shūzō Naka, "Shorōki utsuyūshō" [Presenile depression], *Shikeigaku Zasshi* [Journal of neurology] 34 (1932): 53–77.

15. Mitsuzō Shimoda, "Sōutsubyō no byōzen seikaku ni tsuite" [On premorbid personality of the manic depressive], *Seishin Shinkeigaku Zasshi* [Journal of psychiatry and neurology] 45 (1941): 101; see also Shimoda, "Sōutsubyō ni tsuite" [On manic depression], *Yonago Igaku Zasshi* [Yonago medical journal] 2 (1950): 3–4.

16. Hubertus Tellenbach, *Melancholy: History of the Problem, Endogeneity, Typology, Pathogenesis, Clinical Considerations* (1961; repr., Pittsburgh: Duquesne University Press 1980).

17. Shin Iida, "Sōutsubyō no jōkyōron to kongo no kadai" [Situational cause of depression and new issues], *Seishin Shinkeigaku Zasshi* [Journal of psychiatry and neurology] 75 (1973): 274–79; Iida, "Sōutsubyō no jōkyōiron" [Theories of situational cause for manic depression], in *Seishinigaku Ronbunshū* [Papers on psychiatry] (Tokyo: Kongō Shuppan, 1978). See also Margaret Lock, "Protests of a Good Wife and Wise Mother: The Medicalization of Distress in Japan," in *Health, Illness, and Medical Care in Japan*, ed. Norbeck E. and Margaret Lock (Honolulu: University of Hawaii Press, 1987), 130–57.

18. Tokyo Kōsai [Tokyo High Court], Songai baishō seikyū kōso jiken [Appeal for compensation for damage], case 1647/4089, 1997.

19. Saikōsai [Supreme Court], Songai baishō seikyū kōso jiken [Appeal for compensation for damage], case 218, 2000.

20. Kitanaka, "Suicide of Resolve."

21. Nobuo Kuroki, "Rōsai nintei ni okeru hannōsei seishin shōgai no kangaekata [Perspectives on reactive mental disorder in terms of workers' compensation], *Seishinka Chiryōgaku* [Journal of psychiatric treatment] 15 (2000): 843–49.

22. "Jisatsu no rōsai nintei kanwa: Taishō 'kokoro no shippei' mo" [Relaxed regulations for work-related suicide compensation: Broader inclusion of "mental illness"], *Asahi Shimbun*, July 31, 1999.

23. Chikanobu Okamura, *Karōshi karōjisatsu kyūsai no riron to jitsumu* [Theory and practice of providing relief to overwork death and overwork suicide) (Tokyo: Junpōsha, 2002).

24. Hiroaki Fujikawa, "Iwayuru karō jisatsu to anzen hairyo gimu hōri" [So-called overwork suicide and the obligation of safety doctrine], *Bessatsu Jurist: Shakai Hoshō Hanrei Hyakusen* [Jurist supplement: Social security 100 precedents)] 153 (2000): 150–51.

25. "Shokuba no 'jakusha' ni hikari, karō jisatsu ni rōsai nintei hanketsu" [Light on the "weak" in workplaces: Workers' compensation granted in overwork suicide lawsuit], *Asahi Shimbun*, June 18, 2001.

26. Yoshihiro Nomura, Naoki Kinomoto, Takaharu Hiranuma, Masahiko Sugita, Nobuo Kuroki, Masaharu Katō, Fumio Itō, et al., "Karōshi to kigyō no songai biashō sekinin: Dentsū karōshi jisatsu jiken" [Overwork death and corporate liability: Dentsū overwork suicide case] *Baishō Kagaku* [Journal of compensation science] 30 (2003): 115–36. See also Kitanaka, "Suicide of Resolve."

27. Tsuneko Hirata, "Hanpukusei utsubyōsei shōgai de atta rōdōsha ni yoru jisatsu to gyōmukiinsei" [A suicide by a worker who was suffering recurrent depressive disorder and its causal attribution to work], *Chingin to Shakaihoshō* [Wage and social security] 1435 (2007): 33–42; "Kiōreki ga aru masuikai no utsubyō jisatsu" [Suicide of an anesthesiologist], *Rōdō Keizai Hanrei Sokuhō* [Law reports on labor and economy] no. 1981 (2007).

28. Nao Okada, "Gyōmu kankyō ga gen'in no utsubyō ni rōsai nintei: Tenkyo kyohi de shigoto o ataerarezu shikiri de kakuri" [Workers' compensation granted for depression caused by work environment: Refusal of transfer led to deprivation of job, secluded by partition], *Rōdōhōgaku Kenkyū Kaihō* [Labor law research report] 54 (2003): 1–35.

29. "'Pawahara jisatsu' rōsai nintei: Jōshi kara bōgen 'kyūryō dorobō' 'mezawari, kiete kure'" ["Power harassment suicide" to receive workers' compensation: Insulted by boss "goldbricker" "eyesore"], *Asahi Shimbun*, October 16, 2007; Masashi Hozumi, "Rībokku Japan rōsai nintei jiken: Otona no ijime taishoku kyōyō de utsubyō wa rōsai" [The Reebok Japan workers' compensation case: Workers' compensation for depression caused by bullying and coerced resignation], *Rōdōhōritsujunpō* [Labor law report] 1650 (2007): 51–53.

30. Nobuo Kuroki, "Shokuba no mentaru herusu to shūrō shien" [Mental health in workplaces and job assistance], *Kenkōkanri* [Health management] 6 (2007): 6–33.

31. "Mottomo omoi yōin ni pawahara tsuika e" [Power harassment added to the severest factor], *Asahi Shimbun*, March 20, 2009.

32. "'Utsu hyakumannin' kage ni shinyaku? Hanbaidaka to kanjasū hirei [New medication behind "one million people in depression"? Ratio of sales to number of patients], *Yomiuri Shimbun*, January 6, 2010.

33. "Seishin shōgai no rōsai nintei saita: kōrōshō matome, sakunendo 130nin" [130 cases approved for workers' compensation: The biggest number last year, says the Ministry of Health, Welfare, and Labor], *Nihon Keizai Shimbun*, June 18, 2005; "Kokoro no yamai rōsai saita" [The highest number of worker's compensation ever granted for mental illnesses], *Asahi Shiumbun*, June 9, 2009.

34. Ivan Illich, *Medical Nemesis: The Expropriation of Health* (London: Calder and Boyars, 1975); Ian Hacking, *The Social Construction of What?* (Cambridge, MA: Harvard University Press, 1999).

35. Rabinbach, *Human Motor*.

36. Mary Douglas, *Risk and Blame: Essays in Cultural Theory* (London: Routledge, 1992): 230.

37. "Tōshiba shain utsubyō kajūgyōmu ga geiin" [Toshiba employees depressed: Overwork is the cause], *Asahi Shimbun*, May 19, 2009.

38. Allan Young, "The Discourse on Stress and the Reproduction of Conventional Knowledge," *Social Science and Medicine* 14 (1980): 133–46.

39. Young, *Harmony of Illusions*.

40. Ibid.; see also Margaret Lock, *Twice Dead: Organ Transplants and the Reinvention of Death* (Berkeley: University of California Press, 2002).

41. G. Nigel Gilbert and Michael Mulkay, *Opening Pandora's Box: A Sociological Analysis of Scientists' Discourse* (Cambridge: Cambridge University Press, 1984).

42. Lawrence Cohen, *No Aging in India: Alzheimer's, the Bad Family, and Other Modern Things* (Berkeley: University of California Press, 1998).

Part Five

Managing Stress

Chapter Nine

The Invention of the "Stressed Animal" and the Development of a Science of Animal Welfare, 1947–86

Robert G. W. Kirk

In Britain, as elsewhere in the 1950s, it had become "fashionable to assert" that there was "an increase in the incidence of mental disorders and that the cause of this is the increased stress of modern life." Some medical professionals feared this trend to be self-fulfilling, warning that "mental health propaganda" was "instilling a phobia for the inevitable stresses of life."[1] The language of stress was certainly ubiquitous at this time, not least within the various branches of the biomedical sciences. In the wake of Hans Selye's general adaptation syndrome, stress had quickly become a conceptual space in which the study of clinical medicine, biology, physiology, endocrinology, neurology, biochemistry, psychology, psychiatry, and behavior, among many other fields, could enter into dialogue. This is not to suggest that there was agreement on the nature of stress or even the meaning of the term. On the contrary, across these disciplines stress was invoked in different ways, according to different models. Arguably, it was the very flexibility of the concept that accounted for its prevalence.

In July 1958, for example, the Mental Health Research Fund organized a conference with the aim to "arrive at a synthesis of the concepts used in different branches of the behavioral sciences when discussing stressful effects."[2] Held at Oxford University, the conference hosted prominent participants, including the psychiatrists Aubrey Lewis, W. Linford Rees, and Martin Roth; the psychiatrist, psychoanalyst, and ethologist John Bowlby; ethologist and animal behaviorist Robert A. Hinde and Oliver L. Zangwill; the Pavlovian psychobiologist Howard S. Liddell; the cyberneticians William Ross Ashby and W. Grey Walter; and Hans Selye himself. It is no coincidence that the majority of participants resist categorization within a single discipline. As the conference progressed, the neurochemist Derek Richter noted, with increasing awe, the multiplicity of meanings that stress held across "common language," "physics," "biology," "physiology," and "psychology." Though finding a shared language had proved far from simple, participants concluded that the practice of differentiating and synthesizing understandings of stress was nonetheless productive.[3]

Bowlby, too, had sought commonalities in the differing meanings of stress employed across the diverse disciplines represented at the conference. Noting common characteristics in the different understandings of stress, he resolved that all presumed that

> an organism lives by maintaining a variety of relationships, external and internal. To define its state at any time we must define the relations which it is set to attain, maintain and escape, and the course of its current activity in regard to those relationships. In "relationships" I include those which serve both physiological needs, like the need for nutrition and psychological needs, like the need for status and success. These relations are maintained by constant activity, e.g., nutrition by an endless succession of meals, "success" by an endless series of successful performances. None can be attained once for all.

Stress discourses, then, were capable of representing the dynamic organism in all its complexity. Stress could capture relational responses to change across sites where interactions had hitherto proved difficult to integrate. Bowlby, therefore, came to believe that all applications of the term addressed the process of adapting to challenge. When challenged, organisms would change along four dimensions, physiologically, emotionally, behaviorally, and structurally. At the end of this process the organism would regain its original state or enter a new one. Change, in any or all of these dimensions, could be attributed to stress. Hence the utility of the concept as a vector of communication across disciplines. For Bowlby, stress "connotes a degree of challenge sufficient to evoke the kind of change or behaviour which interests the particular observer. Its meaning, therefore, depends not only on the 'dimension' in which he is interested but also on the threshold above which appear the kind of phenomenon which he finds interesting."[4] In other words, stress was general enough to be found anywhere yet specific enough to give structure to the chosen object of study. Above all else, then, the concept of stress was epistemologically and ontologically *relational.*

This chapter explores how stress provided a language capable of structuring dynamic and always-active relations, rendering them comprehensible and thereby opening them up to intervention and management. The argument is developed through three parts, beginning with an analysis of the introduction of Selye's concept of the general adaptation syndrome into the regulatory landscape of British animal-dependent science. Here, it is shown how ecological investigations of population decline challenged the regulatory definition of "pain" by invoking stress as an explanatory concept. Regulatory understandings of animal pain, which were conventionally restricted to surgical interventions into the body, were subsequently widened so as to include mental suffering, a condition of possibility for the emergence of the "stressed animal."

The second section unpacks the implications of the "stressed animal" within the laboratory, showing how stress facilitated the emergence of a "science" of animal welfare. In the 1950s stress was mobilized to reveal the complex interdependencies a living organism shared with its physical and social environment. It provided a model that, by including the experimenter, placed knowing human scientist and animal object of knowledge within an interdependent relationship. Though the implications of this move took some time to become explicit, this was nonetheless the originary moment of the ethical framework known as "humane experimental technique" (or the 3Rs) which today governs animal experimentation across the developed world. Finally, the trajectory of the stressed animal is traced from the laboratory to sites of intensive (or "factory") farming. By emphasizing relationality, the conceptual landscape of stress engendered a form of reflexive thought that brought all relationships within its remit, including that between human and nonhuman animal. Consequently, this chapter argues that stress facilitated a fifth dimension of change: *that of the ethical orientation of living organisms to one another*. By rendering relationships knowable, thus manageable, stress provided a language by which traditionally moral notions such as "well-being" could be reconfigured from political philosophical rhetoric to become objects of scientific and economic knowledge materialized in physical spaces, scientific practices, and legal regulations.

The Stressed Animal and the Regulatory Landscape of British Science

The Cruelty to Animals Act (1876) established an elaborate licensing system for the regulation of animal experimentation, through which the Home Office governed animal experimentation in Britain for over a century.[5] The spirit of the act was taken to be the prevention of the infliction of unnecessary pain on animals subjected to experiment. By the mid-twentieth century Home Office inspectors had accrued extensive knowledge regarding the best practices in animal experimentation, together with a considerable body of precedent. Consequently, in most cases civil servants were capable of determining which scientific practices required licensing. Whether or not a given procedure formed an experiment, and if so whether it caused pain, could nevertheless be contentious. In the early years of the act, for example, there was considerable confusion about whether the use of animals in the production of sera and antitoxins fell under the act. Eventually, this question was resolved by legal opinion having determined that the injecting of animals for production purposes did not fall under the act, as the practice was not an experiment (though it may cause pain). Subsequent injection of products into small mammals for the purposes of standardization, however, was judged an experiment and therefore required licensing under the act. Both practices involved similar invasive manipulations of the animal body, but it was intent as opposed to practice that determined legality.[6]

Practices thought to come under the act by some and not by others were conventionally determined in an ad hoc manner, often through consultation with a sitting Advisory Committee whose remit was to advise the Home Office on novel or complicated applications. The status of a given practice might occasionally change over time. The use of mice in the Zondek-Aschheim pregnancy test, for instance, was ruled not to fall under the provisions of the act in 1944, as it had been refined not to involve the infliction of pain and, moreover, having become established as a routine medical test was no longer thought of as an experiment.[7] Importantly, over this period, one aspect of interpretation remained consistent: pain was understood physiologically, that is, as the result of physical (generally surgical) interventions into the animal body.[8]

In day-to-day practice individual scientists were expected to recognize their experimental work as being "calculated to give pain" and thus apply for licensing under the act. In 1949, for this reason, Dennis Chitty and John Clarke applied to the Home Office for a license. In doing so they introduced the concept of stress to the regulatory landscape of British animal experimentation. Furthermore, they inadvertently challenged the long-held definition of pain as being the result of surgical interventions into the animal body. Chitty, a British-born Canadian ecologist, and Clarke, a Australian doctoral student, were members of Charles Elton's Bureau for Animal Population at the University of Oxford.[9] From the 1930s Elton and his small team of researchers had worked to establish population cycles as an economically crucial yet little-understood phenomenon. The promise of being able to predict and control periods of scarcity and abundance in wild populations of animals with economic value attracted the support of numerous parties. Imperial Chemical Industries (ICI), for instance, sponsored research into game populations. Similarly, the Universities Federation for Animal Welfare (UFAW), a self-styled "scientific" animal welfare society, supported an investigation into wild rabbit populations in the hope of demonstrating them to be detrimental to British agricultural production (as opposed to a useful source of food).[10] By pioneering new methods of conducting censuses of wild populations, such as Chitty's methods of trapping, ringing, and recapturing live mammals, the bureau had become a leading center for research into population density and mortality in natural habitats by the 1940s.[11]

The formative work of the bureau was synthesized in Elton's *Voles, Mice and Lemmings: Problems in Population Dynamics* (1942). This book established the reality of cycles in populations of small, wild mammals, as well as the economic importance of understanding such cycles and the inadequacy of current explanations for the phenomenon. Elton contended that none of the four main explanatory hypotheses—food shortage, predation, weather, and epidemic disease—adequately explained sudden population collapses.[12] This led Chitty to develop a controversial, yet latterly influential, hypothesis. He proposed that individuals born into dense populations differed congenitally from those born into growing populations. Such qualitative change, he suggested, provided a self-regulatory mechanism by which populations could control their number.[13]

This theory was first articulated in a manuscript prepared in the late 1940s and submitted to the *Journal of Animal Ecology*. Chitty explained how natural population crashes might be caused "primarily due to adverse conditions to which the parents were subjected in the previous breeding season." Despite Elton and Chitty having founded the journal in 1932 and having served as editors until 1950, the newly appointed editor rejected the paper. At best, Chitty's "vague speculation" was judged to go against the grain of ecological thinking by proposing internal as opposed to external regulatory factors for a population. At worst, it could be read to imply a form of inheritance of acquired characteristics (i.e., Lamarckism). Had it not been for the intervention of Peter Medawar, a past colleague and supporter of the work of the bureau, the paper may not have been published at all. Medawar encouraged Chitty to press on, recommending the article to the *Philosophical Transactions of the Royal Society of London*, where it was published in 1952.[14] For Chitty, this proved to be a formative experience. Subsequently, he became vehemently committed to ecology as an *experimental* science. Indeed, throughout his career he remained suspicious of ecological theories based on observation, descriptive reasoning, or mathematical modeling alone.[15] To be taken seriously, Chitty believed, a hypothesis required replicable experimental evidence.

In 1949, therefore, Chitty challenged John Clarke to provide the evidence through a series of laboratory-based experiments using the short-tailed field vole (*Microtus agretis*). Voles had long served as the favored model for population density research at Oxford because they were readily available in local woods and, anecdotally, were known to increase by dramatic proportions before suddenly disappearing. In the 1930s, Richard M. Ranson and John R. Baker had developed methods for domesticating and maintaining wild voles in the laboratory.[16] Because voles were known to fight with remarkable ferocity in threatening scenarios, fighting was chosen as the object of study. Chitty and Clarke reasoned that increased fighting within a dense population could cause physiological disturbance in pregnant animals capable of creating abnormalities in their progeny. Such abnormalities, it was thought, could be responsible for increasing mortality over generations. But without a mechanism capable of connecting behavior at the level of the population to physiological change at the level of the individual, it was unclear how this could happen or what should be measured as evidence of the process. As ecologists, neither Chitty nor Clarke possessed the necessary pathological expertise to compare whole organisms for abnormalities. They required what Clarke later described as a "quick, uncomplicated measure of the physiological state of the animals, which would be at once meaningful."[17] Stress, as set out in Hans Selye's general adaptation syndrome, proved a perfect fit for this job. Stress not only provided a mechanism by which behavioral change in the population could be related to physiological change in the individual but also suggested an efficient biological marker for the measurement of bodily change.[18]

With an experiment planned, Chitty and Clarke applied to the Home Office for a license, including dispensation from anesthetics, as they believed their experimental design to be "calculated to give pain." They explained their desire "to keep voles under conditions likely to result in fighting for the establishment of social hierarchy" to study the "effect of social stress upon longevity and reproduction with particular reference to the adaptation syndrome (Selye)."[19] But there was no precedent for such a request because "no certificate has previously been submitted to the Secretary of State to allow such experiments to be made in this country." The Home Office was uncertain as to how to respond because "no actual operative procedure" was intended, and it was unclear how the work could be calculated to inflict pain.[20] Importantly, analogous experiments *had* been undertaken in 1930 by Francis A. E. Crew and Ljuba Mirskaia at the Animal Breeding Research Department within the University of Edinburgh. Investigating the effects of density on mouse populations, they described how "mouse differed from mouse temperamentally. . . . The males fought desperately and without respite and . . . the commonest form of injury was partial or complete castration. Such mutilated males as survived were permitted by their masters to re-enter the community. . . . Certain boxes had to be withdrawn from the experiment, for . . . the original occupants had provided a group which spent all their time killing new members and replacements. . . . These were death traps for the new-comers."[21] No license had been requested for this work. Yet there was no question of Crew and Mirskaia having been in the wrong for not having applied to the Home Office.[22] Rather, the Home Office wrote to Chitty asking why he thought a license was required for the proposed experiment.

At no point was the scientific worth of investigating correlations between population density and Selye's general adaptation syndrome questioned.

The singular difficulty, in the view of the Home Office, was how to fit Chitty's understanding of pain within current regulative practices. In a detailed explanation, Chitty described why he believed that "animals subjected to the stress of fighting" should be understood to "suffer." The proposition that "fighting upsets maternal physiology" implied that "the resulting progeny suffer permanent disability to grow and/or reproduce." In addition, there was a risk "some animals may be physically injured or killed by fighting."[23] As was customary in difficult cases, the Home Office called on the Advisory Committee on the Administration of the Cruelty to Animals Act, an expert group consisting of scientists and lawyers, to adjudicate.

All permissions to dispense with anesthesia had hitherto been accompanied by a standard limiting condition, stating that "no operative procedure more severe than simple inoculation or superficial venesection may be adopted in any of the said experiments." This clause formed part of the "pain condition," the intent of which was to ensure that no animal suffered severe pain.[24] In this case, no operative procedure was planned and so such a caveat made little sense. Moreover, it did nothing to address the possibility of "severe injuries" occurring as a consequence of fighting.[25] The Advisory Committee therefore asked Chitty how he intended to meet the "Pain Condition," to which he explained injured animals would be removed and painlessly put to death. Satisfied, the committee concluded that "the experiments were potentially valuable and no undue suffering was likely to result. In effect the experiments would reproduce conditions that occurred in nature, but whereas under natural conditions animals maimed in fighting would die a lingering and often painful death, in this case serious casualties would at once be removed and painlessly destroyed."[26] The moral deference to "nature" is itself worthy of note. However, of most significance is how stress challenged the conventional regulatory understanding of pain. In the event, the full extent of the challenge was evaded.

Chitty and Clarke were granted their license. As their proposed work would not violate the standard limiting condition, it was appended despite its irrelevance. Nonetheless, this episode marked the beginning of a major redefinition and extension of the regulatory understanding of pain. Suffering could no longer be viewed as solely deriving from physical interventions into the body. While stress-induced suffering continued to be predominantly framed in terms of physiological change, the capacity of animals to experience pain had widened far beyond physical interventions into the body. Animal sociality, for example, could now be recognized as capable of causing suffering by altering behavior and detrimentally effecting physiology. The implications of this new model of suffering was quickly mobilized and deployed by those who sought to make animal welfare a foremost concern of animal-dependent experimental science.

Materializing Well-being in the Laboratory: A Science of Animal Welfare?

In 1949 Chitty briefly toured the United States, discussing his World War II development of economic methods of pest control.[27] At Johns Hopkins, he met with Curt Richter, David E. Davis, John B. Calhoun, and John J. Christian, all of whom were undertaking analogous work on population density with a view to controlling rat infestation in Baltimore.[28] In quite distinctive ways the Baltimore group was investigating relations between population density, environment, behavior, and stress.[29] Richter, for example, was investigating how the stress of domestication might alter laboratory rats through a process he thought may "parallel the development of man in society."[30] Though Chitty must have discussed their mutual interests, he failed to make explicit connections between his encounters in Baltimore and his vole work at Oxford. In 1950, when Christian published a paper that effectively preempted his and Clarke's investigation, Chitty was "temporally devastated."[31] It was not in Baltimore, therefore, that Chitty was introduced to the work of Selye but rather at a meeting of the Society for Experimental Biology that Chitty attended on his return to the United Kingdom.

At this meeting Michael Robin Alexander Chance suggested that Selye's ideas "might provide the theoretical framework" for Chitty's "otherwise bald and unconvincing narrative" regarding the regulation of populations.[32] Chance was a zoologically trained pharmacologist, who had worked in industry (Glaxo Laboratories, 1938–46) before joining the University of Birmingham as lecturer in pharmacology (1946–82). His real interest, however, was the new behavioral science of ethology, which is conventionally understood to have methodologically prioritized the relationship between environment and behavior, emphasizing the study of animals in nature as opposed to in the laboratory.[33] Chance, however, applied ethology to the study of domesticated laboratory animals. Reasoning that the "natural" environment of laboratory animals was, in fact, the laboratory, Chance deployed ethological techniques to identify the "normal" species-specific behavior of common laboratory animals (so as to render them more reliable experimental tools).[34] He was among the first to demonstrate that social behavior could alter physiological reactions to pharmaceutical drugs, a discovery that had crucial implications for experimental design and later directly informed experimental studies of stress.[35] For Chance, ethology provided a means to capture the complexity of living organisms within their environment. Ethological techniques could chart interactions between the wider physical and social environment on the one hand and individual physiology, emotion, and behavior on the other. Structural changes in the individual body could thereby be related to behavioral changes in the population. Stress, therefore, was a useful conceptual resource for ethological studies, as it provided a theoretical framework to relate phenomena across psychosomatic and psychosocial territories.

This conceptual orientation, which was shared by many who were influenced by ethology and psychosomatic approaches in the 1950s, situated the knowing subject within the environment of, and therefore in relation to, the object of (or means to) knowledge. Consequently, it encouraged reflective thought. One example of this trend was a tendency toward explicit consideration of the methodological difficulties in the production of objective knowledge. Chance, for example, developed a course for medical students titled "How to Observe," consisting of practical exercises in behavioral observation of laboratory animals. The intention was to demonstrate to students that what they *looked for* in a given situation often had little to do with what they *looked at*.[36] Placing the knowing subject in relation to the object of knowledge also accentuated the subjective relations between the two. Accordingly, in his work Chance emphasized how researchers, animal caretakers, and animal technicians formed part of the social environment for laboratory animals. From this perspective humans were understood as agents in the psychosomatic and psychosocial processes that shaped the animals.[37] This view had clear implications for experimental design—psychosocial spaces now had to be controlled if verifiable experimental knowledge was to be produced. Moreover, this approach also opened up the relationship between experimental scientist and laboratory animal as a new territory for ethical intervention, within which the well-being of laboratory animals came to the fore.

In the 1950s, Chance's studies of laboratory animal well-being were supported by the Universities Federation for Animal Welfare (UFAW) as part of a wider research program to develop "humane experimental technique." UFAW was unique among animal advocacy groups in that it sought to recruit the intellectual elite to develop a "science" of animal welfare.[38] Rather than appealing to popular politics, UFAW worked with scientists and veterinarians in an attempt to pragmatically "reduce the sum total of pain and fear inflicted on animals by man."[39] From the 1940s UFAW had considerable success appropriating a then prevalent concern over the reliability of experimental animals as a means to turn scientific attention to questions of animal welfare.[40] By arguing that the welfare of laboratory animals was the starting point in the production of standardized, and thus reliable, laboratory animals, UFAW encouraged the consideration of laboratory animal well-being as a key methodological concern in the design of experiments. UFAW funded Chance's research, for instance, as his ethological studies were thought to demonstrate "the importance of a happy home life (cage design, nature, and number of companions) in producing uniform results in test animals."[41] In this way, animal well-being was reconfigured and transitioned, moving from a language dominated by moral rhetoric into a new form of specialist expertise grounded in pragmatic science. Within this logic, ethical concern became scientific necessity.

The UFAW Handbook on the Care and Management of Laboratory Animals (1947) did much to establish the new science of laboratory animal welfare (as well as UFAW's credibility within scientific circles). It was the first general handbook providing standard methods of animal care for all the major laboratory animal species. Animal-dependent experimental scientists responded positively to the *Handbook*, one reviewer describing it as "a very practical blend of economics and humanitarianism . . . indispensable to all concerned in any way with the production and use of animals in laboratories."[42] The style of the *Handbook* was strongly practical, providing standard species-specific approaches to animal housing, breeding, feeding, handling, and general husbandry. Yet emphasis was also placed on the sometime subjective and always relational aspects of *working with animals*. For example, the *Handbook* described how "animals may suffer acutely from boredom, and they certainly need exercise, companionship and opportunity for play." As little was known about these needs, much more had to be learned about the "psychological conditions that make for a happy and contented stock."[43] Consequently, UFAW focused a good deal of attention and financial support on such research.[44] Within this work the concept of stress came to play an important role.

In 1954, UFAW funded a new research project intended to develop humane approaches to experimental science. Peter Medawar was appointed to guide the work, chairing UFAW's Scientific Advisory Committee, which also included William Lane-Petter, then head of the Medical Research Council's Laboratory Animals Bureau. Medawar enthusiastically supported what he saw as "research on methods of research," providing space in his laboratory at University College London (UCL) for two researchers, William Moy Stratton Russell and Rex Burch.[45] Russell took the lead in shaping the conceptual development of what became *The Principles of Humane Experimental Technique* (1959).[46] Russell had recently completed a D.Phil at the Department of Zoology at Oxford. While there he had become enamored by ethology, the principles of which he synthesized with cybernetics and systems theory to form what he termed a "psychosomatic" approach to animals. His aim was to develop an approach to laboratory animals about the principle of "*mens sana in corpore sano* [a healthy mind in a healthy body]." What became "humane experimental technique" emphasized that the experimenter would not "get one without the other."[47]

Drawing directly on the work of Chitty and Clarke, Russell presented his psychosomatic approach as a refinement of stress research.[48] It was "regrettable alike on humane and scientific grounds that so large a proportion of the study of psychosomatics in animals has so far been carried out with the bludgeon of 'stress' of the more severe kinds." Russell went on to explain that "everything about the rich physiological network suggests the possibility of much more refined effects of behavioural upon internal states." Here again, stress provided a theoretical approach capable of integrating physiological, psychological, and behavioral change across the levels of individual and population. Russell believed that domesticated animals appeared less able to cope with stress because of the restraints placed on their range of responses by the controlled environments in which they lived. "Conflict states never persist in nature," Russell claimed, because "while lower animals have no direct control over their moods, automatic mechanisms ensure that distressing ones do not persist." However, this "natural sequence is disturbed in captive and domesticated animals."[49] Consequently, those who worked with laboratory animals were under a moral obligation to ensure environments met the welfare needs of animals, either by allowing automatic mechanisms to operate as in nature or by compensating in some way if they could not. The physical environment, thereby, became a site mapped and shaped by ethical considerations.

To understand the "refined effects" of psychosomatic interactions, Russell made "distress" (as opposed to stress) the central concept and object of humane experimental technique. Distress gave notions of "humane" and "inhumane" a practical meaning embedded in quantifiable properties. It was defined as a state that "if protracted, would lead to the stress syndrome." Humane experimental technique demanded not only the removal of negative scenarios but the provision of positive ones. Science was expected to "aim at well-being rather than the absence of distress."[50] The laboratory animal was portrayed as existing on a scale with one end being "distress" and the other "well-being." Russell outlined various promising lines that might provide criteria to quantify distress. Again, stress was the model. The advancement and refinement of endocrinology, for example, promised a reliable approach to the biological measurement of distress. Following the work of Chitty, the measurement of breeding productivity could also serve as a general indicator of well-being, with any decline indicating an increase in distress. Finally, albeit a somewhat subjective indicator, "the animal's behaviour *toward the experimenter*" was suggested as an "extremely pertinent and valuable criteria" of laboratory animal well-being.[51] Within humane experimental technique, well-being became a variable within a new science of animal welfare, which served to reconfigure moral values from political-cum-philosophical concepts to quantifiable material states.

Today, codified as the "3Rs" or the refinement, reduction, and replacement of animals in experimental science, humane experimental technique provides the ethical framework governing animal experimentation in the developed world. Yet few have read *The Principles of Humane Experimental Technique.* Unlike the *UFAW Handbook,* it was poorly received and quickly dropped out of print.[52] The conventional history assumes the 3Rs to have been ignored until they were "rediscovered" in the late 1980s. However, alongside the wider work of UFAW and others, the *Principles* formed an important contribution to the reimagining of the laboratory animal. No longer could animals be approached as mere tools. Not only had recognition of their experiential capacities broadened, but it had vastly escalated in practical as well as ethical importance.

Moreover, animal well-being was gradually reconfigured from a political-cum-philosophical ideal to a set of practices grounded in the material cultures of science. The concept of stress was a critical mechanism within this transformation. In the work of Russell, for instance, stress helped to imbue laboratory animals with mentality, and thus the capacity for mental suffering, recognition of which was cast as simultaneously having ethical significance and scientific consequence (as mental suffering brought physiological change, it had to be controlled to produce replicable experimental results). This new, largely materialized approach to, and understanding of, animal well-being went on to inform the development of "laboratory animal science," the growth of the laboratory animal industry, and the professionalization of the role of animal attendants and technicians in the post–World War II period. Accordingly, laboratories and animal houses were extensively redesigned to provide an environment more conducive to the laboratory animal "welfare," a process that encompassed everything from the design of cages and the development of pathogenically secure buildings to the provision of "silent" fire alarms operating at a range inaudible to common species of laboratory animals. The logic governing these transformations latterly became known as the science of animal welfare.

In this way, stress also contributed to the wider transformation of the ways in which animals were commonly understood to experience pain. The Departmental Committee on Experiments on Animals, for example, which was appointed by the Home Secretary in 1963 "to consider the present control over experiments on living animals," reported that "many scientific witnesses suggested that the concept to be controlled by the Act should be expressly expanded from 'pain' to comprise 'any interference with or departure from the animal's normal state of health or well-being,' and that this larger concept should be termed 'discomfort' or 'distress.'"

Changing understandings of the experiential capacities of animals were not solely driven by the intellectual concept of stress. Rather, they were equally a response to the experimental practices that produced such knowledge:

> Other witnesses reminded us that mental illness and neurosis are largely problems in modern civilisation, and drew attention to increasing interest in states of animal behaviour and psychological experiment designed to find forms of treatment for disordered states in human patients. . . . These

> witnesses told us that manipulation of environment was likely to be much more widely used as an experimental technique in the future, and urged that any procedure designed to produce the equivalent of stress in man should be subject to statutory control.[53]

Recognition that the environment could be used as an experimental tool to impact negatively on the physical and mental health of animals brought with it an obligation to ensure that the everyday environments experienced by animals be designed to maximize well-being. The report of the Departmental Committee recommended the expansion of the regulatory definition of pain to encompass at least three states of incrementally increasing suffering: "discomfort," "stress," and "pain." The emergence of the "stressed" animal had implications far beyond laboratory animal production, provision, use, and welfare. A key site of related transformation was the increasingly industrialized farm.

Materializing Well-Being on the Farm: An Economics of Animal Welfare?

Agriculture and industrialized farming provided a second interrelated discourse within which stress again emerged in conjunction with ethical reflections on animal well-being. For instance, the model of animal suffering developed within the laboratory sciences and expressed by the Departmental Committee on Experiments on Animals directly influenced the report of the concurrent Technical Committee to Enquire into the Welfare of Animals Kept under Intensive Livestock Husbandry Systems.[54] The latter formed a response to Ruth Harrison's *Animal Machines* (1964), an "exposé" that drew on the language of stress to represent modern methods of industrial farming as inherently "cruel."[55] Harrison, like Russell, emphasized relationships, in her case that between stockmen, livestock, and the environment. She lamented that within industrial factory farming, "the domesticated animal is very dependent on those who look after it. . . . In the agricultural world drugs have taken the place of stockmanship, but it is difficult to blame the stockman entirely for this. When he has vast numbers of animals to look after he cannot be expected to have the same feeling and instinct for their needs as he did with relatively few."[56]

Throughout *Animal Machines* dynamic psychosocial relations were presented as the territory through which health and welfare were determined. Improperly structured relations, whether between human and animal, or animal and animal (e.g., population densities), were described as stress situations that led to disease. Wherever possible, the concerns of industrial farmers were quoted verbatim. For instance, the words of K. M. Smith, head of the Veterinary Division of Associated Broiler Breeders, were used to reveal the inhumane consequences of industrial broiler production: "When animals are subjected to adverse conditions a chain of events was initiated in the body, irrespective of the nature of the stress and, if this continued long, the animal developed clinical signs of disease."[57] Harrison blamed industrial practices for the increased suffering inflicted on animals by modern farms. For her, industrialized "factory farming" was incompatible with the well-being of animals because it maximized profit at their expense. Others, however, believed the two to be perfectly compatible, arguing that productivity relied on health and welfare. Here, ethology played a central role, much as it had in the laboratory, by making well-being a condition of productivity. Though agricultural discourses focused on economic as opposed to scientific productivity, in practice this reconciliatory logic again placed emphasis on a material approach to farm animal welfare.

When appointing members to the Technical Committee, the Ministry of Agriculture, Fisheries, and Food was anxious to have "someone on the Committee who is an authority on the reactions of animals to conditions that man imposes upon them" and who was also experienced in questions of "animal mentality." Initially, Phyllis Croft, a veterinarian who had investigated neurosis in farm animals, was the preferred appointee. She was recommended as "a world authority on consciousness in lower animals."[58] Working with Grey Walter at the Burden Neurological Research Institute, and later with Derek Richter at the Neuropsychiatric Research Centre (at the Whitchurch Hospital in Cardiff), Croft, with support from UFAW, had also studied the effects of electrocution, electric stunning, and electric anesthesia on animals. Her work on the electrical activity of the heart as a measure of consciousness and sensibility to pain directly informed the development of humane experimental technique.[59] However, her association with UFAW made it "doubtful farming circles would regard her as an independent member."[60] Consequently, the Cambridge ethologist William H. Thorpe was selected in her place. Thorpe was highly successful in convincing the committee that stress, encompassing mental stress, was incompatible with both the welfare of farm animals and their overall economic productivity. In a detailed analysis titled "The Assessment of Pain and Distress in Animals," included as an appendix to the committee's report, Thorpe explained the experiential capacities of agricultural animals and the utility of ethology for gauging suffering. In doing so, he drew widely on work funded by UFAW, for instance, citing John R. Baker (on *The Scientific Basis of Kindness to Animals*) and referring to Lord Russell Brain's address to a UFAW symposium on "The Assessment of Pain in Man and Animals."[61] Brain's reasoning so swayed the committee that it was quoted verbatim to justify their acceptance that "animals can experience emotions such as rage, fear, apprehension, frustration and pleasure, though they do display different degrees and types of intelligence which may affect the reaction to particular stress-causing circumstances."[62]

Through his experience chairing the Technical Committee, Francis W. Rogers Brambell, a veterinarian by training, became a leading proponent of ethology's potential to provide a scientific approach to animal welfare. He believed ethology opened a window into "the feelings of animals . . . derived from their structure and functions and also from their behaviour." Echoing Russell, Brambell also identified a moral obligation toward animals as a condition of their domestication. Placing animals "wholly and continuously under human control," he argued, would "markedly increase the responsibility of those who use them towards the animals in their charge."[63] In practice, this translated into a series of detailed species-specific recommendations specifying the types of environments and, crucially, population densities, thought to be concordant with maximizing animal welfare.

Animal well-being was elided with efficiencies of livestock production, for example, through the widespread assumption that stress impaired breeding and growth rates. The report described how "cattle of all ages kept indoors become very accustomed to their immediate environment and routine and that a change, even to another house, unsettles them and tends to set up a temporary state of stress which is reflected for a week or two by decreased growth."[64] This was a highly instrumental form of animal ethics; the provision of adequate environments was driven as much by the desire to maximize animal productivity as to preserve animal well-being, so much so that the committee entertained the idea of breeding animals better suited to economically designed environments as opposed to altering industrialized farms to suit the needs of existing animals. The geneticist, Kenneth Mather, for example, assured the committee "it was possible deliberately to breed birds with temperaments or mental attributes suitable to specialised types of keeping." Evidently, by this point, the category of "mental stress" had become broadly accepted, although there was little consensus on "how important a part of the animal's existence this represented."[65] In its conclusion, the *Report of the Technical Committee* made clear that animal welfare, grounded in scientific information on the behavioral needs of domestic animals, "could be of great economic value to the industry."[66]

By the late 1960s the stressed animal had become prominent across veterinary literature. In 1967, for instance, the *Veterinary Record* published an extensive review of research on the effects of domestication on behavior and health, which explained how "overcrowding in many species . . . acts as an adrenal stress and may cause sudden death (Selye's syndrome)."[67] The work of John B. Calhoun, Heini Hediger, Konrad Lorenz, Curt Richter, and William H. Thorpe, among other ethologists, was deployed to argue that the "relationship between social stress and the incidence of certain mental disorders in humans" should now be extended (or returned) to the study of domesticated animals. Problems such as cannibalism in poultry would then be reimagined as forms of "paraneurosis" caused by social stress.[68] Elsewhere, stress-related research, including that by John J. Christian, David E. Davis, and Vero Copner Wynne-Edwards, was mobilized to transform veterinary responsibilities as well as knowledge and practice. "Stress manifestation . . . is a confession of failure on our part to give guidance to the animal husbandman" claimed a 1969 article in the *British Veterinary Journal*.[69] Such a conclusion was far from unique. As in human medicine a decade before, stress was becoming ubiquitous within the veterinary literature almost as though Selye was being discovered anew.

In May 1973 the Royal Society for the Prevention of Cruelty to Animals (RSPCA), in conjunction with the recently established Society for Veterinary Ethology (1966), organized a symposium to discuss growing concerns about "Stress in Farm Animals." The meeting was notable on several counts, not least that it was the first scientific meeting the RSPCA had organized in its near-150 years of existence.[70] The move to court scientific expertise was indicative of the growing influence of a new pragmatic "middle ground" within animal advocacy politics, which promised to reconcile animal suffering with utility. The landscape of the "animal question" was changing. Traditional antagonism over animal use was moving from a focus about a rhetorical dichotomy grounded in a language of moral values to a pragmatic, quantifiable science, expressed in material practices. Without literacy in the new scientific language, animal advocacy groups—even those as preeminent as the RSPCA—risked becoming sidelined. Put another way, the UFAW model of animal advocacy was quietly gaining ground where it mattered, shaping policy and practice. At a time when philosophies influenced by radicalized animal liberation and direct action were gaining widespread public attention, a pragmatic scientific approach to animal welfare appeared increasingly valuable to industries finding themselves newly under siege.

Papers presented at the 1973 meeting attempted to formulate a general concept of stress as well as find pragmatic methods of identifying, preventing, controlling, and understanding stress in domesticated animals. Several themes discussed at the Mental Health Research Fund's 1958 conference were replayed, not least the problem of the multiple meanings of stress. "Although Hans Selye gave stress its medical meaning he did not deprive the word of its broad meaning to the layman," complained one participant. Consequently "those . . . who would study stress in animals have been hampered by an inadequate vocabulary."[71] The 1973 meeting struggled to formulate a general concept of stress. Having "left the meeting with confused thoughts and suffering from mental constipation," one attendee reported that "the concept of stress seems to have taken on misleading connotations. Stress is a convenient shorthand term which describes a number of incomprehensibles. As yet, it does not explain a mechanism."[72]

Such views, however, were held by a minority. General veterinary opinion acknowledged that the stress concept was "not, apparently, open to easy definition" yet was nonetheless highly useful (particularly when "Selye's original terminology" was remembered).[73] The vagueness of the term was understood to be productive. It allowed stress to serve as a vector by which what had been individual, ephemeral, and often subjective observations of animal ill health could be codified within a new language of disease. The stress concept allowed subjective observations to be communicated and widely understood. In this way, the "isolated point of view of a veterinary surgeon" could be translated into a new "terminology of what is all too obviously a disease syndrome." Increasing veterinary use of the stress concept "could not be otherwise," one surgeon concluded, because "all practicing veterinary surgeons know these factors exist, most of them suffer from the symptoms!"[74]

This, again, indicates how the conceptual landscape of stress encouraged reflective thought. Stress situated all living organisms, including human and animal, within interdependent relationships. Accordingly, the adoption of the language of stress was often followed by the recognition of moral and ethical obligations. Throughout the 1973 meeting, for instance, stress was understood to be a problem of veterinary health with corollary significance to animal well-being (hence the RSPCA's interest). In closing the symposium, P. L. Brown concluded that all agreed that "animal behaviour may well prove to be the best indicator that we have of the animal's wellbeing and welfare."[75] Yet, in an analogous way to how laboratory animal welfare had become amalgamated with the needs of experimental science, here farm animal well-being was equated with productive economies. If stress could explain sudden animal death in transportation, for example, it had clear economic significance in terms of preventing the loss of "product."[76] More subtly, the stress concept was increasingly employed to make animal productivity a marker of well-being. Here, the work of John J. Christian, who had shown that both growth and reproduction rates could be suppressed by stress, was invoked to establish "economic performance" as an indicator of animal well-being.[77] In this way the stress concept facilitated a rapprochement of the economic priorities of intensive farming and the welfare needs of agricultural livestock.

Reflections: The Materialization of Well-Being

The stress concept served a comparable role within laboratory animal science and factory farming, operating to reconfigure the problem of animal well-being from a political-cum philosophical critique to a set of scientifically grounded materialized practices linking welfare to productivity. In doing so, stress transformed what had been a problematic site, that of animal suffering in the laboratory and the farm, into a newly productive space for interventions by new forms of expertise. Ethology, for instance, has developed as an applied science, a science of animal welfare. Applied ethology as expert knowledge increasingly polices a new, and latterly influential, middle ground, where rhetorical debates between animal use and animal ethics are reconciled by reforming practice to enhance productivity.

Concurrently, the stress concept has incrementally widened understandings of the experiential capacities of animals, encouraging, for instance, a wider recognition of their capacity for mental suffering. Although legislative change to place animal "distress" on a par with "pain" within the regulatory landscape of British animal experimentation was not enacted until the Animals (Scientific Procedures) Act of 1986, this understanding was nonetheless widely entrenched by the early 1960s. On the farm the legislative extension of animal suffering to include distress occurred much earlier, incorporated within the Agriculture (Miscellaneous Provisions) Act of 1968 (a direct response to the 1965 *Report of the Technical Committee*). While the credibility of Selye's general adaptation syndrome had declined within human psychiatric and medical thought by the 1980s, it remained a useful tool with which to frame and problematize human-animal relations. For instance, stress, as structured by Selye's general adaptation syndrome, was presented as a reliable indicator for measuring animal suffering by Marian Stamp Dawkins in *Animal Suffering: The Science of Animal Welfare*, published in 1980.[78]

As a concept, stress drew much of its utility from its flexibility of meaning. The multiple meanings inherent to the language of stress allowed ideas and dynamic processes that had been unhelpfully separated to be systematically and scientifically related to one another. Indeed, stress was so effective that it could act as a vector of communication across disciplines, specialisms, and even long-polarized political positions on the politics of human-animal relations.

In contrast to terms such as "psychosomatic," which instantiated through their construction the historical legacy of the separation they were intended to overcome, stress appeared to provide a scientific language capable of capturing the ethereal and subjective relational experiences that hitherto could be represented only in common language. Within animal-dependent science, stress provided a language through which laboratory animals could be situated within, and understood to interact with, the complex physical and social environment of the laboratory. Stress made the physical and social environment determining factors of the physiological state of the laboratory animal under study. Furthermore, stress relocated the human subject within that environment, making the researcher integral to, controller of, and obligated to, the laboratory animals' well-being. This logic also gave new importance to the role of animal caretakers and technicians, as well as the work and structure of the animal house. Stress provided a language that resonated with a fundamental, yet not systematically articulated, aspect of animal experimentation: the relational, epistemological, and ontological interdependence of the knowing human and the animal object of (or means to) knowledge.[79]

Experiences previously expressed in common language could be codified within an apparently scientific language, and subjective states such as pain and suffering could now be quantified, each of which in turn allowed ethical concerns previously limited to the realm of political-cum-philosophical rhetoric to be reconfigured as material practices within, and of importance to, the experimental work of the laboratory. This accounts for how and why the language of stress proved capable of bridging the gulf between practices of animal use and moral arguments for animal well-being. Perhaps of most significance was that the invention of the stressed animal allowed the explicit recognition of the mentality of animals and their capacity for mental suffering. This, more than any other consequence, had radical implications for our understandings of, and relations to, nonhuman animals in the material cultures of the laboratory and elsewhere.

Notes

1. I. Atkin, "Stress and Mental Disorders," *Lancet* 2 (July 6, 1957): 44.

2. Special Correspondent, "Adaptation to Stress Conference of Behavioural Scientists," *British Medical Journal* 2 (August 9, 1958): 382; see also James M. Tanner, ed., *Stress and Psychiatric Disorder Proceedings of the Second Oxford Conference of the Mental Health Research Fund* (Oxford: Blackwell, 1960).

3. Derek Richter, "Current Usage of the Word 'Stress' in Different Fields," PP/BOW H 223, John Bowlby Papers, Contemporary Medical Archives Centre, Wellcome Library, London, UK (hereafter cited as PP/BOW); Special Correspondent, "Adaptation to Stress," 382.

4. John Bowlby, "Research on Stress in Relation to Mental Health and Mental Illness," PP/BOW H 223, p. 1.

5. Richard D. French, *Antivivisection and Medical Science in Victorian Society* (Princeton, NJ: Princeton University Press, 1975).

6. See E. M. Tansey, "The Wellcome Physiological Research Laboratories 1894–1904: The Home Office, Pharmaceutical Firms, and Animal Experiments," *Medical History* 33 (1989): 18–19.

7. "Pregnancy Tests Legal Opinion as to the Necessity for License," HO 45/251/45, National Archives (hereafter cited as NA), Kew. The Friedman test, which involved surgically opening rabbits to assess their suitability, was thought to cause pain but was also judged not to require a license as it was not an "experiment."

8. For an account of the transformation of pain in nineteenth-century British culture, see James Turner, *Reckoning with the Beast: Animals, Pain and Humanity in the Victorian Mind* (Baltimore: Johns Hopkins University Press, 1980).

9. Peter Crowcroft, *Elton's Ecologists* (Chicago: University of Chicago Press, 1991).

10. A. D. Middleton, "Periodic Fluctuations in British Game Populations," *Journal of Animal Ecology* 3 (1934): 231–49; Charles W. Hume, *Some Facts and Queries relating to the Wild Rabbit Problem*, UFAW Monograph 4F (London: UFAW, 1938).

11. Dennis Chitty, "A Ringing Technique for Small Mammals," *Journal of Animal Ecology* 6 (1937): 36–53.

12. Charles Elton, *Voles, Mice and Lemmings: Problems in Population Dynamics* (Oxford: Clarendon Press, 1942); Dennis Chitty, "Mortality among Voles (Microtus agrestis) at Lake Vyrnwy, Montgomeryshire in 1936–9," *Philosophical Transactions of the Royal Society of London Series B, Biological Sciences* 236 (1952): 505–52.

13. Dennis Chitty, "Population Processes in the Vole and Their Relevance to General Theory," *Canadian Journal of Zoology* 38 (1960): 99–113.

14. Chitty, "Mortality among Voles," 506.

15. Dennis Chitty, *Do Lemmings Commit Suicide?* (Oxford: Oxford University Press, 1996), 114–15.

16. The vole's comparatively recent domestication was described as an advantage because existing laboratory stocks have been living under artificial conditions for only a few generations. The usual types of laboratory rodents (white mice, rats, guinea pigs, etc.) have been domesticated for such countless generations that they have developed a number of characteristics by artificial selection. There is little possibility of such selection having had much effect on the vole stocks yet. This overcame those who argued for behavioral and physiological differences between laboratory and wild animals, such as Curt Richter, making the Oxford stock of laboratory voles a reliable model for their wild relatives in Wytham Woods. See Richard M. Ranson, "The Field Vole (Microtus) as a Laboratory Animal," *Journal of Animal Ecology* 3 (1934): 71; cf. Curt P. Richter, "Domestication of the Norway Rat and Its Implications for the Problem of Stress," in *Life Stress and Bodily Disease: Proceedings of the Association for Research in Nervous and Mental Diseases*, ed. Harold G. Wolff, Stewart G. Wolf, and Clarence C. Hare (Baltimore: Williams and Wilkins, 1950), 19–47.

17. John R. Clarke, "The General Adaptation Syndrome in the Study of Animal Populations," *British Journal for the Philosophy of Science* 3 (1953): 351.

18. For instance, Seyle's general adaptation syndrome had established the enlargement of the adrenal glands and the involution of the thymus as quantifiable reactions of an organism to stress; see Hans Seyle, *The Physiology and Pathology of Exposure to Stress: A Treatise Based on the Concepts of the General-Adaptation-Syndrome and the Diseases of Adaptation* (Montreal: Acta, 1950).

19. "Experiments on Living Animals Licence no. 11364," July 31, 1950, H0 285/13, NA, 2.

20. "Advisory Committee on the Administration of the Cruelty to Animals Act, 1876," H0 285/13, NA, 2.

21. Francis A. E. Crew and Ljuba Mirskaia, "The Effects of Density on an Adult Mouse Population," *Biologia Generalis* 7 (1931): 241–42.

22. Crew's Home Office file contains several minor infringements but shows no record of an application for the population density investigations, see file 45 24715, NA.

23. "Supplementary Statement by Applicant," n.d., H0 285/13, NA.

24. The "pain condition" was attached to all certificates in line with recommendations of the Second Royal Commission (1912). It read, "If an animal, at any time

during any of the said experiments is found to be suffering pain which is either severe or is likely to endure and if the main result of the experiment has been attained, the animal, shall forthwith be painlessly killed: if an animal at any time during any of the said experiments is found to be suffering severe pain which is likely to endure, such animal shall forthwith be painlessly killed; if an animal appears to an Inspector to be suffering considerable pain, and if such Inspector directs such animal to be destroyed, it shall forthwith be painlessly killed." See "Advisory Committee on the Administration of the Cruelty to Animals Act, 1976," H0 285/13, NA, 2.

25. "Advisory Committee on the Administration of the Cruelty to Animals Act, 1986," H0 285/13, NA, 3.

26. "Advisory Committee on the Administration of the Cruelty to Animals Act, 1876: Note of a Meeting held at the Home Office, 11th October 1950," HO 285/13, NA, 1.

27. This work revealed how little was known about common vermin, how inefficient the current methods of trapping and poisoning were, and how quickly practices could be improved when properly studied, demonstrating the economic utility of applied population density research. See Dennis Chitty, ed., *Control of Rats and Mice* (Oxford: Clarendon, 1954).

28. David E. Davis, "Early Behavioral Research on Populations," *American Zoologist* 27 (1987): 827.

29. For the Baltimore Rodent Ecology Project, see Edmund Ramsden, "Rats, Stress and the City: Rodent Models and Built Environments," *History of the Human Sciences,* 25 (2012): 123–47; for Calhoun's later work on population density, see Edmund Ramsden, "From Rodent Utopia to Urban Hell: Population, Pathology, and the Crowded Rats of NIMH," *Isis* 102 (2011): 659–88.

30. Richter, "Domestication," 44.

31. Crowcroft, *Elton's Ecologists,* 83; John J Christian "The Adreno-Pituitary System and Population Cycles in Mammals," *Journal of Mammalogy* 31 (1950): 247–59.

32. Chance, quoted in Chitty, *Lemmings,* 99.

33. Many ethologists, famously Lorenz, believed that domestication corrupted behavioral patterns. See Richard W. Burkhardt Jr., *Patterns of Behaviour: Konrad Lorenz, Niko Tinbergen, and the Founding of Ethology* (Chicago: University of Chicago Press, 2005).

34. Robert G. W. Kirk, "Between the Clinic and the Laboratory: Ethology and Pharmacology in the Work of Michael Robin Alexander Chance, c. 1946–1964," *Medical History* 53 (2009): 513–36.

35. Michael Robin Alexander Chance, "Aggregation as a Factor Influencing the Toxicity of Sympathomimetic Amines in Mice," *Journal of Pharmacology and Experimental Therapeutics* 87 (1946): 214–19. For relevance to stress, see David A. Hamburg, "Crowding, Stranger Contact, and Aggressive Behaviour," in *The Psychosocial Environment and Psychosomatic Diseases,* vol. 1 of *Society, Stress and Disease,* ed. Lennart Levi (London: Oxford University Press, 1971), 209–18.

36. Michael Robin Alexander Chance and D. A. Humphries, "Medical Student's Powers of Observation," *British Journal of Medical Education* 1 (1967): 141–34.

37. Michael Robin Alexander Chance, "The Contribution of Environment to Uniformity," in *Collected Papers: Laboratory Animals Bureau* 6 (1957): 59–73.

38. Charles W. Hume, "Science and Animal Welfare," *Animals' Friend* 45 (1939): 110–12.

39. UFAW, "The Aims and Methods of UFAW," *24th Annual Report*, September 30, 1950, 2.

40. Robert G. W. Kirk, "'Wanted: Standard Guinea Pigs': Standardization and the Experimental Animal Market in Britain, ca. 1919–1947," *Studies in the History and Philosophy of the Biological and Biomedical Sciences* 39 (2008): 280–91.

41. UFAW, "Laboratory Animals," *31st Annual Report*, June 30, 1957, 4.

42. Alfred L. Bacharach, "Laboratory Animals: The UFAW Handbook on the Care and Management of Laboratory Animals," *British Medical Journal* 2 (1949): 20–21.

43. Charles W. Hume, "Law and Practice: The Rights of Laboratory Animals," in *The UFAW Handbook on the Care and Management of Laboratory Animals*, ed. Alastair N. Worden (London: UFAW, 1947), 19.

44. "UFAW," *Lancet* 2 (1958): 632.

45. Peter B. Medawar, foreword to *Humane Technique in the Laboratory*, vol. 6 of *Laboratory Animals Bureau Collected Papers* (London: HMSO, 1957), 5. This period overlapped with the most significant decade of Medawar's scientific career, during which he consolidated the work on acquired immunological tolerance that won him the 1960 Nobel Prize.

46. Burch, a microbiologist, acted primarily as a data gatherer, touring British laboratories in an effort to understand current practice and needs. He left the project early to take up a job in industry.

47. William M. S. Russell and Rex L. Burch, *The Principles of Humane Experimental Technique* (London: Methuen, 1959), 13.

48. Russell may have encountered Chitty and Clarke at Oxford. Medawar, as noted, certainly knew of their research. He also served as the external examiner of Clarke's D.Phil thesis (Niko Tinbergen, the renowned ethologist, was the internal).

49. Russell and Burch, *Principles of Humane Technique*, 12, 22.

50. Ibid., 24, 23.

51. This suggestion was made by William Lane-Petter; see Russell and Burch, *Principles of Humane Technique*, 28; italics in the original.

52. "Review: The Principles of Experimental Technique," *Lancet* 1 (1959): 34.

53. Sydney Littlewood (chair), *Report of the Departmental Committee on Experiments on Animals* (London: HMSO, 1965), 56, 57.

54. The Departmental Committee on Experimental Animals' statement on "pain" was quoted in full as an appendix; see W. Rogers Brambell (chair), *Report of the Technical Committee to Enquire into the Welfare of Animals kept under Intensive Livestock Husbandry Systems* (London: HMSO, 1965), 80–81.

55. For the antecedents of factory farming, see Abigail Woods, "Rethinking the History of Modern Agriculture: British Pig Production, c. 1910–65," *20th Century British History* 23 (2012): 165–91.

56. Ruth Harrison, *Animal Machines* (London: Stuart, 1964), 151.

57. Ibid., 19.

58. Phyllis G. Croft, "Some Observations on Neurosis in Farm Animals," *Journal of Mental Sciences* 97 (1951): 584–88; "Cruelty Committee," April 23, 1964, MAF 121/267, NA. At this time, a full decade before Donald Griffin's controversial argument for animal mentality as an object of ethological study, to be an authority on animal consciousness was a dubious accolade within most scientific circles.

59. Phyllis G. Croft, "The Criteria for Humane Technique," in *Humane Technique*, 19–22; Russell and Burch, *Principles of Humane Technique*, 26.

60. "Cruelty Committee."

61. Lord Russell Brain, "Presidential Address," in *The Assessment of Pain in Man and Animals, Proceedings of an International Symposium held under the Auspices of UFAW, 26th–28th July 1961*, ed. C. A. Keele and Robert Smith (London: E & S Livingstone, 1962), 3–11.

62. Brambell, *Report*, 71–79, 10; John R. Baker *The Scientific Basis of Kindness to Animals* (London: UFAW, 1948). Baker, as noted, began his career working with Elton on voles.

63. Brambell, *Report*, 9, 15.

64. Ibid. 40.

65. Kenneth Mather, "Committee of Enquiry into Intensive Livestock Husbandry Systems, Minutes of Meeting held at 2PM on the 3rd December 1964," MAF 121/267, NA, 1.

66. Brambell, *Report*, 10.

67. Michael W. Fox, "Influence of Domestication upon Behaviour of Animals," *Veterinary Record* 80 (1967): 699. Fox, a British veterinarian and ethologist, was active in promoting laboratory animal welfare during the 1970s before associating himself with American radical animal advocacy groups, such as the Humane Society, in the 1980s.

68. W. Ferguson, "The Role of Stress in Epidimiology," *British Veterinary Journal* 125 (1969): 253–54.

69. T. K. Ewer, "The Assessment of Stress in Farm Animals," *British Veterinary Journal* 124 (1969): 249.

70. John Napier, "Introductory Address: Society for Veterinary Ethology Proceedings of Joint Symposium with the Royal Society for the Prevention of Cruelty to Animals," *British Veterinary Journal* 130 (1974): 85–86.

71. A. F. Fraser, "Ethostasis: A Concept of Restricted Behaviour as a Stressor in Animal Husbandry," *British Veterinary Journal* 130 (1974): 91–92.

72. J. R. Bareham, "The Concept of Stress," *Veterinary Record* 92 (June 23, 1973): 682–83.

73. Roger Ewbank, "Use and Abuse of the Term 'Stress' in Husbandry and Welfare," *Veterinary Record* 92 (June 30, 1973): 709–10.

74. E. M. Pittaway, "The Concept of Stress," *Veterinary Record* 93 (July 21, 1973): 88.

75. P. L. Brown, "Summary: The Synthesis of the Stress Entity," *British Veterinary Journal* 130 (1974): 95.

76. T. N. Allsup, "Welfare Problems Associated with Transport," *British Veterinary Journal* 130 (1974): 92.

77. M. J. Bryant, "The Social Environment: Behaviour and Stress in Housed Livestock," *Veterinary Record* 90 (1972): 355.

78. Marian Stamp Dawkins, *Animal Suffering: The Science of Animal Welfare* (London: Chapman and Hall, 1980), esp. 56–68. Dawkins, an Oxford-trained ethologist, was a student of Tinbergen in the generation following William M. S. Russell.

79. Cf. the notion of "becoming with," in Vinciane Despret, "The Body We Care For: Figures of Anthropo-zoo-genesis," *Body and Society* 10 (2004): 111–34.

Chapter Ten

Memorial's Stress?

Arthur M. Sutherland and the Management of the Cancer Patient in the 1950s

David Cantor

Writing in 1952, Arthur M. Sutherland characterized the psychology of the cancer patient as "the psychology of a person under a special and severe form of stress in which many fundamental underlying emotionally charged convictions are brought to the surface." Sutherland, a psychiatrist at Memorial Hospital in New York, was interested in how patients adapted to the disease and its treatment. In his view people responded to such stresses in ways that were maladaptive in that they undermined successful treatment and recovery. As he noted in the same 1952 article, "Stresses are often met postoperatively by avoidance or denial, or depression and dependence may develop which the patient may not be able to overcome without help."[1] In his view, professional persons, including the social worker, best addressed such problems.[2]

I concentrate on Sutherland because his interest was quite different to that of the bulk of publications on stress and cancer in the 1950s. Whereas most focused on the role of stress as a cause of this group of diseases, or on the body's physiological responses to surgery, Sutherland was more concerned with how it affected people's behavioral and emotional responses to cancer and cancer treatments, especially in postoperative recovery. Put simply, for Sutherland stress offered a means of explaining a variety of emotional and behavioral responses to cancer and provided clues to managing these responses.

Today Sutherland is remembered as a pioneer in the development of what became known as psycho-oncology.[3] His group at Memorial was one of a few that that contributed to a growing interest after the war in the psychological management of cancer patients, alongside other major centers in Chicago and Boston. Yet despite the huge interest in the role of the emotions in shaping recovery, Sutherland's efforts to make stress a central explanation of patients' responses to cancer and treatment largely failed, at least in the 1950s. Most physicians and nurses interested in the subject made little more than passing reference to stress; the growing numbers of patients' groups and the commercial manufacturers or retailers of equipment such as surgical bras or colostomy equipment neglected stress as well. While many of Sutherland's ideas on the management of cancer found a receptive audience, his notion of stress was not among them. This chapter explains why Sutherland turned to the concept of stress, and why his ideas were rarely taken up by others in the 1950s.

My focus is on Sutherland's institutional base—Memorial Hospital—and the growing interest in radical mastectomy within that hospital. Radical mastectomy raised two major issues that worried physicians. The first was a long-standing concern that surgery, the main treatment for cancer, generated such fear among the public that it prompted people to delay seeking appropriate help if they suspected they had the disease. The treatment generated as much fear as the disease itself, and the radical and superradical treatments that developed in the 1950s exacerbated the problem, raising the possibility that patients' tendency to delay might worsen. The second issue was comparatively more recent: a concern about the role of psychological factors in aiding and hindering postoperative recovery and rehabilitation. While interest in postoperative recovery was not new to the 1940s and 1950s, it gained growing attention during those decades as physicians faced mounting criticism from patients about the way they handled postoperative problems and as new professional and commercial groups emerged with an interest in postoperative care, notably specialist cancer nurses, manufacturers of specialist bras and bust forms, and corsetieres who fitted the bras. Sutherland himself argued in a 1952 *New York Times* article that the consequence of surgery was not only physical mutilation but also "psychological invalidism."[4] His turn to the concept of stress, I suggest, was part of a broader effort to understand the problems of delay and psychological invalidism, to speed patients to their physicians, to smooth the path of recovery, and to counter growing criticism of surgeons' attitudes toward postoperative care.

Arthur M. Sutherland, Memorial and Stress

Born in White Plains, New York, and educated at Phillips Academy in Andover, Massachusetts, Arthur M. Sutherland (1910–71) graduated with a BA from Yale University in 1932 and then started medical school at Columbia University College of Physicians and Surgeons.[5] After obtaining his MD in 1936, he did an internship and residency in medicine at New York Hospital (1936–39). There followed wartime service as a commander in the US Navy (1941–46), teaching at Cornell University Medical College (1937–61), and work for the Psychosomatic Clinic at New York Hospital (from 1946), before he obtained the first of a series of appointments at Memorial Hospital in 1949.[6]

When Sutherland arrived at Memorial, the hospital was known for its embrace of radical and superradical surgical treatments of cancer.[7] Yet if Memorial embraced such techniques, its physicians also came to worry about their impact on the public and patients. These operations seemed to exacerbate existing public fears of cancer treatment and so threatened to worsen a tendency among some to delay seeking appropriate medical help. They also seemed to magnify the problem of postoperative depression in their patients. As with concerns about delay, the issue was not new. Physicians had worried about postoperative depression long before they started cutting deeper and further with radical and superradical operations. But the new techniques of the 1940s and 1950s seemed to heighten the problem, and depression seemed a significant complication of surgery.

It was against the backdrop of these concerns that Memorial began to portray the "care of the cancer patient as a whole" as one its guiding principles and to reform medical training to cut across specialty boundaries.[8] Specialists in internal medicine would learn the fundamentals of surgical procedures, and surgeons and radiation therapists would be taught supportive medical techniques for the cancer patient and the new tools of chemotherapy so that each specialist was aware of what others had to offer and could call on them when needed. At the same time teaching and treatment programs were to give more emphasis to social service, physical retraining, vocational guidance, palliative care, and recreational therapy. The goal of treatment came to be more than the eradication of the disease; the hospital strove to return patients to "useful and satisfactory" places within in their homes and communities.[9] The cure or control of the disease was meaningless, it claimed, if the patient was "not returned to a useful and happy existence."[10] Sutherland's appointment to Memorial was part of this new focus of the "care of the cancer patient as a whole."

Stress and the "Patient as a Whole"

During the 1950s Sutherland and his coworkers at Memorial came to see stress as a key to "care of the cancer patient as a whole." From this perspective the treatment of cancer involved much more than the treatment of the biological disease. A holistic approach meant that physicians also had to understand how patients responded emotionally and psychologically to cancer and to develop means of addressing these responses. In Sutherland's view stress was central to an understanding of why even the strongest and most normal of people reacted in unpredictable ways to the prospect of cancer and its treatments and why such responses could undermine efforts on the part of physicians to help them.

The roots of such an approach to cancer and stress can be traced to the wartime work of psychologists on stress. Theodore M. Brown and others have shown that at the start of the war clinical psychologists tended to view stress as a general contextual factor that worked largely as a trigger to neurotic reactions among those military personnel already "predetermined" by their defective personalities to adverse reactions. During the 1940s, however, they increasingly came to see stress not only as something that affected those already sensitive to adverse events but as a major cause of problems in "normal" men that led to disabilities that could significantly affect their capacity to function effectively as military personnel. This wartime experience of healthy young men under stress was, according to Roy Grinker, one of the keys to the rising interest of postwar clinicians in normal psychology and also to a growing attention to the effects of particular situational stresses on normal people.[11]

Sutherland's approach to cancer was part of this new focus on the effects of situational stress on normal men and women. In his view the patient with cancer experienced a special form of stress prompted by the prospect of mutilation or death or both. Patients were caught between a rock and a hard place. They were as fearful of the treatment as of the disease and, Sutherland argued, often harbored unrealistic ideas about the consequences of the operation. He believed that to understand the reactions of patients to an operation one had to know not only the real anatomical and physiological consequences of that operation but also the patient's private physiological and anatomical beliefs about the function, value, and importance of the organ removed. (Responses to the potential loss of an eye, for example, were often very different from responses to the potential loss of a breast, larynx, or rectum.) When organs were compromised or lost such as during surgery, long-term patterns of adaptation were threatened or disrupted. The consequence was anxiety, which mounted before an operation, climaxed during it, and subsiding thereafter.

Responses to cancer might follow such general patterns of adaptation, but Sutherland also argued that they were highly idiosyncratic. People reacted to the disease in a variety of often-unpredictable ways, depending on the type of cancer, the proposed intervention, the imagined consequences of the disease or its treatment, and the phase of treatment. The physician's job was to figure out why individual patients reacted in ways that they did and to develop appropriate means of managing these responses to ensure that patients went to the doctor early, remained compliant, and recovered smoothly. But this was no easy task. Patients, Sutherland explained, often endowed their doctors with magical powers to cause or cure illness or to help or injure them. All too often they identified physicians with unconscious images of parental figures so that the physicians became the object of many confused and conflicting emotions.

The result was that the doctor's relationship with the patient had to be very carefully handled. A casual referral, even to a psychiatrist or social worker, could be resented and interpreted as abandonment, something that happened all too often in modern medicine. In Sutherland's view, some patients established a relationship with their physician only to find that they were discarded later; others had difficulties in establishing any form of relationship and were forsaken almost from the start. He was particularly critical of the sorts of care provided to ward or clinic patients, who often had great difficulty in establishing a relationship with any doctor. These patients, he noted, were aware that house staff were in training, had limited contact with senior staff, and had no choice in the selection of a physician. The right of the private patient to elect or reject a physician was, Sutherland claimed, a powerful defense against fears of incompetence or brutality that was usually denied to the ward patient. The social and economic relations of private medicine thus provided a foundation of holistic cancer care.[12]

A further complicating factor was the often-parlous state of doctor-patient communication. Sutherland argued that physicians sometimes imposed their own values on a patient or mistakenly assumed patients shared their own values. The consequence was that patients often did not understand what their doctors told them, a problem compounded by their anxiety about the disease or the operation, which made them doubly liable to misconstrue what a doctor said.[13] It was, to Sutherland, crucial that physicians do what they could to relieve such anxiety. "If the physician can be seen by the patient as a kindly, protective, and healing figure who is also interested in preventing damage to him, the patient," he noted, "then anxiety can be considerably diminished and the patient approach his treatment with greater equanimity."[14] If doctors failed to do this, the consequences could be disastrous. Physicians who were distant or unable to manage the anxieties of their patients "may be seen unconsciously by the patient as an injuring figure, identified with the punitive, internalized conscience figures, with the result that the patient has difficulty in believing that anything accomplished by the physician can be curative or therapeutic."[15]

In such ways physicians could often be as much a cause of patient delay or noncompliance as a solution to the problem. The American Cancer Society (ACS) and its forerunner, the American Society for the Control of Cancer (ASCC, renamed ACS in 1944), had often blamed "ignorant" physicians for misleading patients with false or misleading information about cancer and cancer treatment and so encouraging them to delay.[16] Sutherland shifted the focus of criticism away from their ignorance of the disease or what could be done about it to their ignorance of the psychodynamics of the doctor-patient relationship. In his view it was not enough for physicians to learn the biology of cancer and the technicalities of diagnosis and treatment. They also had to be aware of the effects of their words and actions on their patients.

Thus, Sutherland portrayed the psychologically informed physician as a key to the problem of delay, much as others argued that a key to solving this problem was to better educate physicians in current knowledge about cancer. At the same time Sutherland also argued that cancer-education programs had an important role in channeling people to their physicians. In a 1958 article he attacked the common criticism that cancer education unnecessarily inflamed public fears of the disease and so promoted delay.[17] Most people, he claimed, did not respond in this way, despite their anxieties about the disease and its treatments. The exceptions were the extremely fearful, those with psychiatric problems in which cancerophobia was the presenting symptom. But true psychotic cancerophobia was rare, he argued, and even in these cases physicians could help if they were psychologically informed.[18] More broadly, the psychologically informed physician could help prevent normal anxieties from turning pathological. In his view a combination of public education about cancer and the psychological training of physicians should work hand in hand—the public education driving patients to their physicians, and the physicians working to ensure that anxieties generated by the disease, by the treatment, or by the education programs themselves did not impede effective medical interventions.

Delay

If Sutherland's holism had roots in transformations in the understanding of stress, it also had roots in a related transformation in understandings of why people delayed seeking what physicians regarded as appropriate medical help. The problem of patient delay was not new: concern about it can be traced back to the beginnings of anticancer efforts in the 1910s. Indeed, early disquiet about delay can often seem very similar to Sutherland's later worries. Like Sutherland, cancer organizations such as the ASCC/ACS argued that fear of the disease and its treatment was a major reason for delay, and also like Sutherland they argued that physicians had to take particular care to understand the psychological responses of their patients to the disease and its treatments. Where they differed from Sutherland was that they tended to argue that the problem of fear was limited to a few psychologically sensitive individuals. Sutherland did not dispute that some people were more sensitive to others. But in general his work on stress and cancer suggested that the psychological motivations behind delay were much more complex and widespread than hitherto realized.

Cancer organizations saw delay as a particular problem because it threatened the mainstay of cancer control efforts, "early detection and treatment." For example, from its foundation in 1913 the ASCC argued that for cancer control to succeed, the public had to be persuaded to abandon past practices and seek qualified medical assistance at the first sign of what might be cancer. In the view of its founding physicians, control depended on identifying the disease as early in its development as possible, while the tumor or a precursor was still a local condition and before it spread to other parts of the body and constitutional complications set in. Yet the early signs of cancer could be subtle and easily missed, and there was often no pain or debility to prompt patients to see their physicians before the disease had spread and become incurable. The consequence was that patients often delayed seeking care until after the best opportunities for successful treatment were gone.[19]

If the natural history of the disease was a cause of delay, so too was the public, the ASCC argued.[20] In its view the public was too often ignorant of the disease and its treatments, and from the 1910s it began educational programs urging people to seek early detection and treatment at the first sign of what might be cancer. Much of this effort involved dispelling myths about cancer that physicians believed encouraged fatalism about the disease (the beliefs that it was hereditary or contagious, for example); teaching the public to recognize and avoid "quacks" and incompetent physicians; educating them about the bodily signs that should send them to their physicians; and encouraging them to go for regular checkups even in the absence of any signs or symptoms. But public ignorance was only part of the problem. To the consternation of the ASCC, the organization came to realize that its educational programs were often undermined by people's emotional reactions to cancer and its treatment. Too often, it seemed, people delayed seeking help not because they were ignorant of the disease and its early warning signs but because they were overwhelmed by fear.

In its efforts to make sense of such responses, the ASCC tended to divide people into two groups: those who were essentially emotionally stable and those who were not. The former tended to respond to fears of cancer by seeking appropriate help from a physician. The others—described by one ASCC official as "certain ill-adjusted or hypersensitive individuals"—responded quite differently.[21] In these individuals fear led not to action but to a paralysis that left its victim not only in a state of inaction but also unable even to face an unpleasant situation. The problem for public-education programs was to ensure that the health messages that worked on the emotionally stable did not harm those in whom it was likely to induce paralysis. This is not to say that it was possible to predict who was likely to be hypersensitive or that otherwise stable individuals might not slide into hypersensitivity. But in general the assumption was that most people were resilient and were unlikely to be paralyzed by the cancer-education messages publicized by the ASCC.

What this meant in practice was that a core task of the ASCC was to ensure that its messages were not likely to turn the emotionally stable hypersensitive and to build into its programs mechanisms to monitor and manage any unwanted public reactions. Thus the ASCC sought to ensure that subjects that might tip the public toward fearful paralysis were omitted from educational literature—subjects such as radical surgery, radiotherapy, rehabilitation, and postoperative recovery were omitted from much early public-education material and only introduced piecemeal by the 1950s as the organization's view of what constituted a sensitive subject gradually changed. At the same time local physicians were often urged to watch for signs of undue anxiety in their patients, and the ASCC would provide doctors with talking points to address any concerns that patients might raise. It also sought to ensure that public gatherings such as movie showings, lectures, and slide shows included an expert (usually a physician), whose role was in part to monitor and address any unwanted reactions in the audience. Such efforts allowed the organization to target those who were hypersensitive or not resilient to the message. "It is because people do react differently to the knowledge that they have cancer and to the various kinds of treatment which may be prescribed for them," noted Eleanor Cockerill, director of Social Service at the Barnard Free Skin and Cancer Hospital in Saint Louis, Missouri, in 1939 "that the 'human equation' is such an important factor in cancer control." In her view it was essential to supplement public education with "a special kind of service for those individuals who cannot benefit from the presentation of facts alone."[22]

Concerns that cancer education might promote cancerophobia gained new attention after the war as the renamed American Cancer Society (ACS) revived older concerns that the organization's educational campaigns exacerbated fears of the disease. The organization had long argued that the inclusion of a modicum of fear within its educational programs was necessary to encourage people to seek early detection and treatment. But deciding how much fear was appropriate was a difficult task. There was always the danger that it might actually have the opposite effect to that desired by the ACS, freezing people into inaction or tempting them to go to quacks or other alternatives. Such concerns were not new. But whereas before the war attention had tended to focus on how physicians might monitor and manage such responses, after the war this approach was joined by a new set of tactics that sought to encourage patients and the public to monitor and manage their own reactions. From this perspective a calm, rational understanding of the self could provide an emotional armament that would help people overcome their fears and so ensure that they responded appropriately to cancer-education messages.

An example of this new approach is the movie *Man Alive* (1952), significant among public health education movies of the 1950s in the depth of attention it gave to the psychology of delay.[23] Like most other films of the 1940s and 1950s, the movie highlighted the early warning signs of cancer, encouraged people to learn them and to go to a physician as soon as possible after spotting any of them. It also sought to encourage people to go for regular checkups from a physician even in the absence of signs or symptoms. But what was new about the film was the way in which it sought to encourage people to overcome any fears that they might have of the disease or its treatment. Whereas many other educational movies acknowledged the role that fear played in encouraging delay and urged audiences to overcome it, *Man Alive* went further. It highlighted *two* sets of warning signs: the warning signs of the disease itself and the warning signs of delay and avoidance—denial, sarcasm, icy disdain, and unreasoning anger, all of which led to delay and avoidance and all beautifully evoked iconographically in the film.

According to the film, all these reactions were the product of fear, and part of the aim of this movie was to help audiences recognize these responses in themselves and combat their inclination to delay by cultivating a healthy, self-controlled fear of the disease. As the narrator noted, "It is foolish to worry day and night about cancer, but it's just as foolish not to worry about it at all. Be on guard. Don't let fear make a mess of your life again. But, use your good common sense." This self-controlled fear was the key to early detection and treatment. If in the 1930s the ASCC had worried about the impact of its message on "ill-adjusted or hypersensitive" individuals, *Man Alive* sought to provide the normal population with a means of maintaining emotional equilibrium by psychologizing their fear in something of the same way fear among servicemen had been psychologized during World War II.

It was in this context that Sutherland's publications on stress and cancer began to appear. In some ways his work picked up on themes that had been evident in debates over ASCC/ACS educational programs since the 1910s. Like the ASCC/ACS, he argued that very few people exhibited cancerophobia and that public-education programs could not be blamed for prompting it. On the contrary, he argued, cancer-education programs did more good than harm: they reduced the problem of patient delay more than they induced excessive fears that led to delay. The psychological responses they induced were of a different order. Sutherland accepted that fear and anxiety induced by stress could affect even the most normal of individuals. Ordinary people could react in a multitude of different ways when faced with the extraordinary situation of cancer, and not always in ways that promoted their own best interests. Despite the ACS's efforts to encourage patients to control their own fears, Sutherland was not convinced that they could do it without professional intervention. If *Man Alive* urged the public to monitor and manage themselves, Sutherland also sought to provide physicians with tools to monitor and manage the public.

Sutherland's interest in stress thus fit into a then existing model of cancer education, in which the role of the physician was to counter any unwanted emotional reactions to cancer-control messages. Since at least the 1910s, the ASCC/ACS had accepted that some aspects of cancer education were best dealt with in the privacy of the doctor-patient consultation, where physicians could deal one to one with their patient. In its view the patient's physician was best placed to deal with any unwanted reactions to cancer-education programs in patients. Ideally, doctors had developed a deep knowledge of individual patients' circumstances over many years; ideally, they were trusted by their patients; and, ideally, they had the best opportunity to talk about their reactions to cancer and its treatments in such a way as to reassure them about the ASCC/ACS's message of early detection and treatment. What Sutherland offered were tools for physicians to understand the nature of their relationship with their patients and to explain the meanings of cancer and surgery for them.

In the first place Sutherland sought to provide a way for physicians to understand their patients' responses to cancer. He argued that the impact of messages about cancer and its surgery depended less on whether the patient was classified as "normal," "neurotic," "psychopathic," a "solid citizen," or with some particular psychiatric diagnosis: it depended more on how the loss of an organ and the whole experience of cancer was integrated with or deranged the patient's major adaptations. The behavior of patients, Sutherland argued, should be considered as designed to prevent, avoid, minimize, or repair injury to their body (or body part) and threats to basic adaptive patterns and social, economic, and cultural life. Their behavior and concurrent emotions, Sutherland claimed, were appropriate to the state they perceived themselves to be in. They may be realistic, inappropriate, or less than optimal; nevertheless they should be regarded as attempts at repairing a perceived threat or state of injury.

More broadly, in Sutherland's view, physicians had to understand that reactions to messages about cancer and its therapy often changed over time, from the first time individuals noticed something wrong, through the climax of hospitalization and treatment, to convalescence and cure, or to recurrence and death. In the preoperative phase, when the problem of delay was most important, the majority of patients with cancer faced the prospect of surgery as the initial phase of their treatment. Sutherland argued that the time between discovery of something wrong and the acceptance of definitive treatment could be thought of as the "preventive" phase, in which actions were designed to prevent or minimize injury by disease or therapy or both. Because of the uniqueness of the threat, he continued, the way that individuals handled it was determined not so much by how they had handled past threats as by how they saw the nature of this particular threat and its magnitude, both the physical injury itself and how it might disrupt existing life patterns. Patients could adopt several courses of action. Some might avoid physicians; others might seek appropriate help. But motivations might be mixed, even among those who sought help. The problem for physicians was that while individuals who came to them for help might appear reasonable and realistic, they might in fact be close to disorganization through fear. Such individuals, Sutherland argued, had to be handled with considerable skill and tact lest they be overwhelmed by anxiety or flee from treatment.

Such arguments provide an insight into Sutherland's view of the relationship between the physician and psychiatrist. On the one hand, it validated the knowledge that ordinary physicians had of their patients. Sutherland argued that the ability to predict patients' reactions was extremely difficult. It required considerable detailed knowledge of the individuals' basic patterns, as well as their capacity for developing compensatory patterns, something that family physicians with a deep knowledge of their patients and their circumstances was best placed to acquire. But, if family physicians had a detailed knowledge of individual patients and their circumstances, they did not necessarily have training in cancer or psychological responses to it. This required the opportunity to observe the responses of many patients to cancer, and most family physicians saw relatively few cancer patients compared to (cancer) hospital-based psychiatrists. The role of psychiatrists, such as Sutherland, was to help physicians embed their deep knowledge of individual patients within the growing knowledge of cancer patients coming out of hospital-based centers such as Memorial.

Recovery

If Sutherland's concept of stress aimed to help physicians manage the problem of delay, it also aimed to help them manage postoperative recovery. Medical interest in postoperative recovery was not new, but it gained greater public visibility after World War II, as more and more patients were "cured" of the disease and as a variety of professional and patient groups emerged that questioned the quality of existing postoperative care. Such questions meant that postwar interest in recovery was quite different to that of earlier decades. Prior to the war the term "recovery" tended to refer to an end state rather than the process or route by which people arrived at that end state: the postwar interest tended to focus on recovery as a process.[24] Sutherland's focus on stress was part of a growing interest in the 1940s and 1950s in understanding and managing this process.

Sutherland's opportunity to work with postoperative patients came about in May 1950, when he was appointed director of Memorial's newly created

Rehabilitation Service, joined later by Ruth Dyk, a psychiatric social worker; Charles Orbach and Morton Bard, both clinical psychologists; Irving Bieber, a consultant in psychiatric research; and Marvin G. Drellich, who assisted Sutherland in psychoanalytic investigation and therapy.[25] Through clinical teaching and conferences, the service aimed to train physicians in rehabilitation and to promote teamwork among the various practitioners involved in the postoperative care of the patient.[26] Its creation built on a growing enthusiasm for physical and psychological rehabilitation as a solution to the war and postwar problems faced by wounded servicemen and veterans.[27] According to Sutherland, the service aimed to promote awareness among team members about the need for both physical and psychological adjustment of cancer patients and about the contributions that each team member could make to this process.

The creation of the Rehabilitation Service should not be read to imply that there were no rehabilitation services at Memorial before 1950. There were, but they tended to be handled by surgeons themselves, scattered unevenly across the hospital or imported into Memorial from elsewhere. In general it was the surgeon who discussed rehabilitation issues with the patient, supported by nurses and social workers who would guide patients in physical exercises prescribed by the physicians, help them choose prosthetic devices, and move from hospital to home.[28] A speech instructor, Willard White, visited Memorial twice a week from the Post-laryngectomy Clinic of the National Hospital for Speech Disorders to teach laryngectomy patients to speak again. Ethel Saltus, a volunteer worker at Memorial Center, constructed prostheses for patients who had radical surgery for breast cancer. Saltus was later made a full-time member of Sutherland's group.[29]

In addition to these services, some physicians also encouraged the creation of patient support groups. For example, in 1948 Bradley L. Coley, chief of the Bone Service, helped to found the Amputee's Alliance, whose membership originally consisted of patients who had lost limbs because of cancer and later expanded to include other amputees, including war veterans. The alliance had some characteristics of a self-help group, with members of the alliance assisting one another in finding suitable prostheses, developing physical skills, and regaining social confidence. But it also served as a patient recruitment device, with alliance members seeking to persuade patients to accept surgeons' recommendations for an amputation.[30]

Part of the impetus behind the creation of Sutherland's Rehabilitation Service was to rationalize rehabilitation provision at Memorial: the new service sought to bring the disparate existing services together; integrate them with new services for patients who underwent operations for colon, stomach, or breast cancer; expand other services such as vocational guidance for all patients; and add psychiatric perspectives to the predominant focus on physical rehabilitation. But if part of the impetus behind the Rehabilitation

Service was to promote rationalization, another impetus was to counter growing discontent among some patients about the quality of postoperative care at Memorial. To some physicians the support groups they wished to encourage seemed to be getting out of hand.

The point can be made by a focus on growing criticism among mastectomy patients about the quality of postoperative care at Memorial. Shortly after the Rehabilitation Service was founded, two women who had undergone mastectomy at Memorial—Helen Radler and Terese Lasser—produced self-help pamphlets for fellow "breast amputees."[31] Both women praised the technical skills of their physicians, but they also criticized their failure to provide adequate aftercare following surgery. Lasser, for example, found her physician, Frank Adair, chief of the Breast Service at Memorial Hospital, unable or unwilling to provide advice on rehabilitation exercises, what she should tell her children, how she might resume sexual relations with her husband, or how to go about getting a prosthetic device. Such criticisms strengthened the case for the newly created Rehabilitation Service. The service was to provide the hospital with a means of countering these allegations by offering practical help to patients, physicians, and other professionals regarding postoperative recovery and rehabilitation.

The case for a Rehabilitation Service was strengthened further in 1953 by the creation of a new organization, Reach to Recovery.[32] Founded by Terese Lasser, Reach to Recovery was a patient's group that encouraged breast amputees to provide support to other, often more recent, mastectomees. Lasser argued that women who had undergone mastectomy were particularly well suited by reason of their experience to provide advice and support to other women who had recently undergone the operation. Indeed, she suggested that male physicians, while often technically very competent in providing therapeutics, were often unable to address all the concerns of their female patients: "Remember that your surgeon is a busy man and being a man, he cannot always foresee the many questions which beset a woman," Lasser noted in 1953.[33] A story goes that Reach to Recovery came about a few months after Lasser's own surgery.[34] Another of Adair's mastectomy patients asked to see her. She was deeply depressed, and Lasser's meeting with her was the beginning of Reach to Recovery.

In this story Adair is generally portrayed as sympathetic to Lasser's efforts: he approved Lasser's visit to the depressed mastectomee patient and later wrote a preface to the first edition of her booklet, *Reach to Recovery*.[35] Other surgeons, however, were not so supportive. As increasing numbers of women visited recent mastectomee patients in hospitals across the country, the tale is told that some were ordered off the premises, sometimes escorted by police or security. But Lasser and her followers did not easily give up, and surgeons found it a difficult task to wish these women away. Many were socially well connected, able to use their connections to counter surgeon opposition.[36]

Faced with the prospect of what they regarded as an invasion of their space by influential laywomen, Memorial's surgeons began to see political and practical value in a Rehabilitation Service as a means of both keeping this emergent problem at bay and assisting the growing numbers of patients through the difficult times after an operation. While the Rehabilitation Service argued that the *laity* was important in promoting healing and recovery, it saw its main role as providing *professional* help, especially from psychiatrists, nurses, and specialists in rehabilitation.

It was in this context that Sutherland turned to the concept of stress to explain the responses of patients after an operation, what he called the reparative phase.[37] In his view the special type of stress that cancer patients experienced during this phase brought a variety of emotions to the surface that were quite different from those experienced before treatment. If patients (or would-be patients) tended to exhibit fear or anxiety before an operation, they tended to exhibit depression afterward, as well as a range of other emotions. Sutherland argued that this depression was the consequence of two factors: the real physical limitations imposed by the operation on the patient and the limitations imposed by the patient's perception of what these changes meant. The role of the physician and psychiatrist was to understand both the real and perceived limitations.[38]

Sutherland argued that patients in the reparative phase exhibited a range of emotional and behavioral patterns, the aim of which—as in the preoperative phase—was to repair injury, restore function, and resume valued life activities. Some were quite realistic, but others were not, and emotional and behavioral disturbances varied in severity depending on patients' perceptions of how difficult it might be to restore successful patterns of adaptation. Sutherland argued that in most cases the level of disturbance was not sufficiently serious to cause gross distortion of emotionality or behavior and was often so mild that it frequently escaped the notice of the physician. Nevertheless, almost all patients showed some disturbance after surgery. Depression was the most common, but patients also exhibited dependency, anxiety, hypochondriasis, obsessive-compulsive reactions, and paranoid reactions, all of which had specific adaptive functions.[39]

Stress thus resulted in a variety of psychological, emotional, and behavioral responses to cancer surgery, with a variety of difficult functions.[40] In the case of dependency, for example, Sutherland argued that it could be seen as an attempt to enlist powerful professional figures because patients felt threatened and unable to function in their own defense or perhaps to fulfill their own basic needs. Anxiety, by contrast, served to alert individuals to dangers in themselves or in the environment and often focused on the possibility that cancer might recur and could occur even among those who were never told that that had cancer.[41] Depression served yet other purposes: of withdrawing individuals from those activities in which they felt they would fail or of coercing the internalized conscience or parent figure to restore the missing part or to give love.[42] In Sutherland's view none of these responses would necessarily become a major problem. Nevertheless, they were also something to watch and manage, warning signs that something worse might come. And they all required intervention, even in the relatively mild or "impure" forms in which they often appeared.

Much the same could be said of other responses. Hypochondriasis tended to occur, he argued, in individuals who seemed greatly preoccupied with self-destructive tendencies and whose pattern of adaptation included masochistic self-punishment or the inhibition of activities for fantasized sins; they often approached surgery with a very lively expectation of serious injury, which turned after the operation into a belief that irreparable damage had taken place. Obsessive-compulsive reactions, Sutherland claimed, were usually seen in patients who had operations on sphincters, commonly the rectal sphincter; usually centered on irrigation; and aimed to gain a measure of control over the colon and to replace the missing rectal sphincter. And finally, individuals with paranoid and delusional reactions frequently believed that they brought the disease on themselves by undertaking some forbidden activity. The resulting guilt, Sutherland noted, was accompanied by strong self-directed rage, frequently suicidal in quality or projected out onto figures in the environment seen as malign, often the surgeon. These reactions were potentially dangerous, but manageable.

Thus, in Sutherland's view stress gave rise to a very wide range of psychological, emotional, and behavioral responses to treatment, most of which were reparative in nature, though some miscarried, hindered recovery, and handicapped the patient. The role of physicians and other specialists more generally was to help patients in their efforts to resume previous activities and to ensure they did this without endangering themselves. In some cases Sutherland argued that this required the specialized help of the physical therapist and psychiatrist. But in general he suggested that surgeons could do much of the work themselves, much as already happened at Memorial. "For the large majority of patients, however, the surgeon is the first choice for assistance," he noted. "When there is a good relationship and easy communication between surgeon and patient, the surgeon knowledgeable in physical medicine and in the human understanding called psychology or psychiatry will materially shorten convalescence. He will easily guide the patient to the resumption of all his valued life activities, which the surgeon's skill has now made possible."[43]

Nevertheless, Sutherland felt impelled to reiterate the point that physicians should not impose their own values or those of their own class or social group on others. The "upper class, white American, Protestant ideal[s]" of many physicians could not be imposed on members of different communities, such as Neapolitan-Sicilian immigrants.[44] The problem was that many physicians continued to impose such values, and it was an open question whether this would change.

The Limits to Stress

Sutherland may have portrayed stress as central to the management of cancer patients, but for much of the 1950s his ideas were not widely adopted. This is not to say that others were not interested in the management of psychological responses to cancer and its treatment. On the contrary, the topic was an increasing focus of attention in the 1950s, and Sutherland himself was a key figure in this work. His group at Memorial was one of the major centers of research on the psychology of cancer, their publications were widely cited by other researchers, and Sutherland was a regular and prominent contributor to discussions on a broad range of psychological issues regarding cancer, both in professional journals and popular media. He also produced a medical-training program on the subject for the pioneering Telecolor Clinics closed-circuit television series in 1954.[45]

But if Sutherland was central to a growing interest in the management of cancer patients, his concept of stress had a more problematic status. Instead of being a regular part of the discourse about patient management, stress tended to be quite marginal, rarely used or mentioned by others. Thus, Sutherland's importance to the growing interest in the psychological management of patients did not open the door to the uptake of his ideas on stress, at least in the 1950s. Others in this volume have shown that stress gained wide currency in the 1940s and 1950s because its meaning was unstable, elastic enough to link together activities in a wide range of fields. Sutherland's stress, however, does not appear to have profited from this. Just because stress had a variety of meanings did not mean it had to be taken up.

Part of the reason for its lack of uptake was that Sutherland's stress often seemed to offer little that was new. Physicians had recognized long before Sutherland that the prospect of cancer or its treatment generated fear and anxiety, that depression was often a consequence of treatment, and that delay and (what came to be known as) noncompliance often resulted. They had consequently developed a variety of methods for speeding people to their doctors and ensuring that patients kept to what could be a difficult course of treatment and recovery. Sutherland argued that the particular stress faced by a cancer patient lay at the root of delay and noncompliance. But these problems could be understood in other ways, and physicians often found it unnecessary to adopt stress as an explanation. There was no necessary antagonism to the idea. It was only one of several possible interpretations of these behaviors and generally failed to displace its rivals.

Nor did Sutherland's stress come to dominate explanations of why cancer brought out deep-seated fears and depression. Sutherland's account was closely related to that of psychiatrists, such as Roy Grinker and John Spiegel, who had written about stress from a psychoanalytic perspective and who conceived their work as an exploration of how preexisting neurotic vulnerabilities could be brought to the surface by conditions of war, resulting in breakdown, maladaptation, and neurosis.[46] Sutherland applied such insights to the problem of how people responded to the condition of cancer: from this perspective the disease and its treatments or their prospect brought to the surface vulnerabilities that resulted in fear, anxiety, depression, and other problems. But such ideas had been prevalent long before stress entered common discourse. It was common to argue, like Sutherland, that cancer and its treatments provoked preexisting fears and anxieties along with a range of other problems. It was common to argue, also like Sutherland, that many of these problems could be tackled by the patient's regular physician rather than a psychologist. But many physicians failed to invoke stress to explain why cancer brought emotional or psychological weaknesses to the surface.

This is not to say that Sutherland's work was not useful to physicians. He had after all been appointed to Memorial to help counter the problems of patient delay and noncompliance, and some of his insights seem to have been adopted. Physicians listened to Sutherland's warnings about the magical powers their patients might accord them, the problems facing the ward patient, the dangers of imposing their own values on their patients, the issues raised by the patient's privately held anatomical and physiological beliefs, and the importance of the psychology of the normal patient. But they tended to use them in piecemeal fashion. Sutherland's hopes that he might offer physicians tools with which to deal with unwanted reactions to cancer or its treatment were fulfilled, but only in part and not on his terms. Physicians rummaged around his insights, picked those that were most useful to them, and ignored or abandoned others. Stress was generally disregarded.

This problematic status of stress is illuminated by the fact that, with the exception of Sutherland and his team at Memorial, the growing number of physicians researching the psychology of the cancer patient in the 1950s rarely invoked the label. For example, Richard Rennecker and Max Cutler in Chicago, while interested in very similar questions as Sutherland—the psychological meaning of the breast and the emotional shock associated with its loss or destruction—tended to view this problem in psychoanalytic terms and rarely (if at all) used the term "stress."[47] And writing on emotional responses to cancer, Jacob Finesinger and his colleagues at Massachusetts General Hospital tended to use the term "distress" rather than stress.[48] All these researchers were aware of Sutherland's work and often cited it, but only infrequently did they take up the language of stress, and where they did they often felt free to use it interchangeably with other terms. Stress may have been widely discussed in the popular and medical literature, but with the exception of Sutherland only some applied the language of stress systematically to the psychology of the cancer patient.

As tellingly, within Sutherland's home institution, Memorial, stress also seems to have been only rarely adopted. Memorial's surgeons do not seem to have used the notion of stress much: it was largely absent from their publications on patient's hopes and fears and on postoperative recovery, despite the fact that Sutherland worked closely with them and that they had turned to Sutherland to counter growing concern about delay and noncompliance. Nor did patients' advocates make use of the concept. Helen Radler's and Terese Lasser's publications on postoperative rehabilitation made no reference to stress in their efforts to promote psychological healing among breast cancer patients, perhaps because stress did little to advance their arguments regarding the value to recovery of patients' experiences of cancer. Sutherland was not hostile to the idea of patient self-help and, indeed, sought to promote it. But he tended to prioritize the authority of the psychologist and surgeon in interpreting patients' responses to cancer and its treatment and in promoting psychological healing. While Radler and Lasser would have welcomed more psychologically aware surgeons, and probably also more interventions by psychologists or psychiatrists, they also argued that the breast cancer patient had a unique insight into the effects of surgery. From such a perspective, Sutherland was a problematic ally, given his dependence on surgical support within Memorial. Surgeons had, after all, turned to the Rehabilitation Service to counter growing patient criticism.

Nor did nurses and social workers deploy stress, despite the fact that both groups were keen for advice on how to manage postoperative psychological problems and were important to the Rehabilitation Service's work. The literature on the new field of oncological nursing in the 1950s made little use of the term, as did the literature produced by social workers or by manufacturers and retailers of equipment intended to aid rehabilitation, such as surgical bras, bust forms, and colostomy equipment.[49] Manufacturers and retailers might seem a surprising inclusion in this chapter, but nurses and social workers worked very closely with these groups to ensure a smooth transition for the patient from hospital to home, and these groups themselves claimed that the products they produced and sold were crucial to the psychological well-being of cancer patients and that the sale of this equipment was as much a therapeutic as a commercial encounter. But stress was rarely mentioned in their publications.[50]

This is not to say that the term was never used in the 1950s. In the course of a discussion on psychological stress and surgery, the psychologist Irving L. Janis invoked Sutherland's study of how people reacted to the discovery that they would be exposed to serious dangers such as surgery and his observations that people were often more concentrated on surgical injuries and the disruption to their daily lives caused by it than about cancer, even if they knew the poor prognosis.[51] Nathan Kline and Julius Sorbin acknowledged that "at a time of stress, it is a consolation to the patient to have present someone, such as a physician, who appears adequate to advise competently what should be done."[52] And in their 1959 review of the psychosomatic aspects of cancer, George Perrin and Irene Pierce acknowledged that "the emotional stress to an individual who learns that he has cancer is inevitably great" in the course of a discussion of the emotional reactions of patients to cancer.[53] But these mentions seem to have been exceptions. Stress was only sporadically invoked, and often mutually substituted with other terms, sometimes seeming to take on the meaning of these terms, sometimes seeming to give them new meanings. Sutherland himself was not consistent in his use of stress, sometimes substituting the terms "threat" or "life situation" for "stress."

The puzzle of stress is thus its simultaneous centrality and marginality to 1950s debates about the psychology of the cancer patient. It was central to ideas of one of the major figures in this growing field, crucial to the way Sutherland conceptualized the response of patients to cancer and to interventions against it, and, in his view, essential to the development of effective means of managing patients through the long uncertain path from home to hospital and back again. Yet if it was central to Sutherland, it was marginal to many others working in this field, even among those who engaged with the work of Sutherland and his colleagues at Memorial. There was no overt hostility to the idea, but equally there was little overt excitement; it was simply one of many ways of thinking about the psychology of the cancer patient, and not the most prominent. Even at Memorial his notion seems to have limited impact. Sutherland may have developed his ideas about the role of stress in cancer at Memorial, but Memorial did not taken up the idea enthusiastically—hence the question mark in my title. It was "Memorial's stress" because Sutherland formulated the idea there, not because others at Memorial were invested in the idea.

It should be clear by now that this chapter seeks to tell a different story to the growing historical literature that documents the proliferation of stress in the 1940s and 1950s. Certainly stress was widely adopted, but there were limitations to its spread, and in the 1950s one of these limitations was the psychology of the cancer patient. By focusing on the one physician who took up the concept of stress—Arthur M. Sutherland—this chapter has sought to explain not only why he turned to stress but also why his notion of stress was not widely adopted by others interested in similar questions about the psychology of cancer patients and their management. For many physicians it was unclear what stress offered in terms of explaining patients' psychological responses to cancer that other ideas did not. Sutherland also offered little in terms of patient management to other ways of intervening, and where he did—such as promoting cultural sensitivity, or in his interventions in the long-standing debates on what to tell patients about their disease—it was quite possible to adopt (or reject) his recommendations without any reference to stress or to substitute other terminology. His notion of stress was occasionally adopted, but more often not. It existed alongside other ways of thinking about the patients and their psychology, sometimes taken up, but frequently neglected, the focus of neither enthusiasm nor antipathy. The balance between adoption and abandonment would shift in the 1960s and 1970s, as stress came to be more commonly used to explain the situation of the cancer patient. But, in the 1950s its time was yet to come.

Notes

1. Arthur Sutherland, "Psychological Impact of Cancer Surgery," *Public Health Reports* 67 (1952): 1143.

2. Sutherland's research on the adaptation and rehabilitation of the cancer patient has been characterized as foreshadowing the emergence of the field of health psychology and of professional interest in the rehabilitation of the cancer patient. Michael Braun, "Portrait of Arthur M. Sutherland, M.D.," *CA: A Cancer Journal for Clinicians* 31 (1981): 156–58.

3. Jimmie C. Holland and Talia R. Weiss, "History of Psycho-Oncology," in *Psycho-Oncology*, ed. Jimmie C. Holland, William S. Breitbart, Paul B. Jacobsen, Marguerite S. Lederberg, Matthew J. Loscalzo, and Ruth McCorkle, 2nd ed. (New York: Oxford University Press, 2010), 3–12. See also Jimmie C. Holland, "History of Psycho-Oncology: Overcoming Attitudinal and Conceptual Barriers," *Psychosomatic Medicine* 64 (2002): 206–21.

4. Arthur Sutherland, "Some Perils Noted in Surgery," *New York Times*, October 21, 1952, 32.

5. Braun, "Portrait."

6. His appointments at Memorial included attending physician and psychiatrist, Medical Service (1949–55); head, Research Psychiatry Division at the Sloan-Kettering Institute for Cancer Research (1954–60); director, Rehabilitation Service, Memorial Center (1950–57); and attending physician, chief, Neuropsychiatric Service at Memorial Hospital (1957–61).

7. Barron H. Lerner, *The Breast Cancer Wars: Fear, Hope and the Pursuit of a Cure in Twentieth-Century America* (New York: Oxford University Press, 2003): 70–77, and more generally on radical surgery, see chapter 4. See also Ellen Leopold, *A Darker Ribbon: Breast Cancer, Women, and Their Doctors in the Twentieth Century* (Boston: Beacon, 1999); James S. Olson, *Bathsheba's Breast: Women, Cancer, and History* (Baltimore: Johns Hopkins University Press, 2002); Robert A. Aronowitz, *Unnatural History: Breast Cancer and American Society* (Cambridge: Cambridge University Press, 2007).

8. Memorial Center for Cancer and Allied Diseases, "Semi-Annual Report to the New York City Cancer Committee, January 1, 1951–June 30, 1951," 1. Bates number

1003072899/2915, accessed September 17, 2013, http://tobaccodocuments.org/pm/1003072899-2915.html.

9. Ibid, 2.

10. Ibid, 1.

11. Brown, "'Stress' in US Wartime Psychiatry," this volume. Ellen Herman, *The Romance of American Psychology: Political Culture in the Age of Experts* (Berkeley: University of California Press, 1995). Roy R. Grinker, *Fifty Years in Psychiatry: A Living History* (Springfield, IL: Charles C. Thomas, 1979), 81.

12. Unlike Jewson's model of bedside medicine, economically powerful patients were not able to define the nature of their illnesses, in Sutherland's view. On the contrary, their understanding of the efforts of illness and its treatment was a problem that had to be overcome. On bedside medicine, see Nicholas D. Jewson, "Medical Knowledge and the Patronage System in Eighteenth-Century England," *Sociology* 8 (1974): 369–85; and Jewson, "The Disappearance of the Sick Man from the Medical Cosmology," *Sociology* 10 (1976): 225–44.

13. Arthur M. Sutherland, "Communication between the Doctor and the Cancer Patient," *CA: A Cancer Journal for Clinicians* 8 (1958): 119–21.

14. Arthur M. Sutherland, "Psychological Impact of Cancer and Its Therapy," *Medical Clinics of North America* 40 (1956): 710.

15. Sutherland, "Cancer and Its Therapy," 710.

16. For further discussions of the ASCC/ACS's position, see David Cantor, "Uncertain Enthusiasm: The American Cancer Society, Public Education, and the Problems of the Movie, 1921–1960," *Bulletin of the History of Medicine* 81 (2007): 39–69. Cantor, "Choosing to Live: Cancer Education, Movies, and the Conversion Narrative in America, 1921–1960," *Literature and Medicine* 28 (2009): 278–332. More generally on the issue of delay, see Robert A. Aronowitz, "Do Not Delay: Breast Cancer and Time, 1900–1970," *Milbank Quarterly* 79 (2001): 355–86; and Aronowitz, *Unnatural History*, chap. 6.

17. Arthur M. Sutherland, "What Price Cancer Education of the Public?" *Acta-Unio Internationalis Contra Cancrum* 14 (1958): 693–97.

18. Sutherland identified three types of cancerophobe: the anxiety neurotic, who could generally be reassured by physicians; the true cancerophobic, who needed psychiatric intervention; and the psychotic delusional (those not subject to phobia but who believed they had cancer despite medical evidence to the contrary), who also needed psychiatric help.

19. Aronowitz, "Do Not Delay"; Aronowitz, *Unnatural History*, chap. 6.

20. Cantor, "Uncertain Enthusiasm"; Cantor, "Choosing to Live."

21. Mary R. Lakeman, "Cancer Education in Massachusetts," in *Cancer and Other Chronic Diseases in Massachusetts*, ed. George H. Bigelow and Herbert L. Lombard (Boston: Houghton Mifflin, 1933), 158.

22. Eleanor Cockerill, "The Human Equation: A Factor in Cancer Control," *National Bulletin of the American Society for the Control of Cancer* 21, no. 6 (June 1939): 6.

23. For discussions of this film, see Cantor, "Uncertain Enthusiasm," 68; Cantor, "Choosing to Live," 299–301; and Leslie J. Reagan, "Engendering the Dread Disease: Women, Men, and Cancer," *American Journal of Public Health* 87 (1997): 1779–87.

24. On the emergence of this new interest in postoperative recovery, see David Cantor, "Before Survivorship: The Moment of Recovery in Twentieth Century American Cancer Campaigns," *Social History of Medicine*, in press.

25. On the Rehabilitation Service, see "Semi-Annual Report."

26. Practitioners included fellows and residents, nurses, medical students, social workers, recreational workers, and volunteers.

27. Richard Verville, *War, Politics, and Philanthropy: The History of Rehabilitation Medicine* (Lanham, MD: University Press of America, 2009); Glenn Gritzer and Arnold Arluke, *The Making of Rehabilitation: A Political Economy of Medical Specialization, 1890–1980* (Berkeley: University of California Press, 1985).

28. A social work department at Memorial Sloan-Kettering was created in 1942; see Patricia Fobair, Naomi Stearns, Grace Christ, Deborah Dozier-Hall, Nancy W. Newman, James Zabora, Heser Hill Schnibber, et al., "Historical Threads in the Development of Oncology Social Work," *Journal of Psychosocial Oncology* 27 (2009): 162. On the history of cancer nursing, see Katherine Nelson, "The History of Cancer in the Nursing Curriculum, 1860–1951," in *Cancer Nurses Make It Happen*, ed. Vera Keare and Videen McGaughey (Wallingford, CT: ACS Connecticut Division, 1987), 1–9; Brigid Lusk, "Prelude to Specialization: US Cancer Nursing, 1920–50," *Nursing Inquiry* 12, no. 4 (December 2005): 269–77; and Lusk, "Nursing Patients with Cancer in the 1950s: New Issues and Old Challenges," in *Nursing Interventions through Time*, ed. Patricia D'Antonio and Sandra Lewenson (New York: Springer, 2010), 123–38.

29. Arthur Sutherland, "Rehabilitation Service," in *Quadrennial Report (1947–1951)* (New York: Memorial Center for Cancer and Allied Diseases, 1951), 71–73.

30. Sutherland, "Rehabilitation Service."

31. Helen B. Radler, *A Handbook for Your Recovery with Exercises* (New York: Society of Memorial Center, 1952); Helen B. Radler, *A Handbook for Your Recovery*, rev. ed. (New York: Women's Society for Memorial Center, 1954); Terese Lasser, *Reach to Recovery* (New York: Lasser, 1953).

32. Lerner, *Breast Cancer Wars*, 143–44; Kirsten E. Gardner, *Early Detection: Women, Cancer, and Awareness Campaigns in the Twentieth-Century United States* (Chapel Hill: University of North Carolina Press, 2006), 148–51; Cantor, "Before Survivorship."

33. Lasser, *Reach to Recovery*, 6–7.

34. Arthur I. Holleb, "Two Decades of Reach to Recovery: A Tribute to the Volunteers," *CA: A Cancer Journal for Clinicians* 40 (1990): 5–7.

35. Lasser, *Reach to Recovery*.

36. At Memorial, for example, Lasser and Radler were members of the Society of Memorial Center, founded by a number of prominent women in 1946 to raise funds for a variety of the hospital's activities and to promote a focus on care for the entire person. Joan Sutton Straus, *A Legacy of Caring: The Society of Memorial Sloan-Kettering Cancer Center* (New York: Society of Memorial Sloan-Kettering Cancer Center, 1996).

37. Arthur M. Sutherland, "The Psychological Impact of Postoperative Cancer," *Bulletin of the New York Academy of Medicine* 33 (1957): 428–45. See also Sutherland, "Psychologic Barriers to Rehabilitation of Cancer Patients," *Postgraduate Medicine* 17 (1955): 523–26; Sutherland, "Psychological Factors in Surgical Convalescence," *Annals New York Academy of Sciences* 73 (1958): 491–99; Arthur M. Sutherland and Charles E. Orbach, "Psychological Impact of Cancer and Cancer Surgery: II. Depressive Reactions Associated with Surgery for Cancer," *Cancer* 6 (1953): 958–62; Morton Bard and Arthur M. Sutherland, "Psychological Impact of Cancer and Its Treatment: IV. Adaptation to Radical Mastectomy," *Cancer* 8 (1955): 656–72; Charles E. Orbach and Arthur M. Sutherland, "Acute Depressive Reactions to

Surgical Treatment for Cancer," *Proceedings of the Annual Meeting of the American Psychopathological Association* (New York: Grune and Stratton, 1954): 237–52; and Ruth B. Dyk and Arthur M. Sutherland, "Adaptation of the Spouse and Other Family Members to the Colostomy Patient," *Cancer* 9 (1956): 123–38.

38. Sutherland and Orbach, "Psychological Impact," 958.

39. Sutherland, "Psychological Impact."

40. Ibid.

41. Anxiety, he claimed, was often aroused by fears of unacceptability to other people, inability to perform well at work, an increase in family tensions, or the abolition of activities through which the patient has regularly discharged anxiety.

42. Sutherland argued that the most common depressive response to surgery was reactive depression (which could persist indefinitely throughout the life of an individual if a basic pattern was disrupted) but also occasionally ruminative or agitated depressions with suicidal trends and very rarely apathetic depressions.

43. Sutherland, "Psychological Factors," 498.

44. Sutherland, "Postoperative Cancer," 441.

45. Arthur M. Sutherland, Morton Bard, and Ruth B. Dyk, *Psychological Aspects of Cancer*, 16 mm. color and sound film (Telecolor Clinics; Professional Education Division, American Cancer Society, 1954). The Telecolor series was a series of thirty closed-circuit broadcasts for the medical profession, produced by the Columbia Broadcasting System for the ACS from October 21, 1953, to June 2, 1954. Arthur I. Holleb and Frances B. Buch, "Color Television in Medical Education: A Report on "Telecolor Clinics," *Journal of the American Medical Association* 156 (September 25, 1954): 298–302.

46. See for example Brown, "'Stress' in US Wartime Psychiatry," this volume.

47. Richard Rennecker and Max Cutler, "Psychological Problems of Adjustment to Cancer of the Breast," *Journal of the American Medical Association* 148 (March 8, 1952): 833–38; Patricia Jasen, "Malignant Histories: Psychosomatic Medicine and the Female Cancer Patient in the Postwar Era," *Canadian Bulletin of Medical History* 20 (2003): 265–97.

48. Ruth D. Abrams, "Social Casework with Cancer Patients," *Social Casework* 32 (1951): 425–32; Ruth D. Abrams and Jacob E. Finesinger, "Guilt Reactions in Patients with Cancer," *Cancer* 6 (1953): 474–82; Jacob E. Finesinger, Harley C. Shands, and Ruth D. Abrams, "Managing the Emotional Problems of the Cancer Patient," *CA: A Cancer Journal for Clinicians* 3, no. 1 (January 1953): 19–31; Harley C. Shands, Jacob E. Finesinger, Stanley Cobb, and Ruth D. Abrams, "Psychological Mechanisms in Patients with Cancer," *Cancer* 4 (1951): 1159–70.

49. For example, the first edition of *A Cancer Source Book for Nurses* (New York, 1950) published by the American Cancer Society made no reference to the concept of stress in its discussion of the psychology of cancer and how to manage patients. By contrast its second edition in 1963 included the phrase "during this period of stress when everything in his environment seems to be conspiring against him" as part of its discussion of the impact of the nurse on patient's adjustment to his (*sic*) problem. American Cancer Society, *A Cancer Source Book for Nurses* (New York: American Cancer Society, 1963), 45. Other 1950s publications on cancer nursing also failed to mention stress; see, for example, National Cancer Institute, Public Health Service, Federal Security Agency, and the New York State Department of Health, *Cancer*

Nursing: A Manual for Public Health Nurses, rev. ed. (1950; repr. Albany, 1955); and Rosalie I. Peterson and Genevieve R. Soller, *Cancer Nursing in the Basic Professional Nursing Curriculum: Suggested Content and Methods*, Public Health Service Publication 147 (Washington, DC: US Government Printing Office, 1952).

50. See, for example, Ella H. Bernhardt, "The Rehabilitation of the Mastectomy Patient," *R.N.—A Journal for Nurses* 16, no. 13 (October 1953): 52–56. There is little or no mention of stress in the many articles on special bras and bust forms for mastectomees in the trade magazine *Corset and Underwear Review* for the 1950s, nor in the collection of trade-related materials—primarily for mastectomies and colostomy patients—in the Virginia Dericks Papers, Center for Nursing Historical Inquiry, Claude Moore Health Sciences Library, Historical Collections, University of Virginia, Charlottesville, Virginia.

51. Irving L. Janis, *Psychological Stress: Psychoanalytic and Behavioral Studies of Surgical Patients* (New York: Wiley, 1958), 5. The reference is to Sutherland and Orbach, "Psychological Impact."

52. Nathan S. Kline and Julius Sobin, "The Psychological Management of Cancer Cases," *Journal of the American Medical Association* 146 (August 25, 1951): 1548.

53. George M. Perrin and Irene R. Pierce, "Psychosomatic Aspects of Cancer: A Review," *Psychosomatic Medicine* 21 (1959): 405. Perrin and Pierce also highlight how stress could come to cover the work that did not invoke the concept. The quotation referred to the work of Sutherland and his team at Memorial and (despite his tendency not to use stress) of Jacob E. Finesinger and his colleagues, the latter also pointing to the disruptions of normal patterns of activity, the difficulty of readjustment, and the use of certain defense mechanisms often classified as neurotic.

Part Six

Surveilling Stress

Chapter Eleven

Stress in the City

Mental Health, Urban Planning, and the Social Sciences in the Postwar United States

Edmund Ramsden

The Study of Mental Health in the City

The city has long been perceived as a pathological space, a cause of deviance, sickness, and delinquency. Its various social and psychological problems have often been associated with its physical structures and conditions. Perhaps the most famous sociological statement on the city, Louis Wirth's "Urbanism as a Way of Life," identified size, density, and heterogeneity as resulting in superficiality, alienation, anomie, and various forms of social and psychological breakdown.[1] This chapter focuses on a diverse group of social and behavioral scientists, biologists, psychiatrists, architects, and planners concerned with rectifying the problems associated with urban life. From the mid-1950s they were united in a series of conferences supported by the National Institute of Mental Health (NIMH), to better understand and control the influence of the environment on mental health and illness. The Committee on Physical and Social Environmental Variables as Determinants of Mental Health, nicknamed the "Space Cadets," met for two and a half days, twice a year, for twelve years from 1956.[2] The meetings, which were fully transcribed, allow us to examine how diverse scientific and professional communities sought to develop a common language and a degree of unity of purpose in addressing the issues of slum clearance and urban renewal. Many of those involved saw the meetings as having significantly influenced their future research, as John B. Calhoun suggested: "I will leave it to historians to start with the stenotype transcripts of the twenty-three 2½-day sessions and follow them outward."[3] Contributions from the participants were collected in the influential text, *The Urban Condition*, edited by the conference chair, the social psychiatrist Leonard Duhl.[4]

Participants were also drawn together because of their concern that the influence of environmental factors on mental health and behavior had not been properly considered by their parent disciplines. For Duhl, they needed a truly ecological perspective in its broadest sense: "an interrelatedness of the physical, both natural and man-made, the biological, both human and non-human, the psychological and social factors."[5] While previous students of the city, such as the sociologists of Chicago, had declared themselves "ecologists," they were little interested in humans' relation to the physical environment.[6] The city was divided into sections or zones to examine social and economic interrelations. For human ecologists, space served more as "a stage for behavior—a passive element in social structure and human decision making."[7] Or, in the words of the Chicago School: "The city is, rather, a state of mind, a body of customs and traditions, and of the organized attitudes and sentiments that inhere in these customs and are transmitted with this tradition. The city is not, in other words, merely a physical mechanism."[8]

From the nineteenth century, housing reform and city-planning movements had already made much of the power of improved housing to improve not only physical health but mental health, social integration, and morality. Much of the supposed associations, however, were assumed rather than analyzed—it was intuitive, Gunnar Myrdal declared confidently: "Any common sense evaluation will tell us that the causation, in part, goes *from* poor housing *to* bad moral, mental and physical health." There were only a few limited and scattered studies, the most comprehensive being that of James S. Plant, who spoke of "the mental strain arising from constantly having [to] 'get along' with other people" as a particularly damaging consequence of crowded environments, along with the dissolution of individuality and heightened sexual activity among children. In Robert Faris and Warren Dunham's study of mental disorder in urban areas, the structure of housing was important, but it functioned more as a backdrop, container, or setting; their focus was social and economic factors such as low wages and a high turnover of population in rooming-house areas as causes of mental illness.[9]

Plant's use of the language of strain would, in the postwar era, be succeeded by the language of stress. As we shall see in the Space Cadet meetings, the concept of stress was used to aid communication and understanding between different disciplines and professions whose members often held opposing views over the power of the physical environment to improve the lives of urban citizens. In this sense not only did stress serve as a boundary object that linked systems of the body and population, individual and environment, physiology and behavior; it allowed for disciplinary boundary crossing between various social and biomedical sciences and city planning. It also allowed members to bring together different problems associated with the extensive urban renewal programs that had resulted from the 1949 and 1954 housing acts—be they the loss of community through slum clearance, the lack of support for relocation, the poor design of modern housing projects—into a more unified and consistent critique.[10]

After exploring the debates among the Space Cadets, we shall the turn our attention to two general and broadly defined approaches that developed through the meetings. The first focused on the need to identify, isolate, measure, and control key physical variables, most notably that of density, that could be seen to have destructive effects on individual psychologies and social structures. The theoretical framework most commonly applied was that of overload: excessive and unwanted social interaction, mediated through a range of social, psychological, and physical factors, could result in *crowding stress* and its concomitant psychophysiological pathologies. The second again emphasized mediation and adaptation but was focused more on the role of social networks, peer groups, and subcultures attached to urban spaces and territories. Crowding was one of many potential stressors to which human beings could adapt through existent social networks and structures.

While the Space Cadet meetings helped members recognize the similarities between these two approaches, by the early 1970s they were placed in diametric opposition. This chapter, therefore, examines how space and stress were brought together by various critics of urban renewal and then pulled apart as different communities increasingly competed to realize their own visions of science in the service of the city. In doing so, we examine the central role of social and behavioral studies of the environmental determinants of mental health to debates over urban renewal and slum clearance, a subject that requires considerably more attention from historians of medicine.[11]

The Space Cadets

The first Conference on the Physical Environment as a Determinant of Mental Health took place at the American Psychological Association in May 1956. As explained by its organizers, the social psychiatrist Leonard Duhl and the ecologist and psychologist John B. Calhoun, it had emerged from their mutual interest in a subject too often ignored, even at their own institution, the National Institute of Mental Health. Duhl was a member of the Office of Professional Services, which was concerned with long-term planning in mental health. He promoted what he described as an ecological approach to mental health—"the study of the multiple factors of the environment . . . that affect the normal development and behavior of the individual and his society." Mental health was, therefore, no longer "the study of mental disease alone, but the study of man in society."[12] The physical environment was a critical element of ecology. As Duhl emphasized to those present, policy makers, architects, and planners were requesting scientific data to construct healthy buildings and spaces. And yet

> the social scientists, the psychologists and the others have never been able to help them. They want to know something about space. They want to know something about problems of color. What they want to know is do we need free space outside for kids to wander in. Do we need natural areas? Does this have anything to do with people's living qualities or not and on and on you can go. Have we any answers to that?[13]

To provide such answers, Calhoun and Duhl had invited some of the most eminent scientists and planners of the time who were concerned with the relationship between the environment and health. The first meetings included the psychiatrist Erich Lindemann; sociologists Herbert Gans, Erving Goffman, August B. Hollingshead, and John Seeley; planners Catherine Bauer, Richard Meier, Richard Poston, and Melvin Webber; ecologists, ethologists, and comparative psychologists such as T. C. Schneirla and Edward Deevey; the systems theorists Nicolas Rashevsky and John Q. Stewart; social psychologists Marie Jahoda, Daniel Wilner, and Marc Fried; anthropologist Thomas Gladwin; health planner Henrik Blum; and the economist Harvey Perloff. By the time of their conclusion, they had included Ernest Caspari, Albert Deutsch, Joel Elkes, Ian McHarg, Eugene Rostow, Geoffrey Vickers, Michael Young, and even Robert C. Weaver of the Housing and Home Finance Agency, first appointed by President Kennedy to help revitalize and improve the Federal Urban Renewal Program and then serving as the first United States secretary of Housing and Urban Development (HUD) from 1966.

In the first meetings tensions between participants were immediately apparent. These tended to surround two fundamental issues raised by Duhl: What was meant by the "environment" and how was it possible to isolate, measure, and control its effects? What was meant by "mental health," and how did it relate to illness? As we shall see, the flexibility of the concept of stress allowed those present to retain many of their original perspectives, while engineering a compromise that recognized a degree of compatibility with the views of others present. Its use was also pragmatic, helping to realize a degree of unity of purpose in identifying how to correct the problems of the city through the design of physical spaces. Indeed, so central was it that Calhoun commented at the first meeting of his fear that "we might bog down into a conference on stress," and yet, given its generality and usefulness, "perhaps this orientation might give a good focus to the general objective."[14] By the third conference Nicolas Rashevsky warned, "We should never forget that after all the problem of stress is only one of the possible many dozens or hundreds of factors. . . . It would be disastrous, scientifically, if we all concentrate on one thing. . . . But it is natural that one thing catches our attention first. . . . So for the time-being, we will spend two [more] conferences on this discussion of stress. We may spend a third and possibly the fourth."[15] As the conferences progressed, the subject of stress remained central.

The first meeting began with a description by Calhoun of his experiments into the various pathological effects of density among rats. Almost immediately, there was disagreement as to the very definition of mental health. Duhl wanted to keep this out of the discussion until they first addressed the relationship between human behavior and physical environment.[16] Calhoun duly used the most general of definitions: "Mental health here is broadly viewed as any state or change in behavior."[17] Calhoun then described how, as a member of a rodent control project in Baltimore, he had studied the social behavior of wild rats in an enclosed pen over a period of three years. Two different types of animal began to emerge: one a "very highly socially knit stable group" in an interconnecting system of burrows; the other "socially unstable," lacking hierarchy, having low reproduction, and existing in an elongated and divided series of nest cavities that isolated and alienated them.[18] The built environment of the rat reflected, and then reinforced, the mental health of the community. The cause of social instability was high-population density that bombarded the weaker animals with unwanted interactions and prevented them from completing their normal behavioral repertoire. As a consequence there emerged a range of pathologies and stress-related illnesses, deemed consistent with the ideas of Hans Selye.[19] For Calhoun it was necessary to explore the effects of high-density living among humans in the city and, following from his experiments, do so in a way that fully appreciated the effects of the physical environment: "You have to designate two things; size of field, the nature of the field in relationship to how it structures the contact rate. Without specifying these two variables you cannot be sure that group size functions as an independent variable."[20]

Many in the group expressed their support of Calhoun's approach. The human ecologist and medical sociologist August Hollingshead had used an epidemiological approach in understanding the incidence, prevalence, and distribution of psychiatric disorders in urban populations, relying on reported cases of mental illness, which were then correlated to ecological areas: "The poorer the housing, the greater the crowding, that's your density potential, the greater your density the higher rate of commitment is."[21] When it came to his description of pathology, Hollingshead was explicit and dramatic, drawing on not only statistical correlations but observations and interviews. He spoke of the varied kinds of "human rat colonies": "We find there are very definite relationships between the environmental conditions both physical and cultural and social which people live and mental breakdown." Census tract 22 in New Haven had the highest concentration of people, and the most deteriorated tenements: "There maybe one toilet at each end of the hall. . . . This is your long dwelling, Dr. Calhoun, the rat colony, so to speak, you see—these cold water flats along the side; five on a side." The conflict that resulted was only exacerbated by the different "species" competing for territory: "Now you've got Negro rats and you have Puerto Rican rats that are moving in. Then you have Italian rats and you got some Polish rats. Then you go[t] some stranded Irish rats and you may find also there may be a few stranded swamp Yankee rats. . . . Here is social reality; the rats behaving in a social and physical environment."[22]

Hollingshead's description stimulated lively debate. Leonard Duhl and the city planner Catherine Bauer were concerned that he, like many psychiatrists, had focused on a distinct pathological minority at the expense of the general population—ammunition for simplistic, aggressive, and destructive policies of slum clearance as the cure for the sick city. Others were concerned at his characterization of slum life as overwhelmingly negative. John Seeley suggested that while slums may be responsible for much mental breakdown, they also provided their inhabitants with freedom and enjoyment not experienced by the urban middle classes, perhaps even contributing to "high creativity."[23] As Marie Jahoda argued, these differences of opinion were the inevitable result of the lack of an adequate definition of mental health and thus the lack of an ultimate objective. Settling on a definition that satisfied all parties present would be unlikely, as all had different standards, values, and concerns. Some saw health and illness on a continuum, and the majority, Jahoda, Calhoun, Duhl, and Seeley included, argued that mental health was more than the mere absence of illness. Mental health was variously described in terms of "integration," "mastery," "maturity," "satisfaction," "productivity," "creativity," and "happiness." In a later meeting, Jahoda circulated a paper in which she identified the criteria of "positive mental health" for both individuals and groups, which was to be understood relationally to the environment.[24] These consisted of mastery over the environment, autonomy, integration, perception of reality, growth development or self-actualization, and attitude toward the self. Her definition drew mixed support—it would become important to Lindemann but left others unimpressed.[25] The resulting discussion over the definitions of health and illness was repetitive and protracted, that is, until the concept of stress was used to circumvent this problem.

Using the language of systems theory, Meier and Rashevsky provided a series of lengthy presentations on stress that emphasized its uses and power as a concept. Meier was carrying out his own laboratory experiments, identifying the amount of information individuals (or rather, systems) could process before becoming overloaded—what he described as "information" or "communication stress"—and the strategies employed to prevent breakdown.[26] Rashevsky teamed up with Hollingshead, allowing them to test their various theories and mathematical methods "with respect to stresses that operate in the social environment which may result in functional types of mental illness."[27]

Meier first described the concept of stress—the reaction or disturbance of an organized system—as "picayune" when compared to Jahoda's broad framework.[28] Yet as the discussion progressed, attendees were struck by the degree to which the concept was relevant to, and united, her criteria. Deevey observed, "The whole concept of stress seems to be perfectly general."[29] Perception, integration, and mastery of the environment were to be understood in terms of the ability of an individual or group to identify, resist, cope with, and adapt to life's constant stresses. Schneirla spoke of having made sense of Jahoda's monograph, cutting through the sociopsychological jargon by reading it "in terms of the definition of 'stress,' 'stressor,' and 'tension.'"[30] By these definitions a stressor was a change in the environment brought to bear on the organism, stress the immediate effect and significance of the change for the organism, and tension the condition of organization, which in turn affected the organism's adaptive adjustment. While there was much confusion and debate over when, exactly, a stressor became stress, and stress became tension or "strain," these were the definitions that the majority of the group settled on—"we had better use them consistently," Schneirla insisted, "or we will increase our difficulties rather than lessening them."[31] With stress serving as an intervening concept between stimulus and behavioral consequence, mental health now referred to the mode through which an individual coped, or indeed failed to cope, with the various pressures exerted by the social and physical environment. Indeed, the mental health of the individual could be understood, and improved, only through the recourse to environmental factors.[32]

The concept of stress allowed the conference participants to place mental health and illness on a continuum; to establish a common language and more coherent framework that focused on the relationship between individuals and their environment, inferring stress (and stressor) through the measurement of strain; and to focus on the mental health of the entire population rather than an extreme, pathological minority. Indeed, when Hollingshead sought to "defend" himself following his explicit descriptions of behavioral pathology, he used the language of stress. He pointed out that in New Haven they were studying the whole community and provided further examples of mental illness among the wealthy due to various social conflicts. For Hollingshead, while the higher classes suffered stress relating to status and mobility, the problems of those at the bottom "seem to be most directly related to physical environment."[33]

With the concept of stress having allowed them "to continue talking about concrete things," attention now shifted to the problem of defining the environment and identifying the relevant social and physical stressors. To do this Calhoun had suggested that they focus on some of their own research projects that combined city planning with the behavioral sciences: “Each will serve as a sort of laboratory which can focus attention and focus our theoretical and practical questions on.”[34]

The Environments of the Space Cadet Laboratories

In the first conferences some members seemed to interpret the effects of physical environment on behavior as relatively straightforward. This was, in part, driven by a concern to make a social difference through planning and design. Catherine Bauer described the physical environment as “the one variable in the whole picture which is really consciously controllable. Everything else is very, very difficult to do anything about.”[35] Daniel Wilner suggested that when it came to the problem of empowering the lower classes, “It may be cheaper to do it by simply altering the housing.” Of all the physical variables, Bauer specified density and open space to be “most critical,” while Stewart added, “density is the thing that makes a slum.” Duhl also spoke of the need to design smaller communities to avoid having “so many things hitting a person that he becomes completely incapacitated.” Density was also a stressor particularly amenable to measurement, and Calhoun urged participants to focus on those “which we might actually attack . . . so that we could state the situation in the terms of relatively simple formulation. Now this may be an over-simplified approach but . . . I think we could perhaps clarify our general problem . . . to determine the frequency and types of situations which lead to the conflicts.”[36]

Focusing on the significance of housing, they turned to the work of Daniel Wilner, a social psychologist based at the Johns Hopkins School of Public Health.[37] From 1954, supported by the Joint Committee on the Hygiene of Housing of the American Public Health Association (APHA) and the National Association of Housing and Redevelopment Officials, Wilner directed the first systematic survey that analyzed “a discrete quite measurable change in physical environment on behavior and health.” The Johns Hopkins Longitudinal Study of the Effects of Housing in Health and Social Adjustment compared the mental and physical health of those in “very bad slums” of Baltimore with those relocated to new “very good housing.” For Wilner the suggestion was that in the development of neuroses, psychoses, and “the general stresses that we live in . . . the environment plays a role and that somehow it can be manipulated.” Early in the study, however, he expressed some doubt as to whether, “for this group of very low income Negro families that the alteration in housing is necessary. . . . I just wonder at this present stage . . . whether this is really as astonishing a change in their lives as we think it is, and whether this is just another atom floating in space.”[38] Two years later, however, Duhl reported confidently that there "have been some changes in his conclusions . . . that these moves into the new physical environment have in fact resulted in improvement of the mental and physical health of populations."[39] Wilner's ongoing study, regularly presented to the Space Cadets, duly showed how improved housing had led to lower rates of sickness, improved rates of school attendance, and emotional well-being, measured through a series of "psychosocial scales." He identified "space" as a "primary variable" that "had powerful effects upon the families."[40] Its increase allowed for personal privacy and improved relations with family members, rehoused homemakers reporting "reductions in psychological discomfort directly related to space."[41] The design of the housing also encouraged good relations with neighbors through propinquity.

At the other extreme Seeley suggested that the effects of the physical environment were "so trivial that we might turn attention away from them and that subsequently we should discuss the physical environment as socially perceived or psychologically perceived."[42] The physical environment did not exist as an independent reality—it could be understood only sociologically. He continually, in his own words, "refused the whole definition, the name of the meeting and all."[43] Place was to be privileged over space; the physical environment was relevant only to the degree to which it was experienced by people and imbued with social meaning. Seeley lent his support to the findings from an alternative Space Cadet laboratory—a study of the experience and effects of urban renewal in Boston's West End.

The West End project, titled "Relocation and Mental Health: Adaptation under Stress," was directed by Erich Lindemann and funded through the National Institute of Mental Health (NIMH), thanks to Duhl's encouragement and institutional connections.[44] It was based in the Psychiatry Division of the Massachusetts General Hospital in the West End, where Lindemann was chief of the Psychiatry Service. This was a division that he was reorienting toward social psychiatry, by setting up the Center for Community Studies in 1956 and employing the social psychologist Marc Fried as its research coordinator. They were interested in exploring how kinship systems functioned in slum environments to provide social and psychological support and to measure the effects of their disruption. Fried applied Lindemann's conceptualization of "grief," which he developed from the latter's long-term focus on the psychosomatic consequences of crisis and bereavement, to the experience of the physical environment. His Space Cadet paper was later published in Duhl's edited collection as "Grieving for a Lost Home."[45] Through a combination of observation, interview, and survey techniques, Fried was measuring the consequences—social, psychological, and medical—of the Boston Redevelopment Authority's decision to raze a forty-eight-acre portion of the West End, beginning in 1958, and displacing 2,700 families to make way for five residential high-rise and high-rent luxury apartment complexes.[46] The decision was justified through the designation of the West End as a slum, based on the application of the physical housing standards developed by the Committee on the Hygiene of Housing of the APHA (which had also been used by Wilner).[47] One of the most privileged among these standards was density, and the West End project report described the area as "over-populated," "densely covered," and "overcrowded," with a "severe lack of any open space."[48] Among the most advertised qualities of the new Charles River Park development were, in contrast, those of "spaciousness" and "privacy."[49]

The decision to redevelop the West End offered Lindemann's group an opportunity to study the stress-related responses to a changing urban environment over time.[50] Yet to understand the effects of physical change, it was considered essential to gain a better understanding of working-class culture within the cohesive and primarily Italian American community. Fried believed the working class to experience the urban environment in a very different way to the middle class. For the latter the apartment or house was a private space, clearly differentiated from the street outside. For the working classes the boundary between home and street was much more permeable, or rather the concept of "home" was to be extended out into the street, an area of immense importance for social interaction among the closely knit networks of family and friends. Consistent with Hollingshead's observations, the working classes were much more closely tied to, and dependent on, their local physical surroundings.[51] The community was not just a social but a spatial unit, relationships embedded in physical space. Fried interpreted this process in terms of "territoriality." This was a concept central to animal and human ecology and often associated with aggression and segregation, but it was used by Fried as the basis of the mutually supportive community: "We have referred to this way of organizing physical space as *territorial* to distinguish it from the more highly *selective* and individualized use of space which seems to characterize the middle class. And we suggest that it is the territorial conception and manner of using physical space which provides one of the bases for the kind of localism which is so widely found in working-class areas."[52]

Considering the importance of spatial identity—the significance of the physical residential area to interpersonal relationships, social organization, and sense of self—the destruction of the West End produced grief-like reactions and stress-related illnesses. This was further compounded by the failure to provide for relocation. The public housing that was supplied was ill-suited, many associating it in turn with crowding, density, and congestion, with one resident complaining, "It's too congested. The West End was congested, but not like the projects."[53] "These observations lead us to question," Fried and his colleague concluded, "the extent to which, through urban renewal, we relieve a situation of stress or create further damage."[54]

Herbert Gans, a city planner and sociologist, further developed this critique of urban renewal. Through his connection to Duhl, Gans was employed on the project from 1957.[55] His role was that of an observer, interpreting the West End and its various subcultures and informal networks to the other researchers through reports and a field diary, advising on their research strategies, and aiding their communication with residents.[56] He lived among the West Enders from October 1957 to May 1958, prior to their removal, and became sympathetic to their futile struggle against urban renewal.[57] Gans not only questioned the benefits of the renewal program but criticized the very description of the West End as a slum.[58] This had been the consequence of the simplistic application of physical, and supposedly objective, standards provided by the APHA. They had ignored how "stress" was perceived and experienced by people "in terms of their own way of living, and their relation to this environment."[59] It was not the existing housing, but the destruction of "socially and emotionally important social systems" that put the population "under stress."[60] While the area was of high density, it was a healthy community, not a "slum"—a description that had only sociological meaning and was, in any case, better applied to a nearby area that fulfilled the conditions of social disorganization and social pathology.[61] Nevertheless, Gans accepted that there were physical factors that could be universally damaging: "Room overcrowding which forces even people from sociable cultures to live so closely together that they cannot avoid each other . . . is likely to have detrimental consequences."[62] He also accepted that when an area did become an overcrowded slum, it would impact upon the mental health of its inhabitants, making "uncrowding," through renewal and relocation, essential.[63]

Gans's work was very influential. Peter Marris and Michael Young of the Institute of Community Studies in London (both of whom attended Space Cadet meetings) carried out their own studies of family and kinship in London's East End, and they were supportive of Gans's work.[64] Likewise, Jane Jacobs, famed for her critique of urban renewal and her celebration of dense and diverse working-class neighborhoods, was inspired by Gans to visit the West End and the adjacent North End for herself, writing to him about the latter: "here is an area with the highest densities in Boston—above 200 dwelling units per acre—and you get an effect of terrific health and cheer in the place." Nevertheless, she had been informed by the planning board that the North End was also due to be redeveloped in time as "it is a slum": "Oh my. They ought to be down here learning from the area instead of thinking up old, tired garden city things to do with it."[65] The West End study itself helped generate more effective opposition to urban renewal, not only in Boston, where "Remember the West End!" was a rallying call against further redevelopment, but throughout the United States.[66] The work of Gans and Jacobs was commonly combined; the influential planner and architect (and one-time associate of both Gans and Ian McHarg) David A. Wallace summed up, "In general, and with rare exceptions, planning for urban-renewal projects has been poor, execution worse, and the final results decent, safe, and sanitary, but little else." The "sterile, drab, and uninspired physical patterns that replace the slums . . . seem to prohibit any very rich new social textures developing."[67]

Nevertheless, Gans was critical of Jacobs's approach. He had much sympathy for her celebration of diversity of peoples and buildings and for her emphasis on the positive effects of high-density street environments. He agreed with her distinction between urban density and overcrowding in the home. He also thought her to be correct in her criticism of urban renewal for causing "grievous hurt" to the inhabitants of low-rent areas. However, her vision of a healthy neighborhood reflected her values as a middle-class intellectual. It also, paradoxically, relied on a belief in the power of physical design. Jacobs was guilty of the same fallacy of physical determinism that she identified in the planning community: that the built environment and planning principles on which it was based directly shaped human behavior. Her romantic view of the city was no more valid than many of those she criticized, and it ignored the hardship of life in poor neighborhoods.[68] In this respect, it was also dangerous, alienating potential allies in the planning community while turning attention away from real urban problems: "There is much in planning that deserves criticism. . . . But they are not the devils that restrict funds to the North Ends."[69] Rehabilitating older, more attractive buildings was no solution to genuine "overcrowded slums": "These slums are caused not by dullness . . . but by the overcrowding of buildings already old by poverty-stricken and otherwise deprived nonwhites, who have no other place to go."[70] Rehabilitation would have the same consequences as urban renewal, resulting in a population "saddled with social and emotional burdens." Rents would increase, forcing low-income families to relocate and "overcrowd the ghetto even further."[71] He sent her his review of her book prior to its publication, explaining his concern at her failure to consider the "sociological factors" and the need for extensive new housing for low-income families: "I'm afraid that you are going to become the darling of the right wingers, and that is a fate worse than death."[72]

So interconnected was the West End study with the concerns of the Space Cadets that on the publication of two controversial, yet extremely influential, articles on the failures of city planning—written by Gans and Seeley for the *Journal of the American Institute of Planners* in 1959 (and solicited by its new editor and fellow Space Cadet, Melvin Webber)—Duhl described feeling "like a proud parent."[73] While the West End study complicated the relationship between housing and well-being, it was seen to complement that of Wilner's in that both had identified the significance of various physical factors for the increase or mitigation of stress.[74] While the more sociologically minded may have privileged the social over the physical, both elements were recognized to be intertwined and significant to mental health. Calhoun and Duhl continually pushed this point, brokering a compromise reflected in the amended title, "Conference on Physical *and Social* Environmental Variables as Determinants of Mental Health." Calhoun argued, "I realize that the physical situation has no reality without considering the social organization so that we have to consider them both. We can't just consider them completely independently but neither can we just consider social organization because the social organization has no reality in many instances without physical situations."[75] The key was to improve urban renewal, not abandon it, by providing the housing that various population groups wanted—be it urban, suburban, affordable, sanitary, or spacious.[76] While Melvin Webber described how the "simple clarity" of the city planner's role had, with the aid of the social and behavioral scientist, been "dimmed by the clouds of complexity, diversity, and . . . uncertainty," it was also evident that some aspects of the physical environment could bring appreciable benefit or "psychic disturbance" to the city's residents.[77]

Duhl's efforts were rewarded when in 1966 he became a consultant and "special assistant" to Robert C. Weaver at HUD. The new Model Cities program was concerned to correct the previous errors in urban renewal and bring local communities into the planning process. The program was, in part, a consequence of Duhl's work with the Space Cadets (their meetings concluding soon after his departure from the NIMH).[78] When he announced his new role at the Space Cadet meeting of March 1966, he spoke optimistically of the significant changes in the housing agency and the new opportunities for building links between academia, planning, and politics. The client, he suggested, was now "the city"; as it was served by a range of agencies, his task was to "look at how the parts all tie together" to develop a "total program." For the "first time coherent plans for physical planning," would, with the help of scientific expertise, be integrated with those of health, education, and welfare. Even in the mental-health world, he declared, "things have been happening . . . and all the things we have been fighting for for twelve years are suddenly taken for granted, and what Erich Lindemann has screamed and fought and knocked his head against the wall for years is suddenly coming easy."[79]

Duhl's speeches, reports, and correspondence at HUD reflected the ideas developed through the Space Cadets. He argued that the ghetto needed to be understood as more than just a pathological physical space and that to deal with urban "stress and strain" and "confusion and complexity," preventative measures needed to address socioeconomic inequalities and take account of the differing spatial needs and values of population groups in accordance with class, gender, and age.[80] Other Space Cadets also expressed optimism. Gans supported a renewed "war on slums" that would tackle the underlying social as well as physical problems.[81] Urban renewal was "just about dead, whats left of it ought to be put out of its misery and quietly buried. A new baby is being born, and we ought to see that it grows up to be big, strong."[82] They now had an opportunity, declared Weaver, of fulfilling "the promise of science for the city."[83]

The Growing Divergence between Density and Community

The Model Cities legislation was developed as a response to criticisms of urban renewal—those of Fried and Gans prominent among them—but its passing was also the consequence of the rioting that occurred across US cities from the mid-1960s. Many associated the violence with inferior and crowded living conditions.[84] The anthropologist Edward T. Hall went so far to declare the destructiveness of crowded urban environments to be "more lethal than the hydrogen bomb." This was a period of political radicalism, environmental activism, and concern with the so-called population explosion. One of key speakers at the world's first Earth Day in 1970 was the architect and planner Ian McHarg. Invited to Space Cadet meetings, McHarg's contribution to Duhl's *Urban Condition* decried the inhumane physical environment of the modern city: "The epidemiologist speaks of neuroses, lung cancer, heart and renal disease, ulcers, the stress diseases, as the badges of urban conditions. There has also arisen the spectre of the effects of density and social pressure upon the incidence of disease."[85]

This confluence of factors—political radicalism, environmental activism, ecological pessimism, and social anxiety—gave further impetus to ecological studies of the city. A new generation of social and behavioral scientists, often graduate students or recent PhDs, were concerned that they contribute to the resolution of real social and environmental problems. They were also concerned that, while studies such as Daniel Wilner's had provided clear evidence that housing was related to physical well-being, the psychological consequences remained "ambiguous."[86] Further statistical studies correlated density, measured as number of individuals per acre, with a range of variables such as crime and delinquency, alcoholism, suicide, disease, mental illness, divorce, sexual deviance, and poor parental care.[87] Yet results were mixed—density was related to some disorders, but not to others.[88] Social and behavioral scientists now sought to explain these anomalies. As they did so, they developed a more complex and sophisticated approach to the study of the relationship between stressor, stress, and mental health.

Consistent with the studies of the Space Cadets, they recognized that the experience of space, and thus of high-density environments, was influenced by personal experiences, cultural norms, and social values. Nevertheless, they were wary that by going too far in emphasizing subjective factors, they would severely reduce the significance of physical dimensions; as one psychologist declared, "The environment is not in the head!"[89] As a result, they focused on fundamental needs common across individuals and groups: territory, privacy, and personal space. A model of stimulus overload was particularly popular: "the experience of crowding involves an excess of social stimuli, generally in the form of demands on one, combined with an inability to regulate or control."[90] They suggested that human beings "have a need for territory or privacy"; if this was the case, then "overcrowding may, in fact, conflict with a basic (biological?) characteristic of man."[91]

They also focused on sites where individuals would be least able to withstand the various assaults of the urban environment. As Gans had admitted, all people had the need for space and privacy in the home. For the psychologist Daniel Stokols, the household was a "primary" environment where "personal" encounters took place, as opposed to the "secondary" spaces and "neutral" encounters associated with the public realm. This meant that unwanted interaction, excessive levels of stimulation, and restrictions on privacy and behavioral freedom in the household were more likely to result in a state of "general stress."[92] Sociologists also shifted their attention away from simplistic measures of residential and areal density. They turned instead to "overcrowding at the personal, or individual, level."[93] It was in the limited confines of the home where it was possible to find greater degrees of crowding pathology. The data provided by social and behavioral scientists supported increased public-housing provisions. It also emphasized their role in helping to design environments that reduced infringements on behavior and privacy, avoiding, for example, what the HUD assistant secretary Don Hummel described as "monolithic units that result in ghetto-like concentrations of the poor and unfortunate."[94] With its apparent attractiveness to policy and politics, the study of crowding, as Stokols recognized, was "one of the fastest growing areas of psychological research."[95]

Just as the field of crowding research grew, however, the Nixon administration began to slowly withdraw support for Model Cities from 1969, and the program was officially disbanded in 1974. While it was seen to have played a significant role in encouraging political participation among minority populations, its housing program is generally seen to have failed. Duhl left his position for Berkeley in 1968, dismayed at the lack of political will at the city level required to successfully realize the model city.[96] Gans was also perturbed by the lack of political support for the program and criticized the lack of funding to provide the necessary amount of housing for low-income families. However, for Gans, any attempt to resolve the problems of the city, reflected in the rising tide of urban violence, would fail if it did not address the fundamental problems of urban life: social segregation, class conflict, and economic inequality.[97] It was these problems that caused the overcrowding that made the slum, which in turn caused the stress-related illnesses so prevalent among slum dwellers. When it came to priorities, the planner needed to be more concerned with helping to improve the living standards of the people and addressing social inequalities. One of the most important benefits of an extensive housing construction program was, in this regard, the employment that it would provide for poor and minority populations.

In the Space Cadet meetings Gans had described feeling "very skeptical" about the power of the planners to create new social relationships in heterogeneous environments through design.[98] The sociometric tradition, exemplified by Wilner's study, which suggested that better housing, more effectively arranged, could determine friendships and build new and better communities, was naive, and the evidence questionable.[99] Clients did not share the planner's lofty ideals of diversity and heterogeneity but sought social homogeneity according to age, education, and income. Gans described the growing dominance of psychologists in environmental research as "unfortunate," and the "physical approach" to the city as "not v[ery] useful."[100] The increasing focus on architectural solutions was part of the problem, and the subsequent failure of new housing to solve social problems then lent itself to arguments that poor and minority populations were inherently pathological in terms of their behaviors, values, and family life.[101] Gans became more openly critical of the focus on crowding in the 1970s, highlighting the inconsistent evidence generated by density studies. In a presentation on density he described the fascination with the problems of crowding as "really more of anti-poor ideology," and, referring to his experience in the West End, added that "if everybody [was] your buddy, [you] can live easier at high density than when strangers."[102]

Gans's position was complex and seemed at times contradictory.[103] On the one hand, Gans was increasingly critical of architectural determinism; yet, on the other, he did accept that the physical environment, if "substandard and subhuman," could damage mental and physical health.[104] He urged the construction of more and better-designed low-income housing to prevent overcrowding and for the provision of open space for recreation. This complexity was increasingly lost among an emerging community of sociologists critical of the growing obsession with the physical features of the city and hostile to studies of crowding stress. Particularly important was the work of two urban sociologists based at the University of California at Berkeley. Mark Baldassare and Claude Fischer were concerned that ideas such as crowding had become a convenient "nonsocial explanation of the society's social problems; no solution short of a mass urban exodus seemed likely to alleviate the problem."[105] Fischer described the increasingly popular "basic urban alienation thesis": "the urban environment—its overstimulation, density, and complexity—strains individual psyches and social relations." To "moderate these stresses," individuals adapted in a way that led to "interpersonal estrangement" in urban culture and, of course, to violence, withdrawal, and the abuse of drugs and alcohol.[106]

In his own research, supported by grants from HUD and the NIMH Program in Social Structure and Personality Development, Baldassare explored the relations between household density and stress. Through a more refined study of the household, including an analysis of power relations between family members and the use of space within the home, he argued that household crowding could have an adverse effect on the physical and intellectual development of children. This effect, however, was very small and difficult to disassociate from family size.[107] Even in the home, it was possible to use social and personal resources to obtain social goals, use space effectively, and reduce the negative effects of density.[108] Baldassare and Fischer described crowding as one of many physical variables that humans adapted to in their day-to-day lives. What was most critical to the psychological health of individuals was that they be part of a community with shared social values and interests. Drawing on Gans, whom he described as having provided the "definitive statement" on the subject, Fischer argued that the city was not to be viewed as a mass of fearful, confused, and aggressive individuals whose dangerous emotions needed to be managed and controlled through more effective urban designs. Indeed, outside of a comprehensive critique of crowding studies, discussion of the effects of the physical environment on behavior and well-being was conspicuously absent. The city existed as a collection of "small, social worlds . . . so resilient and powerful as to be largely impervious to factors like size and density; . . . there are *no* psychological consequences of urbanization."[109] In spite of the immense effort to provide consistent evidence of hypertension, anxiety, insomnia, alcoholism, mental breakdown, and suicide, it seemed evident, Fischer concluded, that "urbanites do not suffer disproportionately from psychological stress."[110]

Stress, Space, and the City

In 1962 Herbert Gans observed how "American intellectuals have begun to rediscover the city." They had come to appreciate its "physical" features: "the problems of slums and urban renewal, middle-income housing, the lack of open space, the plight of the downtown business district, and the ever-increasing traffic congestion."[111] This was the year that Gans published *The Urban Villagers*, his intimate and sympathetic analysis of Boston's West Enders as they faced the destruction of the neighborhood and, with it, their community.[112] His work generated disquiet among planners and architects, and he described having been "considered a heretic by many of my colleagues in the planning profession."[113] He was seen to attack the very foundation and purpose of city planning and urban design. Gans insisted he was not against planning and was supportive of "more and better housing . . . to rehouse the slum dwellers."[114] But he was opposed to the tendency to assume that all urban problems could be solved by imposing a city planning solution—too often reflecting elitist middle-class values and organized and justified through the simplistic physical standards of space and numbers—on the population in its entirety. The year 1962 was also when Daniel Wilner published his analysis of the positive effects that more spacious housing had on mental and physical health in Baltimore, and John B. Calhoun published his most influential paper in *Scientific American*, describing in graphic detail the stress-related disorders and diseases that had befallen his rats in a crowded environment.[115]

Essays from Gans, Calhoun, and Wilner were included in Duhl's *Urban Condition*, along with those from other Space Cadets. Considering the diversity of disciplines, approaches, and interests represented, this was a text that one reviewer feared would be reminiscent "of the urban sprawl with which it is concerned." And yet he had found himself "heartened that there is more consensus about concepts, goals, and values among experts from a variety of fields in our pluralistic society than his own limited experience had led him to expect."[116] The use of the concept and language of stress played a significant role in creating this consensus. While early attempts to bridge disciplinary boundaries had faltered around definitions of mental health and the physical environment, the concept of stress provided a general, workable, and productive framework that satisfied the majority of Space Cadet members. For their purposes, mental health could be understood in terms of the resources, tools, and methods by which an individual coped with, and adapted to, the various environmental stressors of urban life, along with the consequences of adaptation to psychological, physiological, and social well-being. They agreed that the lower classes, with their lack of resources, were particularly susceptible to the negative consequences of overcrowded environments. This left a considerable role for the planner and designer: adequate housing needed to be provided to low-income families to prevent overcrowding, and environments needed to be designed to limit the impact of various stressors and aid individuals as they attempted to avoid, manage, and adapt to change.

They had also agreed that the physical environment could be understood only in the context of social norms, cultural values, and psychological needs. Lindemann's research project, "Relocation and Mental Health: Adaptation under Stress," established how social identity was directly related to spatial identity in Boston's West End. Central to this was the notion of territoriality—a close social network or peer group bounded by and embedded in physical space. The maintenance of both the social and physical environment was therefore critical to the mental health of the urban working class. While the focus was on the mutually supportive social group, the notion of territory was also used in terms of the individual. The requirements of personal space and privacy could be generalized to the population. Crowding in specific environments, such as the home, generated stress; it was, therefore, a genuine problem that befell many in slums, public-housing projects, and rehabilitated housing. When the two approaches were combined, as in Duhl's *Urban Condition*, they provided a powerful critique of existing programs of slum clearance and urban renewal.

The Space Cadets were, as their name suggests, ahead of their time—at the forefront of an emerging critique of attempts to fix the failing city. Their approaches generated a number of traditions of social scientific research of the urban environment that gathered pace through the 1960s and 1970s. With the growing concern with urban problems, the increased involvement of various social and behavioral scientists in their study, and reduced government support of interdisciplinary planning initiatives, the two broad approaches that had been allied (albeit uneasily) through the Space Cadets, were increasingly placed in opposition. Social and behavioral scientists focused on different elements of the stress process. Some envisaged both crowding stress and many of the methods of coping as pathological, leading at best to a withdrawn and alienated urban dweller and at worst to social, psychological, and physiological breakdown. This justified a close, collaborative relationship between social and behavioral scientists and the planning and design professions. Others, more commonly sociologists, perceived crowding less as a psychological state or stress syndrome and more as a stressor that the individual was able to adapt to in positive and productive ways. Focusing so much attention on the physical environment meant that more significant social and economic factors were being ignored. When stress was mentioned within this literature, it was seen to result from the problems of social inequality, poverty, segregation, and discrimination. Thus, while the fluidity of the concept of stress had provided a means of establishing a degree of unity among the Space Cadets, it could also serve opposing agendas: as a means of establishing objective physical standards for psychological health or, alternatively, as a criticism of such ambitions as damaging to life in the city.

Notes

1. Louis Wirth, "Urbanism as a Way of Life," *American Journal of Sociology* 44 (1938): 1–24.

2. Leonard Duhl explained to an audience of psychiatrists how the name, coined by August Hollingshead, reflected the radical and unconventional nature of their approach to mental health: "several years ago in the middle of one of our way-out discussions, the Russians shot up a Sputnik, and the title of the group became Space Cadets, and it has been that way ever since" Duhl, transcript, Thirty-Ninth Annual Meeting of the American Orthopsychiatric Association, "The Environment of the Metropolis," Biltmore Hotel, Los Angeles, California, March 22, 1962, box 65, accession 2, John B. Calhoun Papers, National Library of Medicine (hereafter cited as NLM), Bethesda, MD, p. 55.

3. John B. Calhoun, "Looking Backwards from 'The Beautiful Ones,'" in *Discovery Processes in Modern Biology*, ed. W. R. Klemm (Huntington, NY: Krieger, 1977), 51. Unfortunately, not all the transcripts were available in the papers of John B. Calhoun. The collection is missing some of those from 1965 and 1966. There are also some closely related conference transcripts available that involved members of the Space Cadets, such as the Conference on Leisure–Outdoor Recreation and Mental Health, Williamsburg, Virginia, June 1, 1961, box 67, Calhoun Papers, NLM.

4. Leonard Duhl, ed. *The Urban Condition: People and Policy in the Metropolis* (New York: Basic Books, 1963). The collection consisted mainly of papers from the Thirty-Ninth Annual Meeting of the American Orthopsychiatric Association in 1962, but both the conference and volume were considered the "culmination" of the Space Cadet meetings (ibid., xiii).

5. Duhl, "Opening Remarks," Thirty-Ninth Annual Meeting of the American Orthopsychiatric Association, p. 7.

6. Emanuel Gaziano, "Ecological Metaphors as Scientific Boundary Work: Innovation and Authority in Interwar Sociology and Biology," *American Journal of Sociology* 101 (1996): 874–907.

7. John S. Pipkin, Mark La Gory, and Judith R. Blau, "The Social Significance of Form," in *Remaking the City: Social Science Perspectives on Urban Design*, ed. John S. Pipkin, Mark La Gory, and Judith R. Blau (Albany: SUNY Press, 1983), 116. Nevertheless, their interest in "natural areas" of the city caused them considerable criticism, reflecting the degree to which the focus on the physical environment was becoming problematic in sociology. Gerald D. Suttles, *The Social Order of the Slum: Ethnicity and Territory in the Inner City* (Chicago: University of Chicago Press, 1968), 6.

8. Robert E. Park, "The City: Suggestions for the Investigation of Human Behavior in the Urban Environment," in *The City*, ed. Robert E. Park, Ernest W. Burgess, and Roderick D. McKenzie (1925; repr., Chicago: University of Chicago Press, 1967), 1. While Park had an enduring interest in the crowd, largely in terms of political action and collective behavior, there was little analysis of the effects of density on health.

9. Gunnar Myrdal, *An American Dilemma* (New York: Harper and Bros., 1944), quoted in Alvin L. Schorr, *Slums and Social Insecurity* (Edinburgh: Nelson, 1964), 143; James S. Plant, "Some Psychiatric Aspects of Crowded Living Conditions," *American Journal of Psychiatry* 9 (1930): 853; Robert E. L. Faris and H. Warren Dunham, *Mental Disorders in Urban Areas* (Chicago: University of Chicago Press, 1939).

10. Federal programs of slum clearance and the provision of public housing first emerged during the New Deal. The approach of the Housing Act of 1937 was reproduced in its essentials in the 1949 act, which intensified the process and focused more attention on housing provision. Eugene J. Meehan, "The Rise and Fall of Public Housing: Condemnation without Trial," in *A Decent Home and Environment: Housing Urban America*, ed. Donald Phares (Cambridge, MA: Ballinger, 1977), 3–42. Local redevelopment agencies were given immense powers of land taking and federal subsidies for redevelopment. While interests in social welfare were prominent, they were combined with business interests, meaning that much of the land was cleared for private entrepreneurs rather than the provision of low-cost housing. Chester Hartman, *Between Eminence and Notoriety: Four Decades of Radical Urban Planning* (New Brunswick: Center for Urban Policy Research, 2002).

11. For work that explores the interest of behavioral scientists in the mental health of urban populations, see Hans Pols, "Anomie in the Metropolis: The City in American Sociology and Psychiatry," in *Science and the City*, ed. Sven Dierig, Jens Lachmund, and J. Andrew Mendelsohn, Osiris 18 (2003): 194–211; and Samuel Bloom's excellent study of medical sociology, *The Word as Scalpel: A History of Medical Sociology* (New York: Oxford University Press, 2002). However, the focus is on mental health and social class. The links between behavioral science, psychiatry, and the professions of architecture and city planning have received little attention from historians.

12. Leonard Duhl, "The Changing Face of Mental Health," in Duhl, *Urban Condition*, 59.

13. Duhl, transcript of Conference on the Physical Environment as a Determinant of Mental Health, Washington, DC, May 28–29, 1956, box 63, Calhoun Papers, NLM, 174.

14. Ibid., 142.

15. Nicolas Rashevsky, Conference on Social and Physical Environment Variables as Determinants of Mental Health, American Psychological Association Building, Washington, DC, May 6–7, 1957, box 63, Calhoun Papers, NLM, 6.

16. Leonard Duhl, conference transcript, May 28–29, 1956, 1–2.

17. John B. Calhoun to Fillmore Sanford of the APA, May 4, 1956, box 63, Calhoun Papers, NLM.

18. John B. Calhoun, conference transcript, May 28–29, 1956, 3.

19. Edmund Ramsden, "From Rodent Utopia to Urban Hell: Population, Pathology, and the Crowded Rats of NIMH," *Isis* 102 (2011): 659–88.

20. John B. Calhoun, conference transcript, May 28–29, 1956, 66.

21. August Hollingshead, conference transcript, May 28–29, 1956, 17. See also August B. Hollingshead and Fredrick C. Redlich, *Social Class and Mental Illness: A Community Study* (New York: Wiley and Sons, 1958).

22. Hollingshead, conference transcript, May 28–29, 1956, 181–85.

23. Ibid., 204–5. Seeley's perspective was shared by Gans, who believed that many of the traits and behaviors that social scientists and psychiatrists (Duhl, Lindemann, and Jahoda included) considered "pathological" were in fact the consequence of differences in culture and goals between classes and communities. Gans, Lindemann Seminar—Notes on Community Policy and Mental Health, February 27, 1957, folder 8, box 2, Herbert Gans Papers, Rare Book and Manuscript Library (hereafter cited as RBML), Columbia University, New York.

24. Marie Jahoda, presentation on concepts of mental health, conference on Social and Physical Environment Variables as Determinants of Mental Health, Washington, DC, October 17–18, 1957, box 63, Calhoun Papers, NLM. This was based on Jahoda's study: *Current Concepts of Positive Mental Health* (New York: Basic Books, 1958). Jahoda had also worked on the social psychology of housing; her study of suburban life was an important influence on Gans's study of Levittown. Herbert Gans to Erich Lindemann, 1957, folder 8, box 2, Gans Papers, RBML.

25. Erich Lindemann, *Beyond Grief: Studies in Crisis Intervention* (Northvale, NJ: Aronson, 1979), 101.

26. Richard Meier, conference transcript, October 17–18, 1957, 5–8.

27. August Hollingshead, conference transcript, May 6–7, 1957, 4.

28. Meier, conference transcript, October, 17–18, 1957, 5.

29. Deevey, conference transcript, October, 17–18, 1957, 14.

30. T. C. Schneirla, conference transcript, October, 17–18, 1957, 9.

31. T. C. Schneirla, conference transcript, October, 17–18, 1957, 26. At times the term "stress" was applied to both stimulus and response. Wilner observed that Meier was using "the same term on both ends. That which you are altering . . . that which you do to bring about something measured by its effect on the individual, you are willing to call by the same essential name, the stressor and the stress." Meier confessed to being pragmatic in his approach: "It is hard to set the dividing point. We are calling these all stress phenomena, and letting it go at that" (ibid., 16–17).

32. Erich Lindemann, "Mental Health and the Environment," in Duhl, *Urban Condition*, 3–10.

33. August Hollingshead, conference transcript, May 28–29, 1956, 187–90, 206, 190.

34. Richard Meier, conference transcript, October 17, 1957, 17; John B. Calhoun, conference transcript, May 28–29, 1956, 270.

35. Catherine Bauer, transcript, Conference on Social and Physical Environment Variables as Determinants of Mental Health, Washington, DC, May 26–27, 1958, box 64, Calhoun Papers, NLM, 22.

36. Daniel Wilner, 171; Bauer, 76; John Stewart, 90; Leonard Duhl, 214; John B. Calhoun, 140; all in conference transcripts, May 28–29, 1956.

37. There were also other examples of planning in relation to mental health that the participants focused on, such as Poston's work in relation to Cairo, Illinois. Poston had been active in attempts to have local communities involve themselves with planning (see Poston's description of this work in ibid., 233–66).

38. Daniel Wilner, ibid., 8–10.

39. Leonard Duhl, conference transcript, May 26–27, 1958, 2.

40. Daniel Wilner, presentation, Conference of Social and Physical Environment Variables as Determinants of Mental Health, May 22, 1959, box 64, Calhoun Papers, NLM, 109.

41. Daniel Wilner, Rosabelle P. Walkley, Thomas C. Pinkerton, and Matthew Tayback, *The Housing Environment and Family Life: A Longitudinal Study of the Effects of Housing on Morbidity and Mental Health* (Baltimore: Johns Hopkins University Press, 1962), 147; cf. Daniel Wilner and Rosabelle P. Walkley, "Effects of Housing on Health and Performance," in Duhl, *Urban Condition*, 215–28.

42. John Seeley, conference, transcript May 28–29, 1956, 127.

43. John Seeley, conference transcript, October 17–18, 1957, 43. He was supported by Gans, who argued, "The physical-social distinction hides the fact that any aspect of the physical environment must directly or indirectly be relevant to what social beings are doing before we need be concerned with it" (ibid.).

44. Duhl was described as "a central person in every phase of the study." As a member of the NIMH, he "encouraged the initial funding of the study and he was, throughout, a model for the effective facilitation of research." Marc Fried, *The World of the Urban Working Class*, with Ellen Fitzgerald, Peggy Gleicher, and Chester Hartman (Cambridge: Harvard University Press, 1973), vii. The editor of Lindemann's collected papers on crisis theory and intervention described how Duhl's Space Cadets had broadened Lindemann's interest in the effect of government policies on coping

patterns in the community and that these meetings had led directly to the West End project. Lindemann, *Beyond Grief*, 138.

45. Marc Fried, "Grieving for a Lost Home," presentation at "Environment of the Metropolis"; Fried, "Grieving for a Lost Home," in Duhl, *Urban Condition*, 151–71.

46. Thomas H. O'Connor, *Building a New Boston: Politics and Urban Renewal, 1950–1970* (Boston: Northeastern University Press, 1993); Lawrence J. Vale, *From the Puritans to the Projects: Public Housing and Public Neighbors* (Cambridge: Harvard University Press, 2000).

47. American Public Health Association, Committee on the Hygiene of Housing, *An Appraisal Method for Measuring the Quality of Housing* (New York: APHA, 1946).

48. "West End Project Report: A Preliminary Redevelopment Study of the West End of Boston," March 1953, folder 3, box 2, Urban Redevelopment Division, Boston Housing Authority, Gans Papers, RBML. See also O'Connor, *Building a New Boston*, 130.

49. "Charles River Park: The Wonderful Experience of Spacious In-Town Living," brochure, folder 2, box 1, Gans Papers, RBML.

50. "Relocation and Mental Health: Adaptation under Stress," folder 13, box 1, Gans Papers, RBML.

51. Duhl noted the difference that also existed regarding noise. He stated that Gans had remarked on the continuous noise that had surrounded him while living in the West End. However, rather than this being a source of stress, it was important to West Enders, connecting them to others and reinforcing "their sense of identity and strength." Conference transcript, May 26–27, 1958, 13.

52. Marc Fried and Peggy Gleicher, "Some Sources of Residential Satisfaction in an Urban Slum," *Journal of the American Institute of Planners* 27 (1961): 314. They also described the observations and experiments of animal ecologists and ethologists as having "considerable bearing on these issues" (311). For another study that took a similar take on "territory" and the slum, see Suttles, *Social Order*.

53. Chester Hartman, "The Limitations of Public Housing: Relocation Choices in a Working-Class Community," *Journal of the American Institute of Planners* 29 (1963): 284. Hartman, a planner who joined the project in 1961, interpreted such a response as reasonable once one considered the social understanding of space. While the projects were physically less crowded, with the lack of structured and meaningful relationships and the absence of control over various personal and spatial elements, the environment would be experienced as more crowded (285).

54. Fried and Gleicher, "Residential Satisfaction," 315.

55. Duhl had first suggested to Gans that he contact Lindemann with regard to the possibility of working on "a cooperative program between a planning group and mental health workers." He described Lindemann as leading "the best preventative mental health program in the country." Leonard Duhl to Herbert Gans, April 5, 1955, folder 2, box 1, Gans Papers, RBML.

56. See correspondence between Gans's and Lindemann's group in folder 2, box 1, Gans papers, RBML.

57. Gans had wanted to circulate early drafts of a paper critical of the redevelopment of the West End to West Enders and members of the Urban Renewal Administration in Washington to improve relocation prospects and then to publish it in the *Journal of the American Institute of Planners*. Herbert Gans to Erich Lindemann,

June 30, 1958, folder 8, box 1, Gans Papers, RBML. The paper was "The Human Implications of Current Redevelopment and Relocation Planning," *Journal of the American Institute of Planners* 25 (1959): 15–26. Lindemann responded, "I am really worried that it would not be compatible with our role as a research organization in the West End to intervene by early publication of our observations in the course of events." Lindemann to Gans, July 7, 1958, folder 2, box 1, Gans Papers, RBML. Gans found himself in a difficult position. On the one hand, he tried to counter antipathy toward Lindemann's group among some key residents due to its lack of political engagement. The writer and West Ender Joseph Caruso wrote to Gans on July 18, 1958: "In fact, I'm going to stop the 'family group' from further contact with me. Anything sponsored by the M.G.H. isn't worth a shit! Anyway, the only reason I refrained from sinking it is you." Gans explained to Caruso that it was the objectivity of Lindemann's study that ensured "they will be listened to. If they come out on one side just as the study gets under way, they will kill off any effectiveness they might have in the future. Thus, I cannot blame Lindemann for what he did; it would have been wrong for him to do otherwise, unless there were some real chance to overturn the West End redevelopment at this time, which you know as well as I there isnt." Herbert Gans to Joseph Caruso, July 21, 1958, folder 1, box 1, Gans Papers, RBML. Gans did provide Caruso and others connected with the West End renewal with a draft of his paper, with the understanding that while the information could be used, it was not to be directly referenced or "used as a political document." Gans to Caruso, June 5, 1958, and cf. Gans to "Joe" Caruso, July 11, folder 8, box 1, Gans Papers, RBML. In a memorandum, Gans expressed his concerns to the project members: "If the team is in the long run concerned with mental health service to the community, it should know the relocation plan problems. . . . It could then decide whether it would be feasible and desirable to take some steps to affect the redevelopment and relocation plans for the area in the interest of contributing to the mental health of the present residents." He recognized that direct involvement would influence the problem being studied and thus the project itself, as well as inciting the opposition of the MGH administration to service activities. But Gans felt they should be more active in community organization or, at the very least, surreptitiously assist certain individuals. "Problems of Relocation and Redevelopment Planning in the West End, as These Affect the Service Function of the West End Research Project," January 23, 1958, folder 8, box 1, Gans Papers, RBML. Duhl also noted the institutional weakness of Lindemann's group. As their aim was to provide mental health, they thus, surely, should help fight redevelopment; however, a lot of the MGH staff did not want a "slum population" in the area at all. Thus, the Department of Psychiatry could not do anything "out of fear of their very existence"; they "can't operate in conflict with the Massachusetts General Hospital's sphere of thinking." Duhl's remarks, Conference on the Physical Determinant as a Determinant of Mental Health, October 11–12, 1956, box 63, Calhoun Papers, NLM, 115.

58. Herbert Gans, "Human Implications"; Gans, *The Urban Villagers: Group and Class in the Life of Urban Americans* (New York: Free Press, 1962); Gans, *People and Plans: Essays on Urban Problems and Solutions* (New York: Basic Books, 1968).

59. Herbert Gans, "Some Notes on a Proposed Participant-Observation Study of the Boston West End," folder 2, box 2, Gans Papers, RBML.

60. Herbert Gans, "An Analysis of Redevelopment and Relocation Planning for the West End of Boston," May 1958, folder 8, box 1, Gans Papers, RBML.

61. Conference, October 17–18, 1957, 59.

62. Herbert Gans, "The Potential Environment and the Effective Environment," paper presented at Space Cadets, 1958, in Gans, *People and Plans,* 9. For example, when studying a community in Park Forest, Illinois, in 1949, Gans wrote to the planner David A. Wallace on the "advisability of backyards." He advised that they needed to be designed to help provide privacy and independence and to reduce crowding in other communal areas. Memorandum, n.d., folder 4, box 38, Gans Papers, RBML.

63. Herbert Gans, "City Planning and Urban Realities," *Commentary* 33 (1962): 170–75.

64. Peter Marris to Herbert Gans, November 19, 1962, folder 6, box 1, Gans Papers, RBML. See also Peter Marris, "The Socials Implications of Urban Development," *Journal of the American Institute of Planners* 28 (1962): 180–86; and "A Report on Urban Renewal in the United States," in Duhl, *Urban Condition,* 113–34; Michael Young, *Family and Kinship in East London* (London: Routledge and Kegan Paul, 1957). For an excellent analysis of the emergence of community and neighborhood studies in sociology, see Christian Topalov, "'Traditional Working-Class Neighborhoods': An Inquiry into the Emergence of a Sociological Model in the 1950s and 1960s," in *Science and the City,* ed. Sven Dierig, Jens Lachmund, and J. Andrew Mendelsohn, Osiris 18 (2003): 212–33.

65. Jane Jacobs to "Herb" Gans, November 24, 1958, folder 4, box 1, Gans Papers, RBML. See Jane Jacobs, *The Death and Life of Great American Cities* (New York: Random House, 1961).

66. Hartman, *Between Eminence and Notoriety,* 9.

67. David A. Wallace, "The Conceptualizing of Urban Renewal," *University of Toronto Law Journal* 18 (1968): 248, 257.

68. In his notes for a seminar talk, Gans explained that while he believed that "most people are quite flexible in adapting to the physical environment," he did not want to "throw [the] baby out w[ith the] bathwater." The physical environment "can have neg[ative] effects, can make people uncomfortable." Most important was the lack of space "inside [the] dwelling" This, he suggested, was "one reason why [there was so] much street life in poor n[eighbor]hoods." "Gettysburg," Gans Papers, folder 4, box 36, RBML.

69. Notes titled "jane," folder 4, box 39, Gans Papers, RBML.

70. Gans, "City Planning," 174.

71. Herbert Gans, "Housing and the Urban Poor," 1965, folder 10, box 38, Gans Papers, RBML.

72. Herbert Gans to Jane Jacobs, January 19, 1962, folder 4, box 39, Gans Papers, RBML. Gans described himself as a "New deal lib. Of which I'm still more or less one." Notes, "iowa, Urb Revit, Dream or Illusion," folder 1, box 37, Gans Papers, RBML.

73. Leonard Duhl to "Mel" Webber, March 24, 1959, folder 8, box 1, Gans Papers, RBML. There was also a third article by Richard Meier. See Herbert Gans, "Human Implications," and John R. Seeley, "The Slum: Its Nature, Use, and Users," *Journal of the American Institute of Planners* 25 (1959): 7–14.

74. While Wilner had identified the benefits to health that could result from improved housing, in Baltimore things hadn't necessarily gone to plan. "I have been in Baltimore sitting on the very edge of a piece of planning which it seems to me has gone totally awry. . . . They tore down . . . block after block of the filthiest slum dwellings imaginable and the rubble has been sitting there for three years. . . . Four or five thousand people have been dispossessed here and they are goodness knows where now. . . . Planning is not well planned." Conference, May 28–29, 1956, 277.

75. John B. Calhoun, conference transcript, May 28–29, 1956, 168.

76. The issue of freedom of choice regarding housing was also critical to the discussions of the Space Cadets, and to the relationship between psychology and planning more generally, but it is beyond the scope of this paper.

77. Melvin M. Webber, "Comprehensive Planning and Social Responsibility: Toward an AIP Consensus on the Profession's Roles and Purposes," *Journal of American Institute of Planners* 29 (1963): 233.

78. President Johnson had established a Task Force on Urban Problems in 1964, chaired by the political scientist and soon to be HUD undersecretary, Robert C. Wood. Duhl and a colleague submitted a two-page memorandum that privileged the "social and psychological" over mere "bricks and mortar." John A. Andrew III, *Lyndon Johnson and the Great Society* (Chicago: Dee, 1998), 135. Duhl suggested that three "demonstration cities" be selected for comprehensive rebuilding, combined with programs of social and economic improvement. Wood had attached it as an appendix to the task force's report, but it later became, he recollected, the basis of the Model City legislation. Wood traced the heritage of the memorandum, in turn, through to "Duhl's own advisory group (dubbed 'space cadets.')." Robert C. Wood, *Whatever Possessed the President? Academic Experts and Presidential Policy, 1960–1988* (Amherst: University of Massachusetts Press, 1993), 79.

79. Duhl, conference transcript, Social and Physical Environment Variables as Determinants of Mental Health, Washington, DC, March 17, 1966, box 67, Calhoun Papers, NLM, 5, 6, 11.

80. Leonard Duhl, "Life Cycle of the Individual," paper prepared for Working Group in US Government in the Year 2000, box 301, RG 207, Records of the Department of Housing and Urban Development, National Archives and Records Administration (hereafter cited as NARA), 14.

81. Herbert Gans, "Housing the Urban Poor," 1965, folder 10, box 38, Gans Papers, RBML.

82. Notes, "NYU-AIP Students," folder 2, box 36, Gans Papers, RBML.

83. Robert C. Weaver, "A Report on the Past, Present and Future of the U.S. Department of Housing and Urban Development," presented at the annual convention of the National Housing Conference, Washington, DC, April 9, 1967, box 306, RG 207, HUD Records, NARA.

84. Edmund Ramsden and Jon Adams, "Escaping the Laboratory: The Rodent Experiments of John B. Calhoun and Their Cultural Influence," *Journal of Social History* 42 (2009): 761–92.

85. Edward T. Hall, *The Hidden Dimension* (Garden City, NY: Doubleday, 1966), 165; Ian L. McHarg, "Man and Environment" in Duhl, *Urban Condition*, 48–49.

86. Omar R. Galle, Walter R. Gove, and J. Miller McPherson, "Population Density and Pathology: What Are the Relations for Man?" *Science* 176 (1972): 24.

87. Robert C. Schmitt, "Implications of Density in Hong Kong," *Journal of American Institute of Planners* 29 (1963): 210–17; Schmitt, "Density, Health, and Social Disorganization," *Journal of American Institute of Planners* 32 (1966): 38–40; Halliman H. Winsborough, "The Social Consequences of High Population Density," *Law and Contemporary Problems* 30 (1965): 120–26.

88. Robert E. Mitchell, "Some Social Implications of High Density Housing," *American Sociological Review* 36 (1971): 18–29; Mitchell, "Misconceptions about Man-Made Space: In Partial Defense of High Density Housing," *Family Coordinator* 23 (1974): 51–56.

89. Joachim F. Wohlwill, "The Environment Is Not in the Head!," in *Environmental Design Research,* vol. 2, ed. Wolfgang F. E. Preiser (Stroudsburg, PA: Dowden, Hutchinson, and Ross, 1973), 166.

90. Walter R. Gove, Michael Hughes, and Omer R. Galle, "Overcrowding in the Home: An Empirical Investigation of Its Possible Pathological Consequences," *American Sociological Review* 44 (1979): 60.

91. Galle, Gove, and McPherson, "Population Density," 28.

92. Daniel Stokols, "On the Distinction between Density and Crowding: Some Implications for Future Research," *Psychological Review* 79 (1972): 276. See also Stokols, "The Experience of Crowding in Primary and Secondary Environments," *Environment and Behavior* 8 (1976): 49–86; Stokols, "In Defense of the Crowding Construct," in *The Urban Environment,* vol. 1 of *Advances in Environmental Psychology,* ed. Andrew Baum, Jerome E. Singer, and Stuart Valins (Hillsdale, NJ: Erlbaum, 1978); Stokols, Walter Ohlig, and Susan M. Resnick, "Perception of Residential Crowding, Classroom Experiences, and Student Health," *Human Ecology* 6 (1978): 233–52.

93. Galle, Gove, and McPherson, "Population Density," 26.

94. Don Hummel, "A Report on the Past, Present and Future of the U.S. Department of Housing and Urban Development," presented at the annual convention of the National Housing Conference, April 9, 1967.

95. Stokols, "Crowding Construct," 111.

96. Joe Flower, "Building Healthier Cities: A Conversation with Leonard J. Duhl, MD," *Healthcare Forum Journal* 75 (May–June 1993): 51. The Model Cities program was also hindered by expansion beyond the recommended three cities, a lack of funding, and ineffective interaction between agencies. See Bernard J. Frieden and Marshall Kaplan, *The Politics of Neglect: Urban Aid from Model Cities to Revenue Sharing* (Cambridge, MA: MIT Press, 1975).

97. Fried expressed his support for Gans's position: "Except for truly degraded housing, however, the consequences of poor physical housing seem to be fairly limited and are, to some degree, compensated by other residential experiences. Poverty and unemployment have wider ramifications." *Urban Working Class,* 232.

98. Herbert Gans, presentation at Ninth Meeting of the Committee on Social and Physical Environment Variables as Determinants of Mental Health, NIH, Bethesda, May 19, 1960, box 64, Calhoun Papers, NLM, 69.

99. Gans often interpreted Wilner's study as having shown little real psychological improvement as a consequence of better housing. See, for example, "The City and the Poor," 1965, folder 10, box 38, Gans Papers.

100. Herbert Gans to Clare Cooper, June 3, 1974, folder 9, box 35, Gans Papers, RBML; Notes, "Future of the City," n.d., folder 2, box 36, Gans Papers, RBML.

101. Gans was very critical of the Moynihan report, for example, for pathologizing the black family. "The Negro Family: Reflections on the Moynihan Report" (1965), in *The Moynihan Report and the Politics of Controversy*, ed. Lee Rainwater and William L. Yancey (Cambridge MA: MIT Press, 1967).

102. Gans referred in particular to the work of Robert Mitchell (see "Some Social Implications of High Density Housing," and "Misconceptions about Man-Made Space"), Rough draft of "Density Talk, 15–20 Min," folder 3, box 36, Gans Papers, RBML. While this talk is not dated, the reference to Mitchell means that it is post-1971.

103. Some of the apparent contradictions in Gans's position, and the problems that it raised for planners, were discussed by the Space Cadets; see, in particular, Ninth Meeting of the Committee on Social and Physical Environment Variables, May 19, 1960, 69–86. Even Peter Willmott, whose studies of Dagenham had influenced, and been influenced by, Gans's studies of suburban life, wrote to him: "You are still so concerned to demolish the 'architectural determinists' that you over-state the case, I think." Peter Willmott to Herbert Gans, April 10, 1962, folder 15, box 36, Gans Papers, RBML.

104. Herbert Gans, "Statement on Urban Renewal and City Planning in New York State," n.d., folder 3, box 36, Gans Papers, RBML.

105. Mark Baldassare, *Residential Crowding in Urban America* (Berkeley: University of California Press, 1979), 7. Baldassare and Fischer's work was also stimulated by a concern of the influence of ethology and animal studies on the social and behavioral sciences; see Ramsden, "Rodent Utopia." The concept of territoriality, having been used by Fried to great effect, also suffered due to its "associations with 'instinctual' or 'innate' theories of human behavior." Richard M. Merelman, "The Political Uses of Territoriality," *Environment and Behavior* 20 (1988): 576–600.

106. Claude S. Fischer, "The Public and Private Worlds of City Life," American Sociological Review 46 (1981): 306.

107. Baldassare, "Residential Density, Household Crowding, and Social Networks," in Claude S. Fischer, Robert Max Jackson, C. Ann Stueve, Kathleen Gerson, Lynne McCallister Jones, with Mark Baldassare, eds., *Networks and Places: Social Relations in the Urban Setting* (New York: Free Press, 1977), 111.

108. Baldassare, *Residential Crowding*, 188.

109. Claude S. Fischer, "Sociological Comments on Psychological Approaches to Urban Life," in Baum, Singer, and Valins, *Advances in Environmental Psychology*, 142.

110. Claude S. Fischer, *The Urban Experience* (New York: Harcourt Brace Jovanovich, 1976), 236.

111. Gans, "City Planning," 170.

112. As Gans explained to Fried, the writing of his book was slow due to his study of the suburban community of Levittown. Herbert Gans to Marc Fried, March 19, 1959, folder 2, box 2, Gans Papers, RBML. In his study of the suburb, he again countered the premise that, due to the environment, suburban life was "so full of stress that it increases psychosomatic illness, divorce, alcoholism, suicide attempts and mental illness generally." See "The Effects of the Move from City to Suburb, and Their Implications for Physical and Social Planning," folder 15, box 38, Gans Papers, RBML. See also Herbert Gans, *The Levittowners: Life and Politics in a New Suburban Community* (New York: Vintage, 1967).

113. His "arguments against renewal were not accepted by them," he went on, "until the ghettoes began to protest effectively against 'Negro removal.'" Herbert Gans to Mark Granovetter, February 7, 1974, folder 3, box 1, Gans Papers. Gans's work was also poorly received by other relevant professionals such as social workers, as a Canadian social worker, Michel Blondin, explained. Letter to Herbert Gans, May 5, 1965, folder 6, box 1, Gans Papers, RBML.

114. Letter to the Editor, *New York Herald Tribune*, September 8, 1962, folder: Letters to the Editor, 1960–2003, box 35, Gans Papers, RBML. He was responding to an article that described him as wholly critical of low-income housing.

115. Wilner et al., *Housing Environment and Family Life*; John B. Calhoun, "Population Density and Social Pathology," *Scientific American* 306 (1962): 139–48.

116. Daniel Adelson, review of *Urban Condition*, by Leonard Duhl, *Community Health Journal* 3 (1967): 410.

Chapter Twelve

Sadness in Camberwell

Imagining Stress and Constructing History in Postwar Britain

Rhodri Hayward

Introduction: Stress and the Problem of Temporality

Implicit within every model of stress is a particular understanding of time. Stress disorders, in their myriad forms, are variously attributed to the fears and terrors of an anticipated future, the pressure of present circumstances, or traumas arising from events buried deep in the individual's past. They are also associated with temporal experience being connected to the increased velocity of life or its slowing down through long episodes of boredom or sensory deprivation. Psychosomatic medicine, in its various forms and iterations over the past two hundred years, has sustained these different temporalities through reference to a rich armamentarium of psychological and physiological objects—ranging from the practices of "expectant attention" described by nineteenth-century mental physiologists through to the hypothalamic-pituitary-adrenal (HPA) axis that plays a central role in twenty-first-century understandings of the stress response.

The sheer number of concepts deployed in descriptions of the stress response and the broad variety of narratives that these make possible have attracted widespread critical comment from anthropologists, historians, cultural critics, and practicing stress researchers. Stress is derided as a sort of "conceptual glue" that can connect forms of physiological and psychological disturbance to any number of experiences and events.[1] While these criticisms are rich and often provocative it is not my intention to rehearse them again here. Rather, I want to concentrate on how stress disorders have been connected to specific life events and ways in which those connections have been stabilized. To explore this process—and the practical and intellectual labor involved in connecting stress to a particular event and particular form of temporality—I offer a close study of the work carried out by the sociologist George Brown and the clinical psychologist Tirril Harris in their landmark study, *The Social Origins of Depression* (1978).[2]

Between 1969 and 1973 Brown and Harris carried out two detailed studies on the relationship between life events and depression. Their work, which focused on depression rates among women in the South London suburb of Camberwell, was remarkable for its high degree of methodological reflection and its theoretical rigor. It made available a new set of conceptual tools—the "index of expressed emotion," "brought forward time," "effort after meaning," and "contextual threat"—that established the grounds for a new program of psychiatric research. At the same time it provided the rationale for a series of political interventions targeting the problems of motherhood and infant care in the 1980s and 1990s.[3] It also, I think, has certain historiographical implications. The psychiatric epidemiology developed by Brown and Harris allows us to think critically about the models of time and causation deployed in contemporary historical writing. In particular their reflections on the associations between events and illness provide a useful counterpoint to the current debates among historians over the limits of historical understanding and the role of neurobiology and evolutionary psychology in the explanation of historical change.

This chapter is organized in four sections. The first sets out to demonstrate the contingency of the temporal assumptions that underlie modern stress narratives. It does so by providing a brief tour of the changing relationship between stress, time, and pathology from the early nineteenth century onward. This short sketch should also serve to demonstrate the changing significance of the different elements in the stress narrative. It illustrates the back-and-forth shift from explanations founded on personal experience to broader sociological accounts that concentrate on such elements as urban organization. The second section introduces the work of George Brown. It focuses on his early research at the Institute of Psychiatry in London and his attempt to develop a metric of stress that could be used in studies of schizophrenia. The third section concentrates on two surveys of life stress and depression that Brown and Harris carried out in Camberwell in 1969 and 1973.[4] It looks at the strategies that they developed to control the meanings attached to stressful events and thereby insulate them from the corrupting influence of autobiographical memory. In particular it raises the problem of the psychological labor involved in producing estimates and etiologies of stress. The final section explores how these etiological narratives were stabilized and rewritten through reference to another order of time—the Pleistocene era held up as the environment of earliest adaptation (EEA) in evolutionary psychology. In examining how the meaning of experience was stabilized and universalized through reference to the EEA, this chapter uses Brown and Harris's work to think critically about the turn to evolutionary neuroscience in recent historical writing.

The Temporal Assumptions of Stress

The contingency of the temporal models that underlie different understandings of stress becomes apparent in even the most cursory historical survey. Whereas twenty-first-century theories describe stress in terms of present experience (in models of cognitive or physical overload) or past suffering and loss (as in post-traumatic stress disorder, or PTSD), early nineteenth-century understandings were structured around the practice of expectation. Informed by Baconian medicine and the growing critical literature on mesmeric practice, medical practitioners claimed that anticipated events inscribed themselves on the body through the powers of imaginative concentration.[5] These anecdotes were formalized in the concept of "expectant attention." Sustained worry or anguish was understood as creating "dominant ideas" that corrupted the action of the lower nervous centers and hence the normal function of the body.[6] Anxiety over future events was thus seen as sustaining a vast range of psychosomatic conditions from heartbreak to hair loss.

By the second half of the nineteenth century the anticipatory model of psychosomatic disorder was being displaced by a new emphasis on the role of memory in the generation of physical and psychological complaints. In the writings of Frederic Myers, Pierre Janet, Jean-Martin Charcot, and Sigmund Freud (among others) the "dominant ideas" that had once orchestrated the body's unconscious responses were now replaced by fragments of memory orphaned from waking consciousness by trauma. In their writings the grounds of unconscious response shifted from the stress of an imagined future to that of a forgotten past.[7]

The break however was not clear-cut. Physiological rationalizations of functional illness, particularly those produced by Walter Cannon, George Crile, and later Hans Selye, played on the disjunction of temporal order as an explanation for pathological response. Thus, Cannon argued that "the persistent derangement of bodily functions in strong emotional reactions can be interpreted as due to the persistence of the stimuli which evoke the reactions. They may persist because not naturally eliminated by the completion of the emotional impulse, or because completion of the stimuli is made impossible by circumstance."[8] Similarly, Selye and others drew from cybernetics the idea that the alarm reaction could be rendered pathological through its extension in cycles of positive feedback. In this cybernetic model physiological routines that had been mobilized to defend the organism against a momentary threat persisted after the threat's removal. This led to a pattern of ulceration and exhaustion that Selye termed the "general adaptation syndrome."[9]

Selye's and Cannon's work located stress in the tension between two different systems: the prehistoric system of evolutionary adaptation and the present environment with its complex and constrained interactions. Through this combination of two different temporalities—the present and the prehistoric—the etiology of stress was extended. There was a movement away from the "family romances" that had been fielded in the psychoanalytic explanations of individual breakdown toward a new recognition of the pathogenic role of social forces. This recognition was partly driven by left-wing dissatisfaction with the Freudian failure to recognize the etiological role of political and economic conditions and by the emergence of new forms of political intervention during World War II.[10]

With the outbreak of World War II, the historical and biographical narratives that had been used to sustain the psychological meaning of illnesses, such as peptic ulcers or minor neuroses, were largely abandoned. The family romances that had been used to explain symptoms in psychoanalytic case histories were now obscured behind the drama of military engagement and civilian bombardment. Government agencies, including the Department of Home Intelligence and the Ministry of Home Security, launched large-scale studies of the "arithmetics of stress" (to use Richard Titmuss's phrase) that mapped changes in behavior and illness rate against the frequency of raids while ignoring, for good practical reasons, any attempt to relate patterns of breakdown to the shape of individual biography.[11] Stress now became visible across the population as a whole, displayed in the patterns of sickness insurance returns or workplace absenteeism, and with this change its etiology shifted from the biographical to the social.[12] It became an environmental illness.

In their effacement of individual history these wartime surveys transformed the social landscape into a field of threats. It was configured as a collection of psychological costs that determined levels of stress and morale but could be controlled through the strategic management of resources and information. As Allan Young noted thirty years ago, "By displacing the human subject from his place in society to a de-socialized and amorphous environment, the discourse banishes the arena of conflicting class and group interests from the real conditions of existence. In its place, the discourse substitutes a *zone of anxiety* within which the power to affect people's well-being is diffuse and subjective."[13] The rich detail of individual history and biography was exchanged for a vision of subjectivity as an elementary collection of psychological resources. Yet this exchange did not lead to the disregard of biographical detail. In the years of postwar reconstruction, large-scale surveys into the relationship between environment and mental health attempted to recover increasingly detailed information regarding the lives of their respondents. Family interactions, domestic arrangements, patterns of leisure, and political attitudes were opened up for psychiatric examination.[14] This information was not treated as a holistic insight that would somehow reveal the full complexity of the respondent's personality; rather, these new findings were presented as series of additional variables that would correct errors in multifactorial analysis. Stress was neither determined by the future nor generated by the buried secrets of the past. It emerged through the complex interaction of present tensions and the failure of the individual to adapt to current circumstances.[15]

George Brown and the Problem of Family Tension

It was this multifactorial understanding of stress that would provide the cornerstone for George Brown's work.[16] His own career began in government work, assessing the efficacy of psychosocial interventions. The son of a Notting Hill lens maker, he graduated in archaeology and anthropology at University College London in 1951 and soon found employment as a social researcher, working on a number of short surveys on the resettlement of mental patients.[17] In 1956 he was approached by George Morris Carstairs, a social psychiatrist with an enduring interest in anthropology, then employed at the Institute of Psychiatry's Occupational Adaptation Research Unit, funded by the Medical Research Council.[18] Carstairs was interested in the social sources of psychological health, and Brown's early work under his direction confirmed the familiar idea that the supportive family served a protective function. Examining the case registers of the Cane Hill and Banstead asylums (London County Council institutions that maintained a close relationship with the Maudsley Hospital), Brown realized that patients who went unvisited for the first eight weeks after committal stood a much higher chance of long-term hospitalization. He argued that it was family pressure on medical superintendents that drove the process of deinstitutionalization at both an individual and community level.[19]

At this stage in his career Brown was convinced that large-scale quantitative surveys could reveal patterns of psychological interaction that went unnoticed in day-to-day conversations. He was, as Tirril Harris later reminisced, "captivated by the ability of Lazarsfeldian-type cross tabulation to open up a complex data set, and the way this could lead to insights about possible mechanisms."[20] This faith was repaid when in 1959 he began a study of patterns of relapse among schizophrenic inpatients returned to the community. Working initially with Carstairs and later with John Wing, he noted that ex-patients who went back to their own families demonstrated a higher rate of relapse than those moving to hostel or halfway house accommodation.

The greatest risk, Brown felt, was carried by those who were out of work and residing with their mothers.[21]

In his reconceptualization of the family as source of stress and tension, Brown found himself allied to a postwar research tradition that had been inaugurated at the Tavistock Institute for Human Relations. In studies of psychiatric disturbance in the families of returned British prisoners of war, Adam Curle (an anthropologist like Brown) and the industrial psychologist Eric Trist described how the home had been transformed into a field of psychological conflict: "The family of today cannot be regarded as a widely ramified system of organized and positive functional relationships, which form of a bridge between the individual (and his family) and society as a whole. . . . For many of those whose restricted pattern of social relationships is associated with feelings of discontent, anger, or bitterness, the marital relationship may be the only social relationship sufficiently real and secure to permit the expression of such hostile feelings to another human being."[22] This reassessment of the family had been made possible by the adoption of detailed interviews and follow-up investigations to uncover the ongoing emotional experience as they readjusted to civilian life.[23] As Curle and Trist noted, this was anthropological fieldwork "performing a psychiatric task."[24]

In his adoption of Curle's method of fieldwork interviews with the families of schizophrenics, Brown hoped to reveal the pattern of present stress that drove patients into relapse. He believed that the probability of relapse was a function of the emotional tension in the household. Thus Brown and his coworkers looked for an instrument that would somehow quantify levels of domestic strain. In detailed interviews with the family as a group, Brown and his colleagues made secondary observations on the number of interruptions and judgmental statements produced in the course of the meeting.[25] As Brown later recognized, the quality of the material produced in these semistructured interviews was very different to that produced in psychiatric questionnaires, such as the Langner's twenty-two-item screening test, the Cornell Medical Index, and the Beck Depression Inventory, which were then employed as the main instruments in epidemiological investigations.[26] The significance of the interviews, he thought, stemmed from their ability to combine two different orders of time. Emotions were made visible, he claimed, because patients and their parents switched when recounting events between the "retrospective" and the "introspective" past.[27]

Brown borrowed this distinction from Robert Merton's work on the focused interview in public-opinion research. Merton and Patricia Kendall had argued that a contrast could be drawn between what a respondent recalled of an event from the vantage point of the present ('the retrospective past') and the kind of feelings turned up through their reliving that event in unstructured conversation ('the introspective past').[28] Encouraging this form of spontaneous expression required a shift from the guided interview to a nondirective practice of minimal intervention.[29] This historical technique for emotional observation, however, faced a number of problems if it was to provide objective knowledge. While Curle had taken emotional expressions as straightforward, Brown (working with the psychiatrist Michael Rutter) recognized that there was widespread disparity between individual judgments of emotional expression—a fact that had been underlined in contemporary anthropological work.[30] Recognizing "expressed emotion," as Brown would make clear, was a practical achievement. It was contingent on a program of training, the refinement of scales, and the ongoing calibration of responses among raters.[31] I will return to this training work in my discussion of the Camberwell studies. Such work was important, for it introduced another temporal dimension into the reconstruction of stress: a dimension far beyond the introspective and retrospective pasts produced in the focused interview.

Brown against Holmes and Rahe

The adoption of the semistructured interview placed Brown in opposition to the vast number of stress researchers. Both sides of the Atlantic had witnessed the rapid development of screening instruments for the refinement of epidemiological surveys, and these in turn had been challenged through the growing literature on illness behavior.[32] Most of these early instruments had been developed in clinical research and focused on obtaining snapshot measures of emotional states or psychological drives to detect hidden forms of psychiatric morbidity. In 1967, however, a new measure, the Social Readjustment Rating Scale, was developed to recover a temporal dimension to psychiatric conditions by tracing the cumulative effect of events across a life course. Devised by Thomas Holmes and Richard Rahe, the scale was inspired by Adolf Meyer's work on the life chart, which correlated personal crises with outbreaks of illness and provided a physiological rationalization through reference to the investigations of Harold Wolff, whose experiments on ulceration promoted a model of illness as a maladaptive response to change.[33] The scale presented a list of forty-three events thought to have an impact on physical and psychological health. The pathological impact of these events was weighted by a panel of respondents in relation to the disruption of marriage, which served as a baseline measure of fifty life-change units (LCUs).

The resulting scale and its derivative, the Schedule of Recent Experience, were remarkably simple to administer.[34] Respondents simply indicated the events experienced over a twelve-month period and the cumulative score of life-change units was read as an index of illness risk. Rahe claimed that those with an LCU score of more than 150 stood a 50 percent chance of serious illness, while those with scores of 300 LCUs stood a 70 percent chance of becoming ill by the end of that period. Moreover, subsequent work indicated an apparent relationship between the strength of the LCU score and the magnitude of any chronic illness suffered.[35] As should be clear by now, the SRRS and SRE embodied a particular understanding of stress. They ignored the personal significance of events in favor of generalized understanding of the difficulties of adaptation.[36] And although they shared with Brown's early work an apparent faith in the powers of quantification and the importance of uncovering historical material, these scales would very quickly become the focus of Brown's criticisms. Indeed, the SRRS and SRE in many ways took on a kind of antitotemic status for Brown. The development of his own research and the refinement of his interview technique were guided by the perceived inadequacies of the Social Readjustment Rating Scale.

Bedford College and Camberwell

In 1969 George Brown took up a new post at Bedford College's Social Research Unit on Harley Street. Under the direction of Margot Jefferys he initiated a survey of 114 diagnosed female depressives (73 inpatients and 41 outpatients) resident in Camberwell, a working-class suburb of South London where, according to the *British Medical Journal*, "depressed women vary from those living in Dickensian conditions to those with titles."[37] The survey was restricted to women, partly because of popular associations between women, depression, and neurosis and partly for ease of access since many respondents would be at home during working hours.[38] Subjects were included only if their first onset or major relapse had occurred in the twelve months preceding the survey date.[39]

Between 1970 and 1971 a comparison group of 220 women randomly selected from the council's list of ratable households was also set up. These women underwent psychiatric screening using the eighth edition of the Present State Examination (PSE), an interview schedule developed by John Wing and others to control and standardize psychiatric judgments.[40] Both groups were subjected to interviews lasting roughly six hours, to elicit a general picture of the life events connected to the illness, the patients' reaction to these events, and the circumstances of their lives. Further studies were carried out on another 238 women in Camberwell in 1974 and North Uist in 1975, using a shortened form of the ninth edition of the PSE.[41]

Brown's work was undertaken with Tirril Harris, a trained clinical psychologist with a background in psychoanalysis (her mother, Penelope Balogh, was a pioneering psychotherapist) and political activism (she was the wife of Nigel Harris, leader of the Socialist International—which would later become the Socialist Workers Party—and a regular contributor to the movement's publications).[42] From the very beginning of their project,

Brown and Harris made clear their rejection of the questionnaire as a technique for making life stress visible. Although they were happy to use the PSE as a screening device, they argued that such techniques could never explain the etiology of an illness. As they made clear, "research workers have almost entirely relied on administering to large numbers of people some form of the standardized questionnaire with its dispiriting pretensions to measure almost anything by means of a few, often fixed-choice, questions."[43]

Brown and Harris shared Ernest Gruenberg's suspicion of the new technologies: "Continuing refinements of the structured questionnaire with efforts to eliminate interviewer bias can lead us up a blind alley." Gruenberg claimed. "When carried to an extreme we will conclude that the best interviewer is a tape recorder containing the questions and the best recorder of replies a second tape recorder. A questionnaire addressed to the subject of the research which becomes very highly refined and standardized in its administration so as to allay our anxieties about interviewer bias may very well throw away the most valuable characteristic of the interviewer, his humanity."[44] It was this humanity, Brown and Harris insisted, that made possible the objective rating of stress. As we shall see, their work was an argument for the replacement of the questionnaire with the interviewer as an effective psychological instrument.

Brown and Harris's dispute with Holmes and Rahe centered on the issues of time and meaning. In their understanding of the relationship between stress and depression, they advanced a similar model to most of the dominant American researchers in which a mixture of *provoking agents* (life events), *vulnerability factors* (long-term difficulties such as losing a mother before the age of eleven) and *symptom formation factors* (events after onset) work together to determine the duration and severity of the depressive episode.[45] Yet they maintained a critical attitude to the model, claiming that it "was best seen as an early and relatively crude theory; it enables us to get some direct sense of what is going on and provides a framework in which we can think and test new ideas." As can be seen, it was distinguished from Holmes and Rahe's theories by its imposition of a different temporal order on the relevant variables. Whereas Holmes and Rahe had included all events in their study within the same series, Brown and Harris sorted individual biography into proximal life events and long-term vulnerability factors. This division was later formalized in their 1978 research instrument, the Bedford College Life Events and Difficulties Schedule.[46]

The Problem of Meaning

Brown and Harris claimed that the SRE was not capable of making sense of individual experience. Like David Mechanic and Robert Lazarus, they insisted that the significance of life changes varied according to the meaning attributed to them.[47] The SRE could not take account of this difference since the questions were open-ended. As Brown and Harris made clear, they were not against the construction of scores; rather, they emphasized: "*Our criticism of the SRE schedule is that it is far too vague in specifying the situations. The way in which each subject understands the brief account of each life event must vary.*"[48] It was not clear from the design of the SRE what should count as a certain illness or who should count as a family member.

Against the catholic models advanced by Holmes, Rahe, and the Dohrenwends, models that presented all kinds of life change as a form of stress, Brown and Harris set a high threshold, arguing,

> It was not just any life event however unpleasant that could bring about depression. Only *severe* events involving long-term threat were capable of doing so. . . . The distinctive feature of the great majority of the provoking events is the experience of loss or disappointment, if this is defined broadly to include threat of or actual separation from a key figure, an unpleasant revelation about someone close, a life-threatening illness to a close relative, a major material loss or general disappointment or threat of them, and miscellaneous crises such as being made redundant after a long period of steady employment. In more general terms the loss could concern a person or object, a role or idea.[49]

Borrowing from the ethological work of their close colleague, Colin Murray Parkes, they argued that a true stressor involved a threat to the subject's "assumptive world."[50] This assumptive world, according to Parkes, included the subjects' understanding of their own identity and relationships across the present, past, and future. The understanding of the past and future promoted in this model of stress was very different, however, from the ideas of threat and trauma contained in the nineteenth-century ideas of expectant attention and the subconscious mind. Past and future were understood as a network of projected ideals that underpinned the subjects' identity and gave it meaning.[51] Meaning rested in the continuity of such projections. As the sociologist of grief, Peter Marris, noted, "it is a structure which relates purposes to expectations so as to organize actions—whether the actions are taken or only thought about. Meaning, that is, makes sense of action by providing reasons for it, and the collapse of compelling reasons to act constitutes the trauma of loss."[52]

This understanding of meaning allowed British stress researchers to emphasize the complexity and particularity of the individual experience of life events in contrast to the generalizing efforts of the questionnaire makers. Yet although they recognized that meaning was relative and reactions varied severely between respondents, they also set a clear limit on the latitude granted to their subjects' reconstructions. As Brown and Harris remarked of their own research,

> The question therefore arises whose perspective do we take about life-events and the changes they entail? Is any perspective more true than another? Much will depend on what we are trying to do but it is difficult to contemplate any way of dealing with such multiple perspectives without the investigator at some stage imposing his *own* viewpoint on the world. He must use his judgment not only for methodological reasons . . . but because the world is capable of having an impact irrespective of the meanings a person brings to it. A widow of forty-five with three children faces a different world, if she wishes to remarry, than one with no children; and the meaning of her widowhood will often only slowly emerge as she faces these contingencies.[53]

There is clearly a certain tension inherent in this model of depression.[54] It was driven by the meanings respondents attributed to events, but this meaning could at the same time be obscured from the subject through some process of repression or false consciousness. The true meaning of stress could be recovered only through the use of trained empathic instruments.

Stress and the Contaminated Past

There was a second reason why the attribution of meaning needed to be grounded through objectifying practices. As Brown had discovered in his work with the families of schizophrenics, attributions of meaning played an active role in the reconstruction of the past. Each element in the process was unstable. As Brown and Harris noted, "The past, present and future are not distinct in their influence on behavior. Past experience can influence the definition of the present: but inferences about the future can also influence an understanding of past events—new meanings may emerge."[55] This contamination of memory, they claimed, was an example of what the Cambridge psychologist Frederic Bartlett had called "effort after meaning."[56] Memories were reworked in the light of current experience and the grief stricken, they believed, were especially likely to engage in this process of gloomy reconstruction.

This process, Brown claimed, was well illustrated by psychosomatic studies of the relationship between stress and Down syndrome. In 1958 the Bristol psychologist Denis Stott had published the results of his survey of the parents of mentally retarded children, arguing that their mothers were repeatedly subjected to stress and shocks during the pregnancy.[57] Over the next two years, however, a number of studies were published providing strong evidence of the condition's link with chromosomal abnormality.[58] Stott's data, Brown and his colleagues suggested, were an illustration of the mother's search "for reasons to explain the birth of her defective child" rather than a demonstration of the effects of maternal stress.

Alongside this active process of narrative reconstruction, Brown also suggested that attempts to map out the provoking agents in the etiology of depression could be complicated by the fact that illness could both bring about life events—the onset of schizophrenia might, for instance, lead to the loss of a job—and would also change the meaning of any events coinciding with an illness episode, imbuing them with a significance that they might previously have lacked. Brown and his colleagues controlled for this by restricting their interview schedule to a series of events that they believed would affect most individuals and over which the subject exercised little or no agency. Questions were restricted to events such as family illness, surgical operations, and career changes.[59] Despite the criticism of SRE's insensitivity to personal meaning, much of the responsiveness of Brown and Harris's own rating scales was compromised in this attempt to control contamination.[60]

The Problem of Temporality

The problem of contamination immediately rendered the content of the questionnaires suspect. To contain the corrosive effects of autobiographical memory, Brown drew on a series of techniques that he had developed in his schizophrenia studies at the Maudsley. These techniques were designed to counterbalance the interviewee's assessment of the life event through the production of a "contextual rating" arising out of a professional team's assessment of the case file: "In our own research we recorded what women said they felt about incidents (including our assessment of any feelings spontaneously expressed at other points in the interview). But for methodological reasons we have placed most weight on 'contextual' ratings which were designed to record what most women would have felt given the particular circumstances—past and present of the individual woman."[61]

These contextual ratings, as previously mentioned, had been developed in Brown and Jim Birley's work on schizophrenia.[62] The procedure involved a form of imaginative identification in which scenarios were rated through objective agreement on the level of threat they contained. As Harris later recalled, these initial investigations into the threshold of threat "involved discussion . . . of hundreds of examples of possible events—often at some length. The seriousness with which this was taken can be gauged by recalling whether to include an eye falling out of a pet goldfish—it was not! The key point is that as with the expressed emotion index, the task of measurement was firmly in the hands of the investigators. It was they, who on the basis of as detailed an account as possible of the event, decided whether or not the incident was to be included."[63]

Brown and Harris legitimated the development of their contextual ratings through reference to the work of Alfred Schutz.[64] Although they resisted the calls of phenomenological sociology, they argued that meaning and motive could be imputed only through close familiarity with the material. Thus, although, following Schutz, they argued that the imputation of meaning and motivations to others was an aspect of everyday life, they also claimed that this process could be refined through the deployment of specific techniques. These included the use of anchoring examples (similar to Schutz's ideal types), the continual rehearsal of case histories, and the correction of deviant interpretations through group discussion.[65] These case histories produced through the Bedford College Interviews were rich enough to sustain a form of empathic identification, and subsequent investigations appeared to demonstrate the persistent achievement of close agreement between raters.[66] As David Mechanic later noted, in this kind of investigation the "qualitative observer is, in a sense, a research instrument, and how he or she is calibrated is an issue of some importance."[67]

Thus the consensus meetings that Brown and Harris organized for their assistants can be understood as a form of imaginative casework in which the raters continually recalibrated their feelings and their imaginations to conceive the depth of threat a patient experienced before the onset of any illness.[68] Through this process the threat of life events was agreed on without the interference of the patient's own assessments: assessments that might always be contaminated by the subject's knowledge of later occurrences. It allowed for the production of a form of historical objectivity, or "intersubjectivity," through the development of specific psychological experiences.[69] It depended, as Brown made clear, on "harnessing the tremendous potentialities of the human mind as a measuring instrument and providing the necessary infrastructure and training for interviewers to do this."[70]

The transformative aspect of this training was brought home by Harris:

> What can be underlined, however, is how much this style of research into the meaning of people's experiences depends on the participation of each member of the consensus group sharing their views. With each programme grant, team members faced different samples and thus different ranges of experiences which required different degrees of empathy to rate. They also had to face different situations in the interview situation, where sometimes respondents became worryingly distressed and sometimes they reported harrowing circumstances with an almost equally worrying calm. Sometimes especially in the later projects where information about childhood was collected, team members would find that material disclosed by interviewees brought back distressing memories of their own past which had to be contained while they finished the interview.[71]

Camberwell and the Environment of Earliest Adaptation

The world of threat, created through the empathic operations of Brown and Harris's rating teams, bore only an oblique relationship to the lived misery of Camberwell in the 1970s. The physical and emotional perils faced by the respondents were not those they described in their interviews but were instead reworked from a pattern of primitive anxieties imagined and calibrated through the raters' empathic group work. At one level, as left-wing commentators noted at the time, this kind of operation ran the risk of substituting the worries expressed by working-class interviewees for the anxious preoccupations of middle-class commentators.[72] Brown and Harris were at pains to avoid this accusation.[73] However, there was another, more profound process of substitution taking place in the production of contextual threat. Although the rating teams sought to adopt the perspectives of their interviewees, the authentic landscape they identified beneath the misremembered and misapprehended narratives of their respondents was the primitive environment described in evolutionary models of clinical depression.

The model of depression adopted by Brown and Harris was drawn from the evolutionary psychiatry of John Bowlby, Murray Parkes, George Engel, and John Price.[74] In their writings, depression was presented as process of surrender—in which the anxious search for or defense of a valued object—was subsumed by hopeless withdrawal. It was a universal process, scripted in Pleistocene episodes of loss and retreat, and it was this evolutionary prefiguration that made the subjects' experiences meaningful. The language of threat that the Bedford College team used to describe the frustrations and humiliations of their respondents located the subjects' reactions in this ethological drama of confrontation and withdrawal.[75] The rating meeting thus became an effective mechanism for rewriting the mundane distress of Camberwell onto the Pleistocene environment of earliest adaptation. True threat, as extracted from the questionnaires and reimagined in the rating meetings, challenged the individuals' biological goals—goals formed in a primitive environment and hardwired into the individual nervous system.

The drawing together of the lived misery of postwar London and the evolutionary challenges of the Pleistocene environment was accomplished by making individual affect the criterion of true experience. As Brown later explained, his investigations had rested on the assumption that emotions provided an insight into the true self that existed beyond the boundaries of social and cultural convention. As Brown later noted, "the most effective way an individual may have of dealing with 'false consciousness' was to pay heed to his own emotional reactions."[76] This model, which insulated affective life from the claims of belief, was drawn from the work of US psychologist Silvan Tomkins, who from early on had argued that emotions could be understood as biological affect programs hardwired into the human system. Although these programs could be triggered by cognitive stimuli, they were essentially independent of them, and intellectual understanding of feelings thus provided a false rationalization of what was, in truth, a discrete biological process.[77] This understanding of emotion introduced the same suspicion of respondent accounts that was raised in the discussion of autobiographical memory earlier. However, unlike the earlier discussions of memory, it opened up the way for the truth of personal experience to be recovered—through an engagement with the individual's evolutionary past.

This systematic rereading of female distress and mental suffering in Camberwell onto an evolutionary past should give historians pause for thought. For the displacement of emotions from a narrative based in the conscious experience of working-class life in postwar Britain to a narrative based on the unconscious adaptations to life in the Pleistocene era mirrors the recent turn to evolutionary psychology in contemporary historiography. Anyone familiar with Lynn Hunt's embrace of the work of Daniel Smail and other "neurohistorians" will recognize this process: a process in which the historian's empathic reconstruction is grounded through reference to evolutionary psychology.[78] Thus, Hunt argues that at the moment in the French Revolution when all our reference points collapsed, a new form of solidarity was made possible by biological categories produced in the environment of earliest adaptation.[79] Those categories, which Hunt holds up as the grounds of historical experience, are used in Brown and Harris's work as a stable point of reference beneath the conflicting temporalities of introspective and retrospective time, the times contaminated through memory and illness, and the times corrupted by the failure of the psychological instrument.

Yet the role that this primitive time serves in stress narratives, or indeed all narratives, can be pushed much further. In a richly provocative but faintly baffling essay on the historical event, Hayden White has suggested that the existence of an event is itself only made possible by the presence of the second order of time behind the flux of modern life. His discussion draws heavily on psychoanalytic ideas of "*Nachträglichkeit*" (deferred action), in which the meaning and significance of an experience is revealed only through later events.[80] Yet although rooted in psychoanalytic thinking, White explores the concept through a language redolent of homeostatic models of stress. "Is it possible," he asks "that the specifically historical event is a happening that occurs in some present (or in the experience of a living group), the nature of which cannot be discerned and a name given to it because it manifests itself only as an 'eruption' of a force or energy that disrupts the ongoing system and forces a change (the direction or trajectory of which is unknowable until it is launched or entered upon), the end, aim, or purpose of which can only be discerned, grasped, or responded to at a later time?"[81]

In his insistence that the significance of an event will be revealed at some later point, White returns to his long-established arguments that events become meaningful only when situated in a narrative.[82] However, he qualifies and to some extent obscures his argument by claiming that this revelation of meaning endows the original event with a prophetic or sacred quality. He claims that the moment at which that meaning is revealed "is not just any old 'later time.' Rather, that later time when the eruption of what seems to be in some way affiliated with an earlier event reveals or seems to reveal in the fact of that affiliation the 'meaning,' significance, gist, even foretelling, though in a masked and obscure way, both of the original event and the later one. Such that the later event can be plausibly represented in a narrative in which it is the fulfillment (or derealization) of the meaning having lain latent and now made manifest retrospectively in the earlier one." As White concludes, "If that turned out to be the case, it would be . . . a miracle."[83]

This is a complex (and fairly gnomic) argument, and it seems there are (at least) two ways of understanding White's claim. The first is that events simply obtain their status and significance through their later narration. This seems fair but I think White also wants to insist on something more interesting. In drawing on the language of biblical typology with its insistence that the events of the Old Testament obtain their significance only when they are revealed as symbolic anticipations of the life of Christ, he advances an argument that experiences become meaningful or historical only through their relationship with another, more profound narrative rooted in an alternative temporality. In this sense, for White, the historical event is miraculous in that it marks the confluence of two forms of time—the sacred and profane.

Although it may seem far-fetched, I want to suggest that this sense of the miraculous can be found in the life events described by George Brown and his colleagues at Bedford College and the Maudsley Hospital. Yet the "Camberwell miracle" (to paraphrase John D. Beresford) is of a very different sort from that imagined in Christian theology.[84] In the work of Brown and Harris the stresses and accidents experienced by the women of Camberwell became meaningful and hence historical events through their location in another order of time: the Pleistocene environment of earliest adaptation. It is the eruption of emotion—scripted in primitive confrontations—that reveals the true threats that confront Brown and Harris's respondents. The transformation of the accidents of everyday existence into the objects of psychiatric epidemiology was predicated not only on this theoretical association between lived and evolutionary time but on a broader edifice built through intellectual, emotional, and practical labor. I'm not sure that this counts as a miracle. If it was, it was a miracle made possible by the different conceptions of temporality inherent in psychiatric ideas of stress and depression.

Notes

1. Andrew Abbott, "Positivism and Interpretation in Sociology: Lessons for Sociologists from the History of Stress Research," *Sociological Forum* 5, no. 3 (1980):

435–58; Grace G. Harris, "Mechanism and Morality in Patient's Views of Illness and Injury," *Medical Anthropology Quarterly*, n.s. 3, no. 1 (1989): 3–21; Betsy Pohlman and Gay Becker, "Stress Knocks Hard on the Immune System: Asthma and the Discourse of Stress," *Medical Anthropology* 25 (2006): 265–95; Kristian Pollack, "On the Nature of Social Stress: Production of a Modern Mythology," *Social Science and Medicine* 26 (1988): 381–92; Russell Viner, "Putting Stress in Life: Hans Selye and the Making of Stress Theory," *Social Studies of Science* 29, no. 3 (1999): 391–410; Allan Young, "The Discourse on Stress and the Reproduction of Conventional Knowledge," *Social Science and Medicine* 148 (1980): 133–46.

2. George W. Brown and Tirril Harris, *The Social Origins of Depression: A Study of Psychiatric Disorder in Women* (London: Tavistock, 1978).

3. Janet Walker, Helen Barrett, Graeme Wilson, and Yan-Shing Chang, *Relationships Matter* (London: Department of Children, Schools, and Families, 2010); Rosalind H. Kirk, "Family Support: The Role of Early Years' Centers," *Children and Society* 17, no. 2 (2003): 85–99.

4. George W. Brown, Maire N. Bhrolcháin, and Tirril Harris, "Social Class and Psychiatric Disturbance among Women in an Urban Population," *Sociology* 9 (1975): 225–54; Brown and Harris, *Social Origins.*

5. Henry Holland, "Effects of Medical Attention on Bodily Organs," in *Medical Notes and Reflections* (London: Orme, Brown, Green, and Longmans, 1839), 64–75; Daniel H. Tuke, *Illustrations of the Influence of the Mind upon the Body, etc.* (London: Churchill, 1884), 1:26–31, 86–87.

6. James Braid, "On the Power of the Mind over the Body: An Experimental Inquiry into the Nature and Cause of the Phenomena Attributed to Baron Reichenbach and Other to the 'New Imponderable,'" *Medical Times* 14 (1846): 214–16, 252–54, 273–74, reprinted as *The Power of the Mind over the Body etc.* (London: Churchill, 1846); William B. Carpenter, "Electrobiology and Mesmerism," *Quarterly Review* 93 (1853): 501–57; Carpenter *Principles of Mental Physiology* (1874; repr., London: Kegan Paul, Trench, Trübner, 1896), 608–10, 561–90. On Carpenter's physiological ideas, see Roger Smith, "The Background of Physiological Psychology in Natural Philosophy," *History of Science* 11 (1973): 75–123; Smith, *Inhibition: History and Meaning in the Sciences of Mind and Brain* (London: Free Association Book, 1992), 41–44; and Kurt Danziger, "Mid-Nineteenth-Century British Psychophysiology: A Neglected Chapter in the History of Science," in *The Problematic Science: Psychology in the Nineteenth Century*, ed. William R. Woodward and Mitchell G. Ash (New York: Praeger, 1992).

7. For a useful survey of the transformation, see Frederic Myers, "The Subliminal Consciousness: Ch. VI: The Mechanism of Hysteria," *Proceedings of the Society for Psychical Research* 9 (1893–94): 3–25; Frederic Myers "The Subliminal Consciousness: Ch. VII: Motor Automatism," *Proceedings of the Society for Psychical Research* 9 (1893–94): 26–128; Pierre Janet, *Psychological Healing* (London: Macmillan, 1925), 590–606.

8. Walter B. Cannon, *Bodily Changes in Pain, Hunger, Fear and Rage* (New York: Appleton, 1929), 261. Cannon's idea of stress as a form of psychological lag was widely picked up by late twentieth-century stress researchers; see Barbara Snell Dohrenwend and Bruce Philip Dohrenwend, eds., *Stressful Life Events: Their Nature and Effects* (New York: Wiley, 1974), 2; and George W. Brown and Tirril O. Harris, *Life Events and Illness* (London: Unwin Hyman, 1989), 5.

9. See Jackson, "Role of Hans Selye," this volume.

10. For notable critiques, see Wilhelm Reich, *The Function of the Orgasm* (1942; repr., London: Souvenir, 1983); and Ian Suttie, *The Origins of Love and Hate* (1935; repr., Harmondsworth: Penguin, 1960). For an overview, see Richard Overy, *The Morbid Age* (London: Penguin Books, 2009), chap. 4.

11. Richard M. Titmuss, *Problems of Social Policy* (London: HMSO, 1950), chap. 16. On these surveys, see Ian MacLaine, *Ministry of Morale: Home Front Morale and the Ministry of Information in World War II* (London: Allen and Unwin, 1979); Robert Mackay, *Half the Battle: Civilian Morale in Britain during the Second World War* (Manchester: Manchester University Press, 2002); and Ian Burney, "War on Fear: Solly Zuckerman and Civilian Nerve in the Second World War," in *History of the Human Sciences* 25, no. 5 (2012): 49–72.

12. Rhodri Hayward, "Enduring Emotions: James L. Halliday and the Invention of the Psychosocial," *Isis: A Journal of the History of Science* 100, no. 4 (2009): 827–38; Hayward, "Psychology and the Pursuit of Serenity in Post-war Britain," in *Clio's Dream: Psychoanalysis and History*, ed. Barbara Taylor and Sally Alexander. Global Intellectual Histories Series (Basingstoke: Palgrave, 2012), 283–304.

13. Young, "Discourse on Stress," 133.

14. Stephen Taylor and Sidney Chave, *Mental Health and Environment* (London: Longmans, 1964); Leo Srole, Thomas S. Langer, Marvin K. Opler, and Thomas A. C. Rennie, *Mental Health in the Metropolis: The Midtown Manhattan Study* (New York: McGraw Hill, 1962). On the turn to interview techniques in postwar sociological fieldwork, see Mike Savage, "Elizabeth Bott and the Formation of Modern British Sociology," *Sociological Review* 56, no. 4 (2008): 579–605; Savage, *Identities and Social Change in Britain: The Politics of Method* (Oxford: Oxford University Press, 2010).

15. Lawrence E. Hinkle and Harold G. Wolff, "Ecologic Investigations into the Relationship of Illness, Life Experiences and the Social Environment," *Annals of Internal Medicine* 49 (1958): 1373–88.

16. Edward H. Hare, "The Distribution of Mental Illness in the Community," in *Aspects of Psychiatric Research*, ed. Derek Richter, John M. Tanner, Lord Taylor, and Oliver L. Zangwill (London: Oxford University Press, 1962), 36–65; Michael Shepherd and Brian Cooper, "Epidemiology and Mental Disorder: A Review," *Journal of Neurology, Neurosurgery, and Psychiatry* 27, no. 4 (1964): 277–90; Hugh L. Freeman, "The Scientific Background," in *Mental Health and Environment*, ed. Hugh Freeman (London: Livingstone, 1984), 23–70; Gerald Grob, "The Origins of American Psychiatric Epidemiology," *American Journal of Public Health* 75, no. 3 (1985): 229–36; Hans Pols, "Anomie in the Metropolis: The City in American Sociology and Psychiatry," in *Science and the City*, ed. Sven Dierig, Jens Lachmund, and J. Andrew Mendelsohn, *Osiris* 18 (2003): 194–211.

17. Tirril O. Harris, *Where Inner and Outer Worlds Meet: Psychosocial Research in the Tradition of George W. Brown* (London: Routledge, 2000).

18. Staff files, FD1/423, Occupational Adaptation Unit, National Archives, Kew; George M. Carstairs, "Perspective," *Bulletin of the Royal College of Psychiatrists* 9 (1989): 110–11.

19. George W. Brown, "Social Factors Influencing Length of Hospital Stay of Schizophrenic Patients," *BMJ*, December 12, 1959, 1300–1302.

20. Harris, *Inner and Outer Worlds*, 4; Paul Lazarsfeld, "Problems in Methodology," in *Sociology Today: Problems and Prospects*, ed. Robert Merton, Leonard Broom, and Leonard Cottrell (New York: Basic Books, 1959), 39–78.

21. George W. Brown, George M. Carstairs, and G. Topping, "Post-hospital Adjustment of Chronic Mental Patients," *Lancet*, September 27, 1958, 685–89.

22. Adam Curle and Eric Trist, "Transitional Communities and Social Re-connection: A Follow-Up Study of the Civil Resettlement of British Prisoners of War," *Human Relations* 1, no. 2 (1947): 283.

23. On the significance of this departure, see Savage, *Identities and Social Change*, 171–72.

24. Curle and Trist, "Transitional Communities," 282.

25. George W. Brown, E. M. Monck, George M. Carstairs and John K. Wing, "Influence of Family Life on the Course of Schizophrenic Illness," *British Journal of Preventive and Social Medicine* 16 (1962): 55–68; George W. Brown, James L. T. Birley, and John K. Wing, "The Influence of Family Life on the Course of Schizophrenic Illness: A Replication," *British Journal of Psychiatry* 121 (1972): 241–58.

26. George W. Brown and Michael L. Rutter, "The Measurement of Family Activities and Relationships," *Human Relations* 19 (1966): 241–63; Michael Rutter and George W. Brown, "The Reliability and Validity of Measure of Family Life and Relationships in Families Containing a Psychiatric Patient," *Social Psychiatry* 1 (1966): 38–53. For an overview of these techniques, see David Goldberg, *The Detection of Psychiatric Illness by Questionnaire*, Maudsley monograph 21 (London: Oxford University Press, 1973), chap. 1.

27. Brown and Rutter, "Measurement of Family Activities," 246.

28. Robert K. Merton and Patricia L. Kendall, "The Focused Interview," *American Journal of Sociology* 51 (1946): esp. 548–52.

29. On the origins of this technique, see Raymond Lee, "'The Most Important Technique': Carl Rogers, Hawthorne and the Rise and Fall of Non-directive Interviewing in Sociology," *Journal of the History of the Behavioral Sciences* 47 (2011): 123–46.

30. Savage, *Identities and Social Change*, 17. For an overview, see Joel R. Davitz, *The Language of Emotion*, New York: Academic Press, 1969.

31. Brown and Rutter, "Measurement of Family Activities," 256–57; Brown, Monck, and Carstairs, "Family Life," 57–58; Joel R. Davitz, *The Communication of Emotional Meaning* (New York: McGraw Hill, 1964).

32. David Mechanic and Eric H. Volkart, "Stress, Illness Behavior and the Sick Role," *American Sociological Review* 26, no. 1 (1961): 51–58; Pierre Pichot, "Quantification of Psychological Stress Responses," in *Society, Stress and Disease*, ed. Lennart Levi (London: Oxford University Press, 1971), 49–52.

33. Thomas H. Holmes and Richard H. Rahe, "The Social Readjustment Rating Scale," *Journal of Psychosomatic Research* 11 (1967): 213–18; Harold G. Wolff, "Changes in the Form and Function of Mucous Membranes Occurring as Part of the Protective Reaction Patterns in Man during Periods of Life Stress and Emotional Conflict," *Transactions of the Academy of American Physicians* 61 (1948): 313–34; Harold G. Wolff and Stewart C. Wolf, *Human Gastric Function: An Experimental Study of a Man and His Stomach* (London: Oxford University Press, 1947), 147–50, 153–84; Harold G. Wolff, "Life Stress and Bodily Disease—a Formulation," in *Life Stress and Bodily Disease:*

Proceedings of the Association for Research in Nervous and Mental Diseases, ed. Harold G. Wolff, Stewart G. Wolf, and Clarence C. Hare (Baltimore: Williams and Wilkins, 1950), 1059–94. On Meyer's life chart, see Ruth Leys, "'Types of One': Adolf Meyer's Life Chart and the Representation of the Individual," *Representations* 34 (1991): 1–28.

34. Richard H. Rahe, "Life Crisis and Health Change," in *Psychotropic Drug Responses: Advances in Prediction,* ed. Philip R. A. May and John R. Wittenborn (Springfield: Charles C. Thomas, 1969), 92–125.

35. Thomas H. Holmes and Minoru Masuda, "Life Change and Illness Susceptibility," in Dohrenwend and Dohrenwend, *Stressful Life Events,* 45–72.

36. Good summaries of these criticisms can be found in Steve D. Brown, "The Worst Things in the World: Life Events Checklists in Popular Stress Management Texts," in *Ordinary Lifestyles: Popular Media, Consumption and Taste,* ed. David Bell and Joanne Hollows (Buckingham: Open University Press, 2005), 231–42.

37. "In Brief," *British Medical Journal,* June 3, 1978, 1477. On the condition of Camberwell, see Harold J. Dyos, *Victorian Suburb: A Survey of the Growth of Camberwell* (Leicester: Leicester University Press, 1966).

38. Ali Haggett, "Housewives, Neuroses and the Domestic Environment in Britain, 1945–70," in *Health and the Modern Home,* ed. Mark Jackson (London: Routledge, 2007), 84–110.

39. George W. Brown, Freda Sklair, Tirril O. Harris, and James L. T. Birley, "Life Events and Psychiatric Disorders," pt. 1, "Some Methodological Issues," *Psychological Medicine* 3 (1973): 74–87.

40. John K. Wing, James L. T. Birley, John E. Cooper, Philip Graham, and Anthony D. Isaacs, "Reliability of Procedure for Measuring and Classifying 'Present Psychiatric State,'" *British Journal of Psychiatry* 113 (1967): 499–515; John K. Wing, John E. Cooper, and Norman Sartorius, *The Measurement and Classification of Psychiatric Symptoms* (Cambridge: Cambridge University Press, 1974).

41. George W. Brown, Sue Davidson, Tirril Harris, Una Maclean, Sue Pollock, and Ray Prudo, "Psychiatric Disorder in London and North Uist," *Social Science and Medicine* 11 (1977): 367–77.

42. See Harris's useful essay on Reich, "WR: World Revolution or Wishful Revisionism," *International Socialism* 54 (1973): 8–10; and her reviews: "Ideology and Insanity," *International Socialism* 72 (October 1974): 30.

43. Brown and Harris, *Social Origins,* 10.

44. Ibid.; Ernst M. Gruenberg, "A Population Study of Disability from Mental Disorders, *Annals of the New York Academy of Science* 107 (1963): 590–91.

45. On the shared understanding of etiological models, see Dohrenwend and Dohrenwend, *Stressful Life Events*; and David Mechanic, "Medical Sociology: Some Tensions between Theory, Method and Substance," *Journal of Health and Social Behavior* 30, no. 2 (1989): 157. For a clear statement of Brown's model see his "A Three Factor Model of Depression," in *Stress and Mental Disorder,* ed. James E. Barrett (New York: Raven, 1979), 111–29.

46. Brown and Harris, *Social Origins,* 281, apps. 2 and 5; Brown and Harris, *Life Events,* 22–29. For the scoring system, see Robert Finlay Jones, George W. Brown, Paul Duncan-Jones, Tirril O. Harris, Elaine Murphy, and Ray Prudo, "Depression and Anxiety in the Community: Replicating Diagnosis of a Case," *Psychological Medicine* 10 (1980): 445–54.

47. David Mechanic, *Students under Stress* (New York: Free Press, 1962); Robert S. Lazarus, *Psychological Stress and the Coping Process* (New York: McGraw Hill, 1966).

48. Brown and Harris, *Social Origins*, 77; italics in the original.

49. Ibid., 274–75.

50. Colin M. Parkes, "Psycho-Social Transitions: A Field for Study," *Social Science and Medicine* 5 (1971): 101–16.

51. George W. Brown, "Early Loss and Depression," in *The Place of Attachment in Human Behavior*, ed. Colin Murray Parkes and Joan Stevenson-Hinde (London: Tavistock, 1982), 236.

52. Peter Marris, *Loss and Change* (London: Routledge, Kegan Paul, 1986), vii. See also the first edition (London: Routledge, Kegan Paul, 1974), 8–10, 33–34.

53. Brown and Harris, *Social Origins*, 273.

54. See George Andrews and Christopher Tennant, "Life Event Stress and Psychiatric Illness," *Psychological Medicine* 8 (1978): 545; and Steven D. Brown, "The Life of Stress: The Saying and Seeing of Dysphoria" (PhD diss., University of Reading, 1997), 235.

55. Brown and Harris, *Social Origins*, 78.

56. Frederic Bartlett, *Remembering: A Study in Experimental and Social Psychology* (Cambridge: Cambridge University Press, 1932), 20–21; Alan Collins, "The Embodiment of Reconciliation: Order and Change in the Work of Frederic Bartlett," *History of Psychology* 9, no. 4 (2006): 290–312.

57. Denis H. Stott, "Some Psychosomatic Aspects of Causality in Reproduction," *Journal of Psychosomatic Research* 3, no. 1 (1958): 42–55.

58. Brown et al., "Life Events," 76.

59. "Socio-Psychiatric Survey on Distribution and Aetiology of Depression in Women in an Urban Population," section 10, Example of Schedules, UK Data Archive Study no. 1571, University of Essex, 1, 3–10.

60. George W. Brown, "Meaning, Measurement and Stressful Life Events," in Dohrenwend and Dohrenwend, *Stressful Life Events*, 217–43.

61. Brown and Harris, *Social Origins*, 273–74.

62. George Brown and James L. T. Birley, "Crises, Life Changes and the Onset of Schizophrenia," *Journal of Health and Social Behavior* 9, no. 3 (1968): 203; George W. Brown and James L. T. Birley, "Social Precipitants of Severe Psychiatric Disorders," in *Psychiatric Epidemiology*, ed. E. H. Hare and J. K. Wing (London: London University Press, 1970).

63. Harris, "Introduction," Brown and Harris, *Life Events*, 6.

64. George W. Brown, "Some Thoughts on Grounded Theory," *Sociology* 7 (973): 1–16; Alfred Schutz, "Concept and Theory Formation in the Social Sciences," *Journal of Philosophy* 51 (1954): 251–73.

65. Brown and Rutter, "Measurement of Family Activities," 249; George W. Brown, "Life Events and Measurement," in Brown and Harris, *Life Events*, 17–18, 25–27; Brown and Harris, *Social Origins*, app. 3.

66. Christopher Tennant, Alan Smith, Paul Bebbington, and Jane Hurry, "The Contextual Threat of Life Events: The Concept and Its Reliability," *Psychological Medicine* 9 (1979): 525–28; Robert Finlay Jones and George W. Brown, "Types of Stressful Life Event and the Onset of Anxiety and Depressive Disorders," *Psychological*

Medicine 11 (1981): 803–15. On empathic identification, see Rachel Cooper, *Psychiatry and the Philosophy of Science* (Durham: Acumen, 2006), chap. 3.

67. Mechanic, "Medical Sociology," 148.

68. George W. Brown, "Teaching Data Collection in Social Survey Research," in "Research Methodology Teaching," special issue, *Sociology* 15 (1981): 550–57; Brown and Harris, *Social Origins*, 133–35. There is an obvious, although unaddressed, parallel with Richard G. Collingwood's advocacy of empathic reconstruction in historical research; see *The Idea of History* (Oxford: Oxford University Press, 1993).

69. The concept of intersubjectivity was drawn from Johann Galtung, *Theory and Method in Social Research* (London: Allen and Unwin, 1967), 28–29; and George Brown and Tirril Harris, "The Sin of Subjectivism: A Reply to Shapiro," *Behavior Research and Therapy* 17 (1979): 10.

70. George W. Brown, "Contextual Measures of Life Events," in *Stressful Life Events and Their Effects*, ed. Barbara Snell Dohrenwend and Bruce Philip Dohrenwend (New York: Prodist, 1981), 201.

71. Harris, *Inner and Outer Worlds*, xv; cf. Lorraine Daston and Peter Galison, *Objectivity* (Brooklyn, NY: Zone Books, 2007), 357–61.

72. Keith Hope, "Critical Note: A Study of Depression in Women," *Sociology* 10 (1976): 321–23; Gareth Williams, "Causality, Morality and Radicalism: A Sociological Examination of the Work of George Brown and His Colleagues," *Sociology* 16 (1982): 67–82.

73. George W. Brown, Maire N. Bhrolcháin, and Tirril Harris, "A Study of Depression in Women: A Reply to Keith Hope's Critical Note," *Sociology* 11 (1977): 527–31.

74. See Frederick T. Melges and John Bowlby, "Types of Hopelessness in Psychopathological Processes," *Archives of General Psychiatry* 20 (1969): 690–99; Parkes, "Psycho-Social Transitions"; John Bowlby, *Attachment and Loss 2: Separation, Anxiety and Anger* (London: Hogarth, 1973); Bowlby, "The Making and Breaking of Affectional Bonds: I. Aetiology and Psychopathology in the Light of Attachment Theory," *British Journal of Psychiatry* 130 (1977): 201–10; George L. Engel, "A Psychological Setting of Somatic Disease: The 'Giving Up–Given Up' Complex," *Proceedings of the Royal Society of Medicine (Section of Psychiatry)* 60 (1967): 553–55; John S. Price, "Neurotic and Endogenous Depression: A Phylogenetic View," *British Journal of Psychiatry* 114 (1968): 119–20; Price, "The Ritualization of Agonistic Behaviour as a Determinant of the Variation along the Neuroticism/Stability Dimension of Personality," *RSM (Section of Psychiatry)* 62 (1969): 1107–10. For the use of these accounts, see Brown and Harris, *Social Origins*, 233–49; and George W. Brown, Tirril O. Harris, and John R. Copeland "Depression and Loss," *British Journal of Psychiatry* 130 (1977): 1–18; Brown, "Three Factor Model."

75. Brown and Harris, *Social Origins*, 90–93; "Reported Chronic Difficulty Lasting at Least One Month," qs. 3–6, section 12, Examples of Schedules, UK Data Archive Study no. 1571, qs. 28, 29 (listed on 28).

76. George Brown, "Accounts, Meaning and Causality," in *Accounts and Action: Surrey Conferences on Sociological Theory and Method*, ed. Nigel Gilbert and Peter Abell (Aldershot, UK: Gower, 1983), 1:38. See also Brown and Harris, *Life Events*, 4–5.

77. Silvan S. Tomkins, *The Negative Affects*, vol. 2 of *Affect, Imagery, Consciousness* (London: Tavistock, 1963).

78. Daniel L. Smail, *On Deep History and the Brain* (Berkeley: University of California Press, 2008). On this trend, see William Reddy, "Neuroscience and the Fallacies of Functionalism," *History and Theory* 49 (2010): 412–25; Jeremy T. Burman, "History from Within? Contextualizing the New Neurohistory and Seeking Its Methods," *History of Psychology* 15, no. 1 (2012): 84–99; and Joelle Abi Rached and Nikolas Rose, "Birth of the Neuro-Molecular Gaze," *History of the Human Sciences* 23 (2009): 1–26.

79. Lynn Hunt, *Measuring Time, Making History* (Prague: Central European University Press, 2008); Hunt, "Experience of Revolution," *French Historical Studies* 32 (2009): 671–78.

80. Jean Laplanche and Jean-Bertrand Pontalis, *The Language of Psychoanalysis*, trans. Donald Nicholson-Smith (London: Hogarth, 1987); Jean Laplanche, "Notes on Afterwardsness," in *Essays on Otherness*, ed. John Fletcher (London: Routledge, 2002), 264.

81. Haydn White, "Historical Event," *Differences* 19, no. 2 (2008): 33.

82. See, for instance, White, "The Question of Narrative in Contemporary Historical Theory," *History and Theory* 21 (1982): 1–33.

83. White, "Historical Event," 30.

84. John D. Beresford, *The Camberwell Miracle* (1933; repr., Harmondsworth: Penguin Books, 1939).

Contributors

THEODORE M. BROWN is professor of history and of public health sciences and medical humanities at the University of Rochester. He is also the Charles E. & Dale L. Phelps Professor of Public Health and Policy. His research falls into several areas: the history of US and international public health; the history of US health policy and politics; and the history of psychosomatic medicine, "stress" research, and biopsychosocial approaches to clinical practice. He is a contributing editor of the *American Journal of Public Health* and editor of *Rochester Studies in Medical History*, a book series of the University of Rochester Press. He coedited and substantially coauthored *Making Medical History: The Life and Times of Henry E. Sigerist* (Johns Hopkins University Press, 1997) and, with Anne-Emanuelle Birn, recently published an edited collection of essays, *Comrades in Health: American Health Internationalists, Abroad and at Home*, which was published in 2013 by Rutgers University Press. He is also a coauthor of *The Quest for Health Reform: A Satirical History*, a history of health reform in the United States as seen in political cartoons, which was published by the American Public Health Association in the fall of 2012.

DAVID CANTOR is the acting director of the Office of History at the National Institutes of Health, Bethesda, Maryland. His scholarly work focuses on the twentieth-century history of medicine, most recently the histories of cancer and medical movies. He is the editor of *Reinventing Hippocrates* (Ashgate, 2002) and *Cancer in the Twentieth Century* (Johns Hopkins University Press, 2008) and coeditor (with Christian Bonah and Matthias Dörries) of *Meat, Medicine, and Human Health in the Twentieth Century* (Pickering and Chatto, 2010). He is a series editor (edited collections) of Studies for the Society of the Social History of Medicine, published by Pickering and Chatto.

OTNIEL E. DROR is the Joel Wilbush Chair in medical anthropology and head of the section for the history of medicine in the Medical Faculty at the Hebrew University of Jerusalem. His research focuses on the history of the study of emotions during the nineteenth and twentieth centuries. His coedited book on *Knowledge and Pain* is forthcoming with Rodopi Press, and his book manuscript *Blush, Flush, Adrenaline: Science, Modernity and Paradigms of Emotions, 1850–1930* is under revision for the University of Chicago Press. He is currently working on the history of the study of pleasure during the post–World War II period. His publications have appeared in *Isis*, *Social Research*, *Science in Context*, and *Configurations*.

RHODRI HAYWARD is a senior lecturer in the history of medicine at Queen Mary, University of London. He has published on the history of dreams, Pentecostalism, demonology, cybernetics, and the relations between psychiatry and primary care. His current research examines the rise and political implications of psychiatric epidemiology in modern Britain. His book *Resisting History: Popular Religion and the Invention of the Unconscious* was published by Manchester University Press in 2007. His new books, *Psychiatry in Modern Britain* and *The Transformation of the Psyche in British Primary Care, 1870–1970*, will both be published by Bloomsbury in 2014.

MARK JACKSON is a professor of the history of medicine and research theme leader for the medical humanities at the University of Exeter. He has served as chair of the Wellcome Trust History of Medicine Funding Committee and the Wellcome Trust Research Resources Funding Committee and is currently senior academic adviser (medical humanities) at the Wellcome Trust. He has taught modules in the history of medicine and the history and philosophy of science for more than twenty years at undergraduate and postgraduate levels to both medical and history students and has also been involved in teaching medical history to GCSE and A-level students. His previous books include *New-Born Child Murder* (Manchester University Press, 1996), *The Borderland of Imbecility* (Manchester University Press, 2000), *Infanticide: Historical Perspectives on Child Murder and Concealment, 1550–2000* (ed., Ashgate, 2002), *Allergy: The History of a Modern Malady* (Reaktion, 2006), *Health and the Modern Home* (ed., Routledge, 2007), *Asthma: The Biography* (Oxford University Press, 2009), *The Oxford Handbook of the History of Medicine* (ed., Oxford University Press, 2011), and *The Age of Stress: Science and the Search for Stability* (Oxford University Press, 2013).

ROBERT G. W. KIRK is a Wellcome Trust Research Fellow at the Centre for the History of Science, Technology and Medicine, University of Manchester. His work examines the role of nonhuman animals in human cultures, particularly within science and medicine, as well as the place of nonhuman animals in historical writing. Rob's contribution to this volume forms part of a wider study examining how, why, and to what consequence animal welfare became integrated within the Anglo-American biomedical sciences in the post–World War II period. Rob is also beginning a new project, examining how human-animal relations shaped twentieth-century psychobiology, psychopharmacology, behavioral science, and medicine.

JUNKO KITANAKA is a medical anthropologist and associate professor in the Department of Human Sciences, Keio University, Tokyo. For her McGill University doctoral dissertation on depression, she received a number of awards including the 2007 Dissertation Award from the American Anthropological Association's Society for Medical Anthropology. This has since been published by Princeton University Press as a book titled *Depression in Japan: Psychiatric Cures for a Society in Distress*, which won the American Anthropological Association's Francis Hsu Prize for Best Book in East Asian Anthropology in 2013. She is currently working on a new project on the psychiatrization of the life cycle.

TULLEY LONG is a postdoctoral research associate and adjunct faculty in the Program in the History of Science, Technology, and Medicine at the University of Minnesota, Twin Cities. She received her PhD in the history of science and technology from the Johns Hopkins University in 2011. Her dissertation, titled "Constituting the Stress Response: Collaborative Networks and the Elucidation of the Pituitary-Adrenal Cortical System, 1930s–1960s," traces the development and deployment of the physiological stress response, the hormonal mechanisms by which the body responds to changes and challenges in its environment.

JOSEPH MELLING is a codirector of the Centre for Medical History at the University of Exeter and a professor of industrial history. He has written widely in the field of medical history with particular reference to occupational and mental health, as well as publishing in economic and labor history. He is currently finishing a book on silicosis and is beginning a second on workplace stress.

EDMUND RAMSDEN is a research fellow at Queen Mary, University of London. His current research, supported by the Wellcome Trust, is focused on the involvement of social and behavioral scientists in architecture, planning, and design in the post-war United States, so as to improve mental health and social well-being. He also continues to work on the history of experimental psychiatry, psychology, and psychobiology in relation to neuroses, emotional disorders, addiction, and suicide. His other research interests include the history of eugenics, the population sciences and policy, and the development of social survey research methods in relation to health, growth, and intelligence.

ELIZABETH SIEGEL WATKINS is the dean of the Graduate Division and a professor of history of health sciences at the University of California, San Francisco. She earned her BA in biology and her PhD in the history of science, both at Harvard University. Watkins is the author of *On the Pill: A*

Social History of Oral Contraceptives (Johns Hopkins University Press, 1998) and *The Estrogen Elixir: A History of Hormone Replacement Therapy in America* (Johns Hopkins University Press, 2007) and coeditor of *Medicating Modern America: Prescription Drugs in History* (NYU Press, 2007) and *Prescribed: Writing, Filling, Using, and Abusing the Prescription in Modern America* (Johns Hopkins University Press, 2012). She has recently published articles on the history of Norplant and the history of male menopause and testosterone replacement. Her work has been funded by the National Endowment for the Humanities, the NIH/National Library of Medicine, the National Academy of Education, the National Science Foundation, and the University of California President's Research Fellowship in the Humanities.

Allan Young is a social anthropologist with special interest in indigenous systems of medical beliefs and practices, clinical psychiatry, psychiatric science, and social neuroscience. His earliest research was conducted in the Gondar region of Ethiopia and focused on indigenous technologies for diagnosing, preventing, and treating medical problems. Subsequent research was conducted in Nepal and focused on the WHO program directed at the integration of Ayurvedic medicine into government-sponsored health care services. In the late 1980s his interests turned to US government-sponsored efforts to diagnose and treat post-traumatic stress disorder (PTSD) among veterans of the Vietnam War. His book, *The Harmony of Illusions: Inventing Posttraumatic Stress Disorder*, was published by Princeton University Press in 1997. His interest in PTSD continues. His most recent research concerns the emergence of the "social brain" as an object of inquiry in neuroscience.

Index

Page numbers in italics refer to figures and tables.

Printed by Libri Plureos GmbH in Hamburg,
Germany

9 781580 464765